Kelly K. Hunt, M.D., Geoffrey L. Robb, M.D.,
Eric A. Strom, M.D., Naoto T. Ueno, M.D., Ph.D.
Editors

The University of Texas M. D. Anderson Cancer Center, Houston, Texas

Breast Cancer

With a Foreword by John Mendelsohn, M.D.

With 127 Illustrations

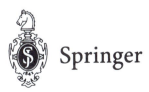

Springer

Kelly K. Hunt, M.D.
Department of Surgical Oncology
The University of Texas
M. D. Anderson Cancer Center
Houston, TX 77030-4009, USA

Eric A. Strom, M.D.
Department of Radiation Oncology
The University of Texas
M. D. Anderson Cancer Center
Houston, TX 77030-4009, USA

Geoffrey L. Robb, M.D.
Department of Plastic Surgery
The University of Texas
M. D. Anderson Cancer Center
Houston, TX 77030-4009, USA

Naoto T. Ueno, M.D., Ph.D.
Department of Blood and Marrow
  Transplantation
The University of Texas
M. D. Anderson Cancer Center
Houston, TX 77030-4009, USA

Series Editors:

Aman U. Buzdar, M.D.
Department of Breast Medical
  Oncology
The University of Texas
M. D. Anderson Cancer Center
Houston, TX 77030-4009, USA

Ralph S. Freedman, M.D., Ph.D.
Immunology/Molecular Biology
  Laboratory
Department of Gynecologic Oncology
The University of Texas
M. D. Anderson Cancer Center
Houston, TX 77030-4009, USA

Library of Congress Cataloging-in-Publication Data
The M. D. Anderson cancer care series : breast cancer / edited by Kelly K. Hunt . . . [et al.].
     p. ; cm. — (Cancer care series)
   Includes bibliographical references.
   ISBN 0-387-95190-3 (s/c : alk. paper)
   1. Breast—Cancer. I. Hunt, Kelly K. II. Series.
   [DNLM: 1. Breast Neoplasms—therapy. WP 900 B8275 2001]
 RC280.B8 B6725 2001
 616.99′449—dc21
                                                                                   200102191
Printed on acid-free paper.

Production managed by Terry Kornak; manufacturing supervised by Erica Bresler.
Typeset by Impressions Book and Journal Services, Inc.
Printed and bound by Maple-Vail Book Manufacturing Group, York, PA.
Printed in the United States of America.

9 8 7 6 5 4 3 2 1

ISBN 0-387-95190-3   SPIN 10789583

Springer-Verlag   New York Berlin Heidelberg
A member of BertelsmannSpringer Science + Business Media GmbH

0974
GM MTZ/Hun

M. D. ANDERSON
CANCER CARE
S E R I E S

Series Editors

Aman U. Buzdar, M.D.   Ralph S. Freedman, M.D., Ph.D.

Springer
New York
Berlin
Heidelberg
Barcelona
Hong Kong
London
Milan
Paris
Singapore
Tokyo

FOREWORD

I am honored to write the Foreword for this first volume of the M. D. Anderson Cancer Care series, because I believe the book represents a milestone not only for M. D. Anderson but also for cancer specialists everywhere. All of us, whether we work in academic medical institutions, medical school hospitals, community hospitals, oncology clinics, or solo practice, have seen remarkable changes in our practice over the recent decades. We know that breast cancer patients live longer, feel better, and look better than ever before, and they face this dreaded disease with more optimism than ever before. Each of us deserves to be proud of this progress. Though I am now primarily a laboratory scientist and administrator, I am proud of my own work on factors that control the growth of tumor cells, most prominently through regulation of EGF receptors and *HER-2/neu*, and the promise that work holds for women who have breast cancer.

The authors represented in this volume have made important contributions to breast cancer care. Likewise, every reader of this book has and will continue to make critical contributions to the health of women with breast cancer. I would like to express the hope here that each of us takes the opportunity to step outside our subspecialties—surgeon, internist, radiation oncologist, pathologist, radiologist, laboratory scientist—and learn how we can better integrate our work with that of other specialists. As evidence of my commitment to that goal, I plan to recommend this book to my colleagues and to every fellow in training at The University of Texas M. D. Anderson Cancer Center, regardless of the specialty boards he or she seeks.

Why do I recommend the book? Because the editors and authors have worked hard to create a complete picture of breast cancer care in a multidisciplinary environment. Their collaborative interactions are apparent in every chapter. So is the willingness of each specialist to approach breast cancer and its sequelae with the perspective of the patient's own primary care physician. I believe the time spent in reading this book will be rewarded many times in the pleasure we can take from working with our colleagues more effectively and in the added hope we can give our patients.

John Mendelsohn, M.D.

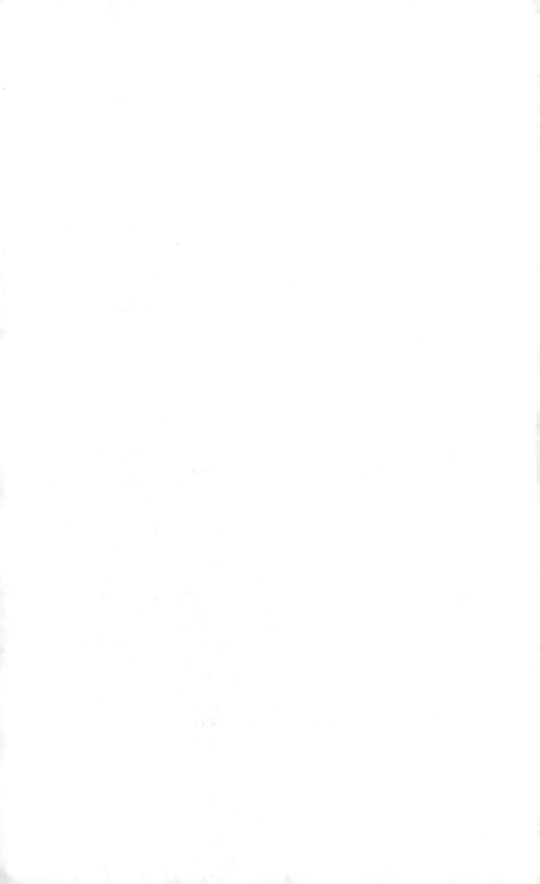

PREFACE

On behalf of the M. D. Anderson Associates and the Division of Academic Programs, we are pleased to present this first volume in the M. D. Anderson Cancer Care series.

Each volume in this series will offer a detailed, comprehensive description of the M. D. Anderson approach to a particular type of cancer. We have chosen to emphasize the day-to-day aspects of practice, minimizing literature review and discussion of approaches not yet incorporated into routine practice. Each volume will describe not just screening, diagnosis, and treatment, but the entire range of related services available for a particular cancer site. Thus this first volume, which is devoted to breast cancer, includes chapters on prevention, genetic predisposition, rehabilitation, postmenopausal health, and management of gynecologic and sexual problems associated with breast cancer.

The care of breast cancer patients at M. D. Anderson has long been based upon a multidisciplinary approach, which involves specialists from multiple disciplines collaborating from the earliest stages of treatment planning to ensure that treatments for each individual patient are integrated in the most effective manner. The first chapter of this volume describes the basic structural framework that facilitates this multidisciplinary approach. In the remaining chapters, the authors have, whenever appropriate, described how specialists from multiple disciplines collaborate at various stages of decision-making and treatment delivery.

We believe that this description of breast cancer care at a major cancer center will be a valuable resource for physicians in other practice settings and an example for other multidisciplinary endeavors.

We thank Mahesh Kanojia, M.D., for his encouragement and support, which were vital to the success of this project. We also thank the Department of Scientific Publications for helping us make this volume and the book series possible, especially Walter Pagel, Director; Stephanie Deming, managing editor for the first volume; Vickie Williams, Scientific Editor; Noelle Heinze, Editorial Assistant; and Rebecca Gershenson Smith, Editorial Assistant.

Aman U. Buzdar, M.D.
Ralph S. Freedman, M.D., Ph.D.

CONTENTS

CONTRIBUTORS

Therese B. Bevers, M.D., Medical Director, Clinical Cancer Prevention; Medical Director, Prevention Outreach Program; Assistant Professor, Department of Clinical Cancer Prevention

Aman U. Buzdar, M.D., Deputy Chairman and Professor, Ashbel Smith Professor in Breast Medical Oncology, Department of Breast Medical Oncology

Richard E. Champlin, M.D., Associate Head, Hematology; Chairman and Professor, Department of Blood & Marrow Transplantation

Beth S. Edeiken-Monro, M.D., Associate Professor, Department of Diagnostic Radiology

Francisco J. Esteva, M.D., Assistant Professor, Department of Breast Medical Oncology

Bruno D. Fornage, M.D., Professor, Department of Diagnostic Radiology; Professor, Department of Surgical Oncology

Ralph S. Freedman, M.D., Ph.D., Director, Immunology/Molecular Biology Laboratory; Professor, Department of Gynecologic Oncology

Herbert A. Fritsche, Jr., Ph.D., Section Chief, Clinical Chemistry; Professor, Department of Laboratory Medicine

Jennifer G. Gotto, M.D., Assistant Professor, Department of Neuro-Oncology

Marjorie Green, M.D., Fellow in Medical Oncology, Department of Breast Medical Oncology

Karin M. Gwyn, M.D., M.Sc., Fellow in Medical Oncology, Department of Breast Medical Oncology

Gabriel N. Hortobagyi, M.D., Chairman and Professor, Nellie B. Connally Chair in Breast Cancer, Department of Breast Medical Oncology

Kelly K. Hunt, M.D., Chief, Surgical Breast Service; Associate Professor, Department of Surgical Oncology

Anne Chmielewski Kushwaha, M.D., Clinical Assistant Professor, Department of Diagnostic Radiology

Funda Meric, M.D., Junior Faculty Associate, Department of Surgical Oncology

Gordon B. Mills, M.D., Ph.D., Medical Director (Ad Interim), Clinical Cancer Genetics; Chairman and Professor, Ransome Horne Professor in Cancer Research, Department of Molecular Therapeutics

Barbara S. Monsees, M.D., Professor, Mallinckrodt Institute of Radiology, Washington University School of Medicine

Pedro T. Ramirez, M.D., Junior Faculty Associate, Department of Gynecologic Oncology

Paula Trahan Rieger, R.N., M.S.N., C.S., A.O.C.N.®, F.A.A.N, Advanced Practice Nurse, Department of Clinical Cancer Prevention

Geoffrey L. Robb, M.D., Medical Director, Plastic Surgery Center; Deputy Division Head, Division of Surgery; Chairman and Professor, Department of Plastic Surgery

Nour Sneige, M.D., Section Chief, Cytopathology; Professor, Department of Pathology

Carol B. Stelling, M.D., Section Chief, Breast Imaging; Associate Medical Director, Breast Center; Medical Director, Julie and Ben Rogers Breast Diagnostic Clinic; Professor, Nylene Eckles Professorship in Breast Cancer Research, Department of Diagnostic Radiology

Eric A. Strom, M.D., Medical Director, Nellie B. Connally Breast Center; Medical Director, Radiation Therapy Technology Program; Associate Professor, Department of Radiation Oncology

Richard L. Theriault, D.O., M.B.A., Medical Director, M. D. Anderson Physicians Network; Professor, Department of Breast Medical Oncology

Anne N. Truong, M.D., Assistant Professor, Department of Symptom Control & Palliative Care

Naoto T. Ueno, M.D., Ph.D., Assistant Professor, Department of Blood & Marrow Transplantation; Assistant Professor, Department of Molecular & Cellular Oncology

Rena Vassilopoulou-Sellin, M.D., Professor, Department of Internal Medicine Specialties

Gary J. Whitman, M.D., Associate Professor, Department of Diagnostic Radiology

1 MULTIDISCIPLINARY CARE OF THE BREAST CANCER PATIENT: OVERVIEW AND IMPLEMENTATION

Eric A. Strom, Aman U. Buzdar, and Kelly K. Hunt

M. D. Anderson Cancer Center has long embraced a multidisciplinary approach to breast cancer care. At M. D. Anderson, multidisciplinary care is defined by consistent use of the best standard of care, collaboration between treating physicians, and coordination of treatment delivery to optimize patient outcomes and convenience. These 3 elements of M. D. Anderson's multidisciplinary approach are exemplified in the Nellie B. Connally Multidisciplinary Breast Center, the Multidisciplinary Breast Planning Clinic, and the institutional Breast Cancer Treatment Guidelines.

NELLIE B. CONNALLY MULTIDISCIPLINARY BREAST CENTER

The Nellie B. Connally Multidisciplinary Breast Center was born of a collaborative attitude combined with a desire to make cancer treatment more convenient for patients. The Breast Center shares a floor of M. D. Anderson's Clark Clinic with the Julie and Ben Rogers Breast Diagnostic Clinic and the Cancer Prevention Center. The Breast Center is staffed by surgical oncologists, medical oncologists, and radiation oncologists; the Breast Diagnostic Clinic is staffed by radiologists and pathologists; and the Prevention Center is staffed by specialists in breast cancer risk evaluation and risk-reduction interventions. Plastic and reconstructive surgeons and physicians from the Department of Blood and Marrow Transplantation work in other areas of the M. D. Anderson complex but are included in discussions of treatment planning when appropriate. Approximately 2000 patient visits occur in the Breast Center each month. In addition to the physicians and nurses, the Breast Center is staffed by research nurses, referral specialists, social workers, business center staff, and volunteers.

The close proximity of the various services involved in breast cancer care allows patients to have all of their clinic visits in one location and encourages collaboration between physicians. Informal and impromptu consultations can occur, and inviting a colleague to examine a patient with you can be as simple as knocking on your neighbor's door. These frequent discussions about a patient's course of treatment help to ensure that everyone on the treatment team is up to date and that all are aware of the patient's overall course of treatment.

This emphasis on each individual patient's overall treatment course also guides the center's day-to-day operations. Whenever possible, appointments with different specialists are scheduled on the same day, and all appropriate tests are ordered before a patient's initial visit so that each physician will have all of the information pertinent to the patient's case when she arrives. As one can imagine, coordinating such a large number of patients, clinicians, support personnel, tests, and treatments requires extensive planning and a certain amount of flexibility. In the Nellie B. Connally Multidisciplinary Breast Center, administrators, clinicians, nurses, and support personnel meet twice a month to discuss problems related to the center's daily operations and their solutions. The ultimate goal is to develop and maintain a system that is consistent and efficient and that frees the center's clinicians from unnecessary paperwork, allowing them to devote more time to the treatment of their patients.

Many aspects of this model can be reproduced on a smaller scale. In some centers, for example, it may be feasible to conduct planning clinics that focus on 1 or 2 common disease sites, such as the breast or lung, and a general oncology clinic for less common sites. In centers where a lower patient volume allows for weekly or twice-weekly planning conferences for each patient, having a centralized location for the delivery of patient care is less critical. Most important is the commitment of the care team to work together, especially during the planning phase, for the benefit of the patient and her family.

MULTIDISCIPLINARY BREAST PLANNING CLINIC

The treatment of patients with breast cancer within the Nellie B. Connally Multidisciplinary Breast Center is generally guided by the institutional Breast Cancer Treatment Guidelines (see the next section in this chapter and appendix 1 at the end of this chapter) or institutional review board–approved clinical trials. Nonetheless, within the context of the general Breast Cancer Treatment Guidelines, decisions must often be made that require consultation between clinicians from different specialties. Since the early 1960s, breast cancer specialists at M. D. Anderson have been holding a regularly scheduled clinic during which patients who require multidisciplinary care are examined and have their treatment plans discussed by a team of physicians.

The purpose of the Multidisciplinary Breast Planning Clinic is to design appropriate, individualized treatment plans for all patients who require coordinated multispecialty care. The physicians in the clinic work together to determine the most appropriate treatments for each patient (combinations of surgery, radiation therapy, and systemic therapy) and the best sequence in which to deliver these treatments.

The Multidisciplinary Breast Planning Clinic is an integral part of M. D. Anderson's multidisciplinary approach to the care of breast cancer patients. The discussions that take place in the clinic not only ensure the highest quality of care for each individual patient but also strengthen cooperation and exchange of information among the various specialties involved in breast cancer care.

Types of Patients Who Are Registered and Discussed in the Clinic

Patients are examined and discussed in the Multidisciplinary Breast Planning Clinic if their disease stage at initial evaluation indicates that a multidisciplinary approach will be required.

Patients with early-stage disease are seen in the clinic if help is needed in determining the appropriate type of surgery and the proper sequence of surgery and radiation therapy. (Patients with early-stage disease who will be treated with surgery alone generally do not require a multidisciplinary evaluation.) Patients with stage II disease who are candidates for preoperative chemotherapy are seen in the clinic to determine the feasibility of breast conservation therapy (surgery plus radiation therapy).

Also routinely discussed in the clinic are patients with stage III disease and all patients with inflammatory carcinoma. These patients are seen in the clinic before preoperative chemotherapy and again after 2 to 4 cycles of therapy to determine the appropriate local therapy. In selected patients with locally advanced breast cancer whose tumors are downstaged by preoperative chemotherapy, breast conservation therapy is feasible.

Patients with treatment-related problems—for example, positive margins after attempted breast conservation therapy or hematoma or infection after biopsy—may be well served by discussion in the clinic. In these cases, the multidisciplinary team can provide clarification of the problems encountered and recommend appropriate interventions.

Schedule and Participants

The Multidisciplinary Breast Planning Clinic is held 2 afternoons per week, and 5 to 8 patients are examined and discussed at each session. Typically, patients are scheduled in advance so that all diagnostic evaluations can be completed before the clinic session.

Each clinic session includes at least 1 breast cancer specialist from each of the following disciplines: surgical oncology, radiation oncology, medical oncology, and diagnostic imaging. Currently, pathologists do not routinely attend. However, before the clinic session, a breast pathologist reviews the patient's pathology slides to confirm the diagnosis. This pathology report is essential to good treatment planning. Faculty attend the clinic on a rotating basis, and the rotation is set in advance to ensure representation from all specialties that may participate in treating the particular patients being discussed.

The patient's primary physician attends, and any physician assuming the care of the patient at any time during treatment is also welcome to attend. In addition, the multidisciplinary planning clinic is open to fellows and trainees doing rotations in the breast service and to visiting physicians.

Clinic Procedures

At the beginning of the clinic, the multidisciplinary team convenes in the conference room, and the first patient is presented to the group by the patient's primary care physician. The physician gives a synopsis of the history and treatments. The current problem is defined, and the patient's radiological studies are reviewed. Then the multidisciplinary team goes to the examination room, where the patient is examined by a surgical oncologist, a medical oncologist, and a radiation oncologist. The diagnostic radiologist also sees the patient to determine if any additional imaging studies may be helpful. After the examinations are complete, the members of the multidisciplinary team return to the conference room, where they deliberate about treatment approaches and formulate a final treatment recommendation. The patient waits in the clinic area during these deliberations. The patient's spouse and other family members or friends are welcome to accompany the patient and to be present during discussions with the primary physician.

Once the team reaches a primary recommendation, the primary physician records the team's opinion in the patient's chart so that the recommendation will be available to all members of the multidisciplinary team who encounter the patient during subsequent treatment. Then the primary physician goes to where the patient is waiting and discusses the findings of the multidisciplinary team. Finally, the primary physician discusses the recommendation of the planning clinic with any other physicians involved in the patient's care.

BREAST CANCER TREATMENT GUIDELINES

For the purposes of discussing treatment, it is convenient to divide breast tumors into the appropriate stage categories (Table 1–1), recognizing that the various clinical presentations represent a continuous spectrum of disease. These categories include the nonmetastasizing in situ lesions (ductal carcinoma in situ [DCIS] and lobular carcinoma in situ [LCIS]); early-stage invasive cancer (stage I and some stage II); operable intermediate-stage disease (stages II and IIIA); inoperable disease; locally advanced disease (stage IIIB, inflammatory, some stage IIIA, and the occasional stage IV disease with only supraclavicular node involvement); and metastatic carcinoma (stage IV). In addition, there are uncommon clinical scenarios that do not fit conveniently into this classification system. These include local-regionally recurrent disease and unknown primary adenocarcinomas involving axillary nodes.

The breast cancer treatment guidelines in appendix 1 at the end of this chapter were developed collaboratively and represent the current standard approach to breast disease at M. D. Anderson. The approach was developed by combining the best current practices with the outcomes of clinical trials at M. D. Anderson and was informed by compelling scientific evidence from other institutions. The most recent version of the breast cancer guidelines can be found at http://www.mdanderson.org. The guidelines are formally reviewed and updated periodically; thus, changes in clinical practice will not immediately be reflected in the guidelines. The breast cancer multidisciplinary group is committed to ongoing collaborative research and makes a point of designing clinical trials for each major category of disease. Ideally, these trials permit the most rapid deployment of promising basic scientific research into the clinical setting. Whenever possible, patients are encouraged to participate in these clinical trials. A

Table 1–1. Staging System for Breast Cancer

Primary Tumor (T)

TX		Primary tumor cannot be assessed
T0		No evidence of primary tumor
Tis		Carcinoma in situ: intraductal carcinoma, lobular carcinoma *in situ* or Paget's disease of the nipple with no tumor
T1		Tumor 2 cm or less in greatest dimension
	Tmic	Microinvasion 0.1 cm or less in greatest dimension
	T1a	Tumor more than 0.1 but not more than 0.5 cm in greatest dimension
	T1b	Tumor more than 0.5 but not more than 1 cm in greatest dimension
	T1c	Tumor more than 1 cm but not more than 2 cm in greatest dimension
T2		Tumor more than 2 cm but not more than 5 cm in greatest dimension
T3		Tumor more than 5.0 cm in greatest dimension
T4		Tumor of any size with direct extension to chest wall or skin
	T4a	Extension to chest wall
	T4b	Edema (including peau d'orange) or ulceration of skin of the breast or satellite skin nodules confined to the same breast
	T4c	Both (T4a and T4b)
	T4d	Inflammatory carcinoma

Regional Lymph Nodes (N)

NX	Regional lymph nodes cannot be assessed (e.g., previously removed)
N0	No regional lymph node metastasis
N1	Metastasis to movable ipsilateral axillary lymph nodes
N2	Metastasis to ipsilateral axillary lymph node(s) fixed to one another or to other structures
N3	Metastasis to ipsilateral internal mammary lymph node(s)

complete listing of clinical trials available at M. D. Anderson can be found at http://www.clinicaltrials.org.

In Situ Lesions (Stage 0)

For in situ (noninvasive) lesions—LCIS and DCIS—careful pathology review is critical to the success of the decision-making processes (see appendix 1, panel 1). For example, distinctions between LCIS and atypical lobular hyperplasia are important for assessing a patient's subsequent risk of developing an invasive carcinoma. Similarly, there is not universal agreement about the dividing line between atypical ductal hyperplasia and well-differentiated DCIS. A clear understanding of the pathological criteria for these distinctions is required before attempts are made to apply

Table 1–1. *Continued*

Distant Metastases (M)	
MX	Distant metastasis cannot be assessed
M0	No distant metastasis
M1	Distant metastasis (includes metastasis to ipsilateral supra-clavicular lymph node(s))
Stage	
Stage 0	Tis N0 M0
Stage I	T1 N0 M0
Stage IIA	T0 N1 M0
	T1 N1 M0
	T2 N0 M0
Stage IIB	T2 N1 M0
	T3 N0 M0
Stage IIIA	T0 N2 M0
	T1 N2 M0
	T2 N2 M0
	T3 N1–2 M0
Stage IIIB	T4 N0–2 M0
	any N3 M0
Stage IV	any M1

Used with permission of the American Joint Committee on Cancer (AJCC®), Chicago, Illinois. The original source for this material is the *AJCC® Cancer Staging Manual*, 5th edition (1997), published by Lippincott-Raven Publishers, Philadelphia, Pennsylvania.

these treatment guidelines. In general, the goal of treatment is to prevent the occurrence of invasive disease while minimizing the side effects of therapy.

Lobular Carcinoma In Situ

Lobular carcinoma in situ is not considered to be a precursor lesion, per se, for invasive cancer. Instead, it represents a histologic finding that correlates with an increased risk for the development of an invasive breast cancer. Typically, LCIS has no clinical manifestations and has no pathognomonic mammographic signs. Although individuals with LCIS are at increased risk for the development of invasive breast lesions, these cancers are more likely to be ductal than lobular, and the risk is the same in the index breast and the contralateral breast. Therefore, no specific treatment of LCIS is indicated, even if the lesion is incompletely removed at biopsy. After adequate work-up, which should include bilateral diagnostic mammography and pathology review, appropriate risk-reduction strategies are discussed with the patient. Patients with a finding of LCIS on biopsy should be approached the same way as patients with a strong positive family history of breast cancer. Lobular carcinoma in situ is a marker of increased risk of breast cancer, and reasonable risk-reduction strategies are appropriate.

Ductal Carcinoma In Situ

Patients with large (≥4 cm) or multicentric DCIS as evidenced by mammography, physical examination, or biopsy generally require a total glandular mastectomy. Although lymph node dissection or sentinel lymph node evaluation is not useful for most patients with DCIS, it may be appropriate for some patients with extensive involvement of the breast with DCIS. Since the risk of occult invasion increases dramatically with the volume affected by in situ carcinoma, it is not unreasonable to perform limited nodal assessment in patients who have extensive disease. Practical considerations also make it difficult to avoid low axillary sampling when a total mastectomy is performed. The lymph nodes of the low axilla are interspersed along the axillary tail of Spence and are therefore frequently removed during total mastectomy. In the rare cases in which tumor metastases are identified in regional lymph nodes, it must be assumed that a small invasive breast cancer is present, and these patients are treated for presumed stage II invasive breast cancer. Patients who require mastectomy are routinely offered the option of breast reconstruction in the absence of anatomic or medical contraindications.

Patients with unifocal DCIS of intermediate size that can be excised with clear margins are generally offered the alternatives of breast conservation therapy or total mastectomy. These alternatives are presumed to be equally effective, although they have not been directly compared in large prospective trials. After providing adequate information about the probable risks and benefits, the physician largely leaves the choice of treatment up to the patient and her family.

On the basis of results from a few small retrospective studies, patients with very small, unicentric, low-grade DCIS may be offered the additional option of excision alone without subsequent irradiation. Since the data about the appropriate management of good-risk DCIS are conflicting, it is preferred that these patients be enrolled in the prospective randomized intergroup trial sponsored by the Radiation Therapy Oncology Group (see http://www.rtog.org/). This and other ongoing prospective studies evaluating the role of local therapy and selective estrogen receptor modulators will be the primary motivators for future modifications to the current guidelines.

Tamoxifen has been demonstrated to reduce the short-term risk of local recurrence for patients with DCIS treated with excision and radiation therapy and has also demonstrated efficacy in preventing contralateral breast disease. The potential benefit of tamoxifen, assessed on the basis of the initial extent of disease, is contrasted with the potential risk of tamoxifen therapy for each individual patient.

In patients with DCIS treated with mastectomy, surveillance after treatment includes annual physical examination and diagnostic mammographic examination of the contralateral breast. In patients with DCIS treated with breast conservation therapy, surveillance includes semiannual physical examinations and annual bilateral mammography.

Early-Stage Invasive Breast Cancer

The standard work-up for patients with early-stage invasive disease (see appendix 1, panel 2) includes bilateral diagnostic mammography, hemogram, liver function tests, and chest radiographs. Sonography of the breast may be done if there are areas that cannot be well defined with mammography (for example, in a patient with radiologically dense breasts). Sonography of the nodal basins may be done if there is suspicion of nodal disease and such disease would affect treatment recommendations. Any pathology reports from other institutions are reviewed by M. D. Anderson breast pathologists. The tumor's size, pathologic subtype, differentiation, and nuclear grade are determined, along with the status of the margins, the presence or absence of vascular lymphatic invasion, and, if appropriate, the status of the regional nodes. Estrogen and progesterone receptors and Her-2/*neu* amplification are also assessed. For most patients, no additional staging is indicated. A baseline bone scan is obtained in patients with stage I disease only when they have skeletal signs or symptoms. Similarly, baseline imaging of the liver is performed in patients with stage I disease only when they have abnormal findings on liver function tests.

Local Treatment

Local treatment is the preferred initial treatment for patients with tumors smaller than 1 cm and a clinically negative axilla. This is appropriate since the risk of systemic disease in most of these patients is not sufficient to warrant the use of cytotoxic chemotherapy. Patients with larger tumors are also referred for initial local treatment if they have significant comorbid illnesses and if histologic evaluation of the axilla will determine recommendations for systemic therapy. Since multiple prospective randomized trials have demonstrated that mastectomy is equivalent to breast conservation therapy, most patients are offered both of these options for primary local therapy. This appropriately requires extensive patient education about the relative contraindications to breast conservation therapy, including prior radiation therapy to the breast (for example, for Hodgkin's disease), evidence of gross multicentricity or diffuse microcalcifications, certain collagen vascular disorders (especially systemic lupus erythematosus or scleroderma), and the inability to obtain clear margins of resection. In patients for whom mastectomy is appropriate, immediate reconstruction may reasonably be considered. For patients who undergo initial breast conservation therapy, lymphatic mapping is considered a reasonable alternative to axillary dissection and is preferred for patients with T1 and T2 tumors that are clinically node negative.

Radiation therapy is used in all patients who undergo breast conservation therapy. Postmastectomy irradiation is recommended for patients with 4 or more positive lymph nodes after mastectomy or advanced stages of disease. Patients with stage II breast cancer and 1 to 3 positive lymph nodes should be offered enrollment in the intergroup trial of postmastectomy irradiation (see http://www.swog.org).

Systemic Therapy

It is ideal to determine recommendations for adjuvant systemic therapy after completion of local surgical treatment. Patients with highly favorable tumors (i.e., tubular, medullary, pure papillary, or colloid) and patients with ductal and lobular carcinomas smaller than 1 cm have a low risk of systemic metastasis and may not require systemic therapy. These patients may consider tamoxifen if their tumor is estrogen receptor positive. The precise role of tumor markers in this most favorable subgroup requires further study. In patients with tumors larger than 1 cm or axillary lymph node metastases, systemic adjuvant therapy is appropriate. Typically, patients with positive lymph nodes are treated with adjuvant systemic chemotherapy using a combination of 5-fluorouracil, doxorubicin, and cyclophosphamide (FAC) and paclitaxel even if the tumor is hormone receptor positive. In this latter group, tamoxifen is recommended after completion of cytotoxic chemotherapy. Postmenopausal patients with tumors between 1 and 2 cm in size and no axillary node metastases may be considered for tamoxifen therapy alone. Patients with T2 primary tumors and all premenopausal patients are treated with cytotoxic therapy.

High-dose chemotherapy with bone marrow or peripheral stem cell rescue may be considered for high-risk patients (i.e., those with 10 or more involved axillary lymph nodes) in the context of a clinical trial. In general, those patients are not treated with bone marrow transplantation outside of an appropriately designed, peer-reviewed clinical trial. The role of those intensive therapies remains controversial and generates considerable discussion at multidisciplinary planning clinics.

When radiation therapy is indicated (see the section Local Treatment earlier in this chapter), it is typically delivered after the completion of systemic therapy.

Surveillance

Follow-up is best performed by the team members who have cared for the patient. Follow-up visits include a detailed patient history and physical examination and selected screening tests. Mammography is performed 6 months after the completion of breast conservation therapy and annually thereafter. Chest radiographs are obtained annually in patients who have undergone breast conservation therapy. The role of more intensive surveillance has been questioned, and the current American Society of Clinical Oncology guidelines suggest that the data are insufficient to suggest the routine use of blood counts, automated chemistry studies, chest radiography, or other imaging studies. These guidelines also state that the routine measurement of CA15-3, CA27.29, or carcinoembryonic antigen for breast cancer surveillance is not recommended.

Wellness is important to all breast cancer survivors but is especially important to those with favorable, early-stage breast cancer. To this end, assessment of the impact of estrogen deficiency is particularly important. Assessment of skeletal and cardiac health is appropriate, particularly in patients with strong family histories of these problems. Quality-of-life issues due to estrogen deprivation, such as depression, hot flashes, weight gain, and vaginal dryness and atrophy, should be addressed symptomatically and preferably without the use of replacement hormones. In patients who have not had a hysterectomy, yearly pelvic examinations are appropriate. Women receiving ongoing tamoxifen therapy may require endometrial biopsies. Ultrasonography may be considered when women have vaginal bleeding or other symptoms.

Intermediate-Stage and Advanced-Stage Breast Cancer

One of the keys to the successful treatment of intermediate-stage and locally advanced breast cancer (see appendix 1, panel 3) is obtaining a detailed and accurate definition of the extent of disease prior to initiation of therapy. Since most patients with intermediate-stage and locally advanced breast cancer will be treated with neoadjuvant (preoperative) chemotherapy, the initial pathologic description of the disease (extent of disease in the breast and the lymph nodes) will not be available to guide the clinician in the subsequent decision-making process. Therefore, the decision whether breast conservation therapy is appropriate is based on a careful breast examination. Subtle skin involvement, attachment of the tumor to the underlying chest wall structures, and the presence of satellite lesions and multicentric tumors can affect whether breast conservation therapy is possible. Radiologic or clinical evidence of tumor in the internal mammary, axillary apical, or supraclavicular nodal basins is important for correct staging of the disease and for planning of local therapy. The systemic staging evaluation for patients with intermediate-stage and advanced-stage breast cancers is similar to that for patients with early-stage disease except that a bone scan and abdominal computed tomography or sonography are performed even in the absence of clinical symptoms or biochemical abnormalities.

Advanced Stage II and Stage IIIA Disease (Operable Disease)

Patients with any T2 tumor larger than 4 cm (IIA) and those with T3 tumors but without fixed or matted axillary nodes (IIB and IIIA) are technically operable by classic criteria. Although total mastectomy with axillary lymph node dissection may be an acceptable initial treatment choice for patients with significant comorbid diseases, neoadjuvant doxorubicin-based or taxane-based chemotherapy is the preferred option for initial treatment. This permits observation for tumor responsiveness to the chosen regimen and allows some patients to subsequently undergo breast conservation therapy. When breast conservation therapy is being considered, it is important to perform percutaneous insertion of radio-opaque markers in the tumor bed (typically using ultrasound guidance) to facilitate future surgical resection. For patients treated initially with mastectomy, adjuvant therapy using a doxorubicin-based or paclitaxel-based regimen is recommended for all patients who are medically fit.

The decision-making paradigm for systemic therapy for stage IIIA breast cancer is similar to that for earlier-stage disease. Tamoxifen is used for 5 years if the tumor expresses hormone receptors. Postoperative radiation therapy is generally employed after the completion of chemotherapy. Breast reconstruction is appropriate for most women treated with mastectomy, although it is preferable to delay reconstruction until after the completion of local therapy for patients who will require irradiation.

Stage IIIB and Selected Stage IVA Disease (Inoperable Disease)

Patients who have classically inoperable breast cancer (inoperable stage IIIA disease, stage IIIB disease, and stage IV disease with involvement of ipsilateral supraclavicular nodes only) will receive neoadjuvant chemotherapy as standard therapy. It is inappropriate to attempt initial mastectomy in this patient group since the risk of positive surgical margins is high and downstaging with neoadjuvant chemotherapy offers numerous advantages. Neoadjuvant chemotherapy using doxorubicin-based or taxane-based regimens is preferred. Patients whose disease responds and becomes operable according to classic criteria (resolution of supraclavicular or matted axillary nodes, normalization of skin changes permitting complete surgical excision) are offered standard mastectomy. In patients whose disease responds rapidly, breast conservation therapy may become possible. Conversely, patients who have little or no response should be switched to a non-cross-resistant regimen before surgical therapy is attempted. Generally, all patients with advanced breast cancer will receive radiation therapy to the breast or chest wall and regional nodes, and thus immediate reconstruction is discouraged. Post-treatment follow-up for patients with intermediate-stage and advanced-stage breast cancer is similar to the follow-up for women with early-stage invasive disease.

Local-Regional Recurrences and Distant Metastasis

The assessment and treatment of patients with local-regional recurrences or distant metastasis (see appendix 1, panel 4) depends in some measure on the particular clinical scenario. Global assessment includes chest radiography, radionuclide bone scan, computed tomography or sonography of the abdomen, complete blood counts, and liver function tests. It is important to have confidence that the diagnosis is correct, so it is usually appropriate to obtain histologic confirmation of the recurrence or metastasis—usually by fine-needle aspiration or core biopsy—and to perform hormone receptor and Her-2/*neu* assays on the specimen.

Local-Regional Recurrence

When the staging work-up fails to reveal any evidence of visceral metastasis and tumor is encountered only in the breast, the chest wall, or the regional nodal basins, it is appropriate to embark on a curative course of therapy. Complete imaging of the disease using mammography, sonography (including regional nodal assessment), and possibly computed tomography should be performed before treatment is initiated. Most patients who have a recurrence after breast conservation therapy will require completion mastectomy as their local therapy. Up-front chemotherapy may be considered in patients with invasive disease whose tumor is not initially resectable. When the breast has not previously been irradiated (usually after surgery alone for DCIS), re-excision of the recurrent lesion followed by irradiation may be considered. Adjuvant systemic therapy is generally recommended after local recurrence of invasive cancer because of the high risk of subsequent metastasis.

While local-regional recurrences after mastectomy can occasionally be managed using initial surgery, it is common to find that the disease is too extensive to be completely encompassed within a reasonable surgical field. In the case of numerous cutaneous nodules, extensive nodal disease, or previous breast reconstruction, initial chemotherapy is the preferred approach. The choice of agents is based on the type of chemotherapy previously used, the interval since prior systemic therapy, and the tumor receptor status. Once a sufficient response is achieved, residual disease is surgically excised. Patients who have not previously had radiation therapy are irradiated.

Systemic Metastasis

The therapeutic goal for patients with documented visceral metastases is prolongation of survival and enhancement of quality of life. Since current approaches do not appear to be curative, it is important to balance therapeutic efficacy with treatment-related toxicity. Thus, when the tumor is positive for estrogen or progesterone receptors and the patient is symptom free, hormonal therapies are the preferred initial therapy. Clinical scenarios especially suited to hormonal therapy include patients with bone or soft-tissue disease only and patients with limited, asymptomatic visceral disease. Tamoxifen is the preferred initial hormonal therapy in patients not previously treated with this agent. In patients with prior tamoxifen exposure, aromatase inhibitors (in postmenopausal women), progestins, or androgens can be employed. When the tumor responds to this initial hormonal maneuver, as evidenced by tumor shrinkage or long-term stabilization of disease, second-line hormonal therapy should be considered at the time of subsequent progression.

Cytotoxic chemotherapy is indicated for patients with hormone receptor–negative tumors, patients with hormone-refractory disease, and patients with symptomatic visceral metastases, regardless of hormone receptor status. A variety of regimens are considered appropriate, including FAC or taxanes in women who have not been exposed to these agents and trastuzumab (Herceptin) in patients whose tumors overexpress Her2/*neu*. Patients should be encouraged to participate in clinical trials when appropriate. Supportive care should be considered when disease fails to respond to 2 sequential chemotherapy regimens or if the patient's performance status deteriorates to Zubrod 3 or greater.

High-dose chemotherapy and bone marrow or stem cell rescue is considered investigational for patients with distant metastases. As is the case for patients with stage II and III breast cancer, patients with distant metastases considering this therapy should be treated in the context of a clinical trial.

Frequently, patients with metastatic breast cancer develop specific clinical scenarios for which surgery, radiation therapy, or regional chemotherapy may be indicated. These include brain metastases, spinal cord compression, painful bone lesions, pathological fractures, plexopathy and radiculopathy, and pleural effusions.

CONCLUSIONS

The M. D. Anderson approach to the treatment of breast neoplasms is centered on optimizing the effectiveness of therapy while minimizing the acute and long-term impact of treatment. Accurate definition of the extent of disease, careful assessment of the treatment options, and consideration of the needs and wishes of the patient and her family are prerequisites to superior care. While the guidelines outlined in this chapter describe the best standard care that we believe can be justified by proven clinical science, many patients at M. D. Anderson elect to have part or all of their care delivered in the context of ongoing clinical trials. Participation in clinical research gives patients the opportunity not only to receive state-of-the-art cancer care but also to potentially be the first to receive tomorrow's treatment today and to contribute to the betterment of breast cancer care for future patients with this disease.

Appendix 1: M. D. Anderson Cancer Center Breast Cancer Treatment Guidelines

Panel 1: Noninvasive Disease

DIAGNOSIS WORKUP LOCAL TREATMENT SYSTEMIC TREATMENT SURVEILLANCE/FOLLOW-UP

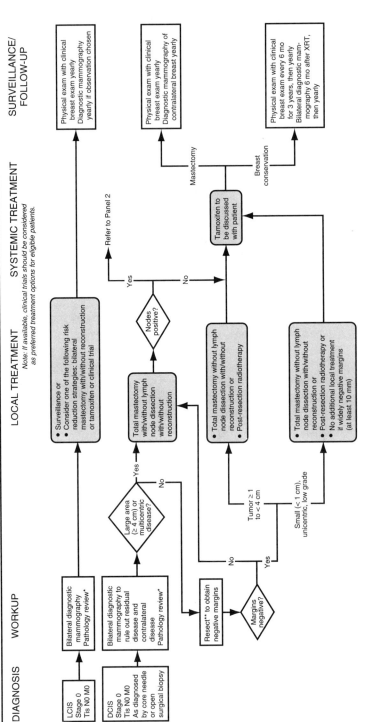

Note: If available, clinical trials should be considered as preferred treatment options for eligible patients.

○ Treatment

Revised 10-25-2000

* Pathology review to include:
- Tumor size
- Differentiation
- Nuclear grade
- Histologic type
- Lymph node status
- Rule out any invasive component

** Patients with breast conservation therapy should have post-resection mammogram to rule out residual mammographic abnormality even if margins are negative.

Panel 2: Invasive Disease*

◯ Treatment

| CLINICAL STAGE | INITIAL EVALUATION | LOCAL TREATMENT*** | SYSTEMIC TREATMENT | SURVEILLANCE |

SYSTEMIC TREATMENT — *Note: If available, clinical trials should be considered as preferred treatment options for eligible patients.*

Clinical Stage

Stage I
T1 N0 M0

Stage IIA
T0 N1 M0
T1 N1 M0
T2 N0 M0

Stage IIB
T2 N1 M0
< 4 cm

Initial Evaluation

CBC, platelets, liver function tests (total bilirubin, alkaline phosphatase, SGPT, LDH)
Pathology review**
Estrogen and progesterone receptors
Her-2/Neu
CXR
Bilateral diagnostic mammography
Bone scan if:
- Stage I and signs or symptoms or
- Changes in liver function tests
CT of abdomen or ultrasound of liver if:
- Stage I and signs or symptoms or
- Changes in liver function tests
ECG if > 60 yr

Local Treatment

Segmental mastectomy (preferred over total mastectomy) with axillary node dissection → Margins negative? → Yes / No → Re-excise → Margins negative? → Yes / No → Completion mastectomy

Total mastectomy with axillary node dissection (MRM) ± reconstruction

Systemic Treatment branches

Node negative and tumor < 1 cm →
- No systemic treatment or
- Based on prognostic factors, consider chemotherapy or
- Consider tamoxifen if ER positive

Node negative and tumor 1 - 2 cm → Patient ≥ 50 yr and ER positive? → Yes / No

Node negative and tumor > 2 cm →
- FAC or
- FEC or
- Paclitaxel followed by FAC or
- FAC followed by paclitaxel or
- Paclitaxel followed by AC or
- AC followed by paclitaxel
(Preliminary evidence does not statistically support added value for sequential paclitaxel in ER-positive patients)
→ FAC or AC

Node positive
≥ 4 positive nodes or tumor ≥ 5 cm or margins positive or extensive lymphatic invasion or extensive extranodal extension

Node negative or < 4 positive nodes →
- Paclitaxel followed by FAC or
- FAC followed by paclitaxel or
- AC followed by paclitaxel or
- Paclitaxel followed by AC
→ Radiotherapy after systemic chemotherapy

Radiotherapy for patients treated with segmental mastectomy

Tamoxifen for 5 yr if ER positive

Tamoxifen for 5 yr if ER positive

Surveillance

Physical exam every 4 mo for 2 yr; every 6 mo for 3 yr; then yearly
Mammography yearly
CXR for patients treated with radiotherapy yearly for 5 yr
Pelvic exam yearly for women on tamoxifen with intact uterus
If adjuvant chemotherapy, CBC, differential, platelets, alkaline phosphatase, SGPT, and LDH yearly

---

* There are special circumstances in which these guidelines do not apply. These include, but are not limited to:
- Sarcoma and lymphoma of the breast
- Special histologies (i.e., tubular-, medullary-, pure papillary, or colloid)
- Patients with gross multicentricity or diffuse microcalcifications
- Patients with lupus, scleroderma, and possibly other collagen vascular disorders
- Patients with limited life expectancy because of comorbid illness
- Cancer during pregnancy

** Pathology review to include:
- Tumor size
- Differentiation
- Nuclear grade
- Histologic type
- Lymph node status
- Extracapsular extension (focal < 2 mm or gross ≥ 2 mm)
- Intramammary vascular/ lymphatic invasion
- Her-2/Neu and receptor status

*** Patients with early-stage (T1, T2, N0, M0) breast cancers will be identified as candidates for participation in the American College of Surgeons 20010/Z0011 trial of lymphatic mapping.
Surgeons with an established record of lymphatic mapping experience for breast cancer may consider sentinel node biopsy as the initial and primary means of evaluating nodal status for selected patients with T1/T2 tumors that are clinically node negative.
A reasonable and acceptable experience with lymphatic mapping would include 30 consecutive cases performed with completion axillary dissection revealing a successful identification rate of at least 85% (26/30) and no more than one false-negative result. These are the skill verification requirements for participation in the American College of Surgeons prospective lymphatic mapping trial.

AC = Doxorubicin and cyclophosphamide
FAC = Fluorouracil, doxorubicin, and cyclophosphamide
FEC = Fluorouracil, epirubicin, and cyclophosphamide

Revised 10-25-2000

Panel 3: Invasive Disease

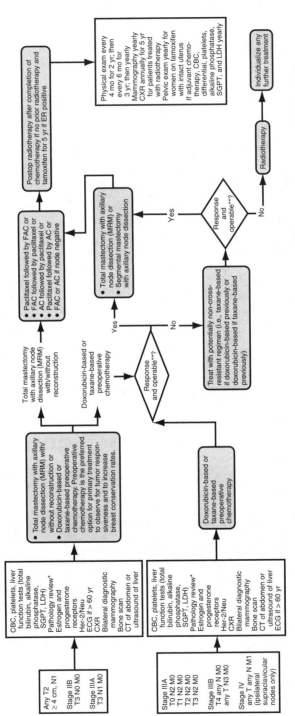

CLINICAL STAGE   **WORKUP**   **LOCAL*** AND SYSTEMIC TREATMENT**

Note: If available, clinical trials should be considered as preferred treatment options for eligible patients.

SURVEILLANCE/ FOLLOW-UP

◯ Treatment

Any T2 ≥ 4 cm, N1

Stage IIB T3 N0 M0

Stage IIIA T3 N1 M0

- CBC, platelets, liver function tests (total bilirubin, alkaline phosphatase, SGPT, LDH)
- Pathology review*
- Estrogen and progesterone receptors
- Her-2/Neu
- ECG if > 60 yr
- CXR
- Bilateral diagnostic mammography
- Bone scan
- CT of abdomen or ultrasound of liver

Total mastectomy with axillary node dissection (MRM) with/ without reconstruction

- Total mastectomy with axillary node dissection (MRM) with/ without reconstruction or
- Doxorubicin-based or taxane-based preoperative chemotherapy. Preoperative chemotherapy is the preferred option for primary treatment to observe for tumor responsiveness and to increase breast conservation rates.

Doxorubicin-based or taxane-based preoperative chemotherapy

◇ Response and operable**? — Yes →

- Paclitaxel followed by FAC or
- FAC followed by paclitaxel or
- AC followed by paclitaxel or
- Paclitaxel followed by AC or
- FAC or AC if node negative

→ Yes →

- Total mastectomy with axillary node dissection (MRM) or
- Segmental mastectomy with axillary node dissection

No → Treat with potentially non-cross-resistant regimen (i.e. taxane-based if doxorubicin-based previously or doxorubicin-based if taxane-based previously)

◇ Response and operable***? — Yes →

No → Radiotherapy →

Postop radiotherapy after completion of chemotherapy if no prior radiotherapy and tamoxifen for 5 yr if ER positive

Physical exam every 4 mo for 2 yr; then every 6 mo for 3 yr; then yearly
Mammography yearly
CXR annually for 5 yr for patients treated with radiotherapy
Pelvic exam yearly for women on tamoxifen with intact uterus
If adjuvant chemotherapy, CBC, differential, platelets, alkaline phosphatase, SGPT, and LDH yearly

Individualize any further treatment

Stage IIIA
T0 N2 M0
T1 N2 M0
T2 N2 M0
T3 N2 M0

Stage IIIB
T4 any N M0
any T N3 M0

Stage IV
any T any N M1 (ipsilateral supraclavicular nodes only)

- CBC, platelets, liver function tests (total bilirubin, alkaline phosphatase, SGPT, LDH)
- Pathology review*
- Estrogen and progesterone receptors
- Her-2/Neu
- CXR
- Bilateral diagnostic mammography
- Bone scan
- CT of abdomen or ultrasound of liver
- ECG if > 60 yr

Doxorubicin-based or taxane-based preoperative chemotherapy

---

* Pathology review to include:
- Tumor size
- Differentiation
- Nuclear grade
- Histologic type
- Lymph node status
- Extracapsular extension (focal < 2 mm or gross ≥ 2 mm)
- Intramammary vascular/lymphatic invasion
- Her-2/Neu and receptor status

** For patients who may become candidates for breast conservation treatment following preoperative chemotherapy, consider percutaneous insertion of radio-opaque markers in tumor bed to facilitate segmental mastectomy, as patients may have complete response of tumor to systemic therapy.

*** For selected locally advanced breast cancers that are clinically node negative (T3N0), consider lymphatic mapping and sentinel lymph node biopsy.

AC = Doxorubicin and cyclophosphamide
FAC = Fluorouracil, doxorubicin, and cyclophosphamide

Revised 10-25-2000

Panel 4: Recurrence or Metastasis

 Treatment

EVALUATION
FOR RECURRENCE
OR METASTASIS

TREATMENT FOR RECURRENCE OR METASTASIS

Note: If available, clinical trials should be considered as preferred treatment options for eligible patients.

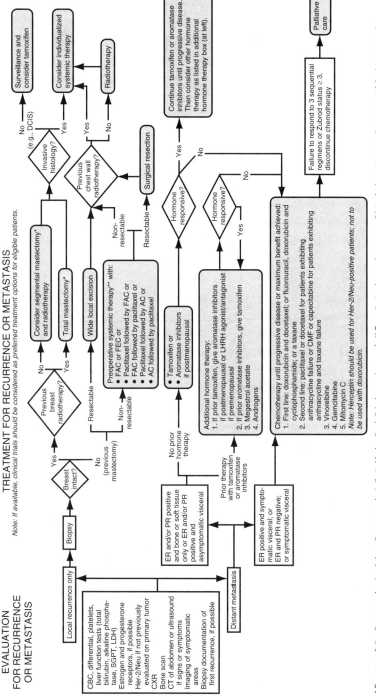

* Surgery, radiation therapy, and regional chemotherapy may be indicated for localized clinical scenarios:

1. Brain metastases
2. Leptomeningeal disease
3. Choroid metastases
4. Pleural effusion
5. Pericardial effusion

6. Biliary obstruction
7. Ureteral obstruction
8. Impending pathologic fracture
9. Pathologic fracture
10. Cord compression

11. Painful lesions
12. Plexopathy/radiculopathy
13. Superior vena cava syndrome
14. Extensive locoregional disease

** For patients who may become candidates for breast conservation treatment following preoperative chemotherapy, consider percutaneous insertion of radio-opaque markers in tumor bed to facilitate segmental mastectomy, as patients may have complete response of tumor to systemic therapy.

Revised 10-25-2000

2 PRIMARY PREVENTION OF BREAST CANCER AND SCREENING FOR EARLY DETECTION OF BREAST CANCER

Therese B. Bevers

CHAPTER OVERVIEW

The paradigm for breast cancer prevention is shifting from a sole focus on screening (breast self-examination, clinical breast examination, and mammography) to an approach that incorporates risk assessment and primary prevention strategies. A computerized breast cancer risk assessment tool that calculates individual women's breast cancer risk is now available for use in the clinical setting.

A critical question is how this risk can be reduced. While lifestyle modification can be suggested as a healthy maneuver, its benefit in reducing breast cancer risk remains uncertain. Prophylactic surgical strategies (mastectomy and oophorectomy) have been demonstrated to significantly reduce breast cancer risk, but because the physiological and psychological consequences can be significant, these surgeries are primarily reserved for women with a known or suspected genetic predisposition to breast cancer.

With the demonstration that tamoxifen can reduce breast cancer risk by almost half, chemoprevention is emerging as the primary prevention strategy of choice for most women at increased risk for the disease. However, tamoxifen is not without significant risks itself, and counseling is imperative so that women understand the potential risks and benefits of therapy and can make an informed decision.

As primary prevention has evolved, so too has breast cancer screening; screening recommendations are now risk based. Diagnostic algorithms are available for clinical and mammographic abnormalities. A key component of the diagnostic evaluation is establishing concordance between radiographic and pathologic findings and the initial clinical examination and level of suspicion.

INTRODUCTION

The Cancer Prevention Center at M. D. Anderson Cancer Center offers a comprehensive array of clinical services and conducts research in the areas of breast, cervical, endometrial, ovarian, prostate, colorectal, skin, lung, and head and neck cancers. Programs include cancer risk assessment and risk reduction counseling, genetic counseling and testing, a multimodality tobacco cessation program, nutrition counseling and health education, chemoprevention, and cancer screening. The Cancer Prevention Center strives to address the cancer concerns of both individuals at average risk for cancer and individuals at high risk. The Cancer Prevention Center serves as a gateway into M. D. Anderson and serves as one of M. D. Anderson's links between healthy individuals and those affected by cancer.

The Cancer Prevention Center's breast cancer program provides risk assessment services, including breast and ovarian cancer genetic counseling and testing, risk reduction counseling, chemoprevention, and screening. Diagnostic services for individuals with undiagnosed breast abnormalities are also offered. In addition, 2 programs have been developed for patients who already have breast cancer. One program provides screening for second primary tumors in appropriately selected breast cancer patients undergoing active treatment, with an emphasis on sites of increased risk determined on the basis of the history of breast cancer and the treatment. The other program combines surveillance for recurrent breast cancer with screening for second primary tumors in selected breast cancer survivors.

EPIDEMIOLOGY

Excluding cancers of the skin, breast cancer is the most common cancer among women, accounting for nearly 1 of every 3 cancers diagnosed in American women. One in 9 women will develop breast cancer by 85 years of age, and 1 in 8 will develop breast cancer by 90 years of age. The United States has the highest crude and age-standardized breast cancer incidence rates in the world. Approximately 192,200 new cases of invasive breast cancer will be diagnosed in 2001 among women in the United States. Breast cancer is the second leading cause of cancer deaths in women, with 40,200 women expected to die of this disease in 2001.

The increase in breast cancer incidence that has been observed over the past 6 decades can be divided into 3 distinct phases. From 1940 to 1982, the incidences of invasive breast cancer and ductal carcinoma in situ (DCIS) increased approximately 1% and 2% per year, respectively. This increase was due to the gradual increase in underlying risk factors for breast cancer, such as delayed childbearing and having fewer children. Between 1982 and 1988, the incidence of invasive cancers increased 4% per year, and the incidence of DCIS increased a dramatic 28% per year. These increases were a direct result of mammographic screening practices. Between 1988 and 1996, the incidence of invasive breast cancer remained level (Figure 2–1). During the same period, the incidence of DCIS continued to increase, but this reflected a shift in the stage of disease at diagnosis toward earlier, more curable cancer rather than a true increase in occurrence.

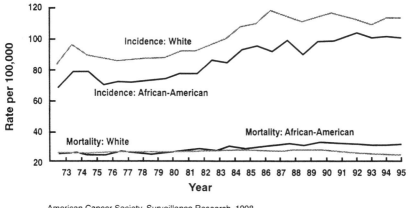

American Cancer Society, Surveillance Research, 1998
Data from SEER, 1998 and NCHS, 1998

Figure 2–1. Incidence and mortality of breast cancer by race.

Breast cancer mortality remained relatively stable between 1950 and the late 1980s. Death rates began to decline beginning in 1989 and have decreased an average of 1.8% per year since then (Figure 2–1). This decline in breast cancer mortality has been attributed both to improvements in breast cancer treatment and to the benefits of mammographic screening. As the percentage of cases diagnosed at the in situ or early invasive stages of disease increases, death rates should continue to decline.

An important paradox is the difference in breast cancer incidence and mortality rates between white and black women (Figure 2–1). Incidence rates are 20% higher in white women than in black women, yet among women diagnosed between 1983 and 1989, the 5-year relative survival rate is 16% lower for black women than for white women. This higher mortality in black women has primarily been attributed to inadequate screening practices in this population, which lead to delayed diagnosis and later-stage disease at diagnosis. However, even when black and white women are compared stage for stage, the mortality in black women is higher. The reasons for this are unknown.

RISK FACTORS

There are a number of established and potential risk factors for breast cancer. These factors can be divided into 7 broad categories: age, family history of breast cancer, hormonal factors, proliferative breast disease, irradiation of the breast region at an early age, personal history of malignancy, and lifestyle factors.

Age

Besides female sex, increasing age is the single most important risk factor for developing breast cancer. Although a woman's lifetime risk of developing breast cancer is 1 in 8, the greatest portion of this lifetime risk is due to the risks at older ages (Table 2–1). An interesting fact is that older women, who are at greatest risk, are the least likely to know that older age is a risk factor for breast cancer. In contrast, women younger than 50 years of age are the most likely to overestimate their breast cancer risk and the benefits of breast cancer screening.

Family History of Breast Cancer

Women with a family history of breast cancer, especially breast cancer in a first-degree relative (i.e., mother, sister, or daughter), have an increased risk of developing breast cancer themselves. The risk is even greater if more than 1 first-degree relative had breast cancer, if the breast cancer occurred before menopause, or if it was bilateral. Table 2–2 illustrates relative risks associated with having a first-degree relative with breast cancer. The relative risk ranges from 1.5 for postmenopausal, unilateral breast cancer to 9.0 for premenopausal, bilateral breast cancer.

Approximately 5% to 10% of breast cancer cases result from inherited mutations in breast cancer susceptibility genes, such as *BRCA1* and *BRCA2*. (For more information about genetic factors, see chapter 3.) It is very important to identify individuals who may have a genetic predisposition for breast cancer because these individuals may have a 40% to 60% lifetime risk of breast cancer, and in some families as high as an 80% lifetime risk, and thus have unique primary prevention and screening needs.

Table 2–1. Age-Specific Probabilities of Developing Breast Cancer[a]

If current age is. . .	Then the probability of developing breast cancer in the next 10 years is:[b]	or 1 in:
20	0.05%	2,187
30	0.39%	258
40	1.48%	67
50	2.67%	38
60	3.42%	29
70	4.01%	25

[a]Among those free of cancer at beginning of age interval. Based on cases diagnosed 1994–1996. Percentages and "1 in" numbers may not be numerically equivalent due to rounding.
[b]Probability derived using NCI DEVCAN software. American Cancer Society, Surveillance Research, 1999.
Reprinted by the permission of the American Cancer Society, Inc., from *Breast Cancer Facts & Figures, 1999–2000.*

Table 2–2. Determinants of Breast Cancer Risk

Factor	Relative Risk
Family History of Breast Cancer	
First-degree relative	1.8
Premenopausal first-degree relative	3.0
Postmenopausal first-degree relative	1.5
Premenopausal first-degree relative (bilateral breast cancer)	9.0
Postmenopausal first-degree relative (bilateral breast cancer)	4.0–5.4
Menstrual History (Age in Years)	
Menarche before age 12	1.7–3.4
Menarche after age 17	0.3
Menopause before age 45	0.5–0.7
Menopause from age 45–54	1.0
Menopause after age 55	1.5
Menopause after age 55 with more than 40 menstrual years	2.5–5.0
Oophorectomy before age 35	0.4
Anovulatory menstrual cycles	2.0–4.0
Pregnancy History	
Term pregnancy before age 20	0.4
First term pregnancy at age 20–34	1.0
First term pregnancy after age 35	1.5–4.0
Nulliparous patient	1.3–4.0

Adapted from Marchant, 1997.

Hormonal Factors

For many years, certain reproductive characteristics have been associated with an increased risk of breast cancer. Early menarche (before 12 years of age), late menopause (after 55 years of age), late age at first full-term pregnancy (>35 years of age), and nulliparity all increase a woman's risk of breast cancer by affecting endogenous reproductive hormones (Table 2–2). Exogenous hormone use has also been linked to breast cancer risk, although the link is more controversial. Recent use of oral contraceptives and prolonged use of estrogen (>8–10 years) have been shown to increase breast cancer risk. This risk seems to disappear 5 to 10 years after the therapy is discontinued. In a recent study, combined therapy with estrogen plus progestin was shown to confer even greater breast cancer risk than estrogen replacement therapy used alone (Schairer et al, 2000). In a woman with an intact uterus, clinical management is especially complex because the risk of breast cancer from combination estrogen-plus-progestin therapy must be weighed against the increased risk of endometrial cancer from use of unopposed estrogen.

The fact that oophorectomy in women younger than 35 years of age is associated with a reduction in the risk of breast cancer by as much as 60%

provides further support for the role of hormones in the development of breast cancer (Table 2–2).

Proliferative Breast Disease

Some women with a history of prior breast biopsy for benign breast disease have an increased risk of breast cancer. The degree of increase in risk depends on the specific epithelial abnormality (Table 2–3). The majority of lesions do not have proliferative changes and are not associated with an increase in breast cancer risk. Proliferative lesions without atypia are associated with a 2-fold increase in risk. Proliferative lesions with atypia (atypical ductal or lobular hyperplasia) confer a 5-fold increase in breast cancer risk. The addition of a first-degree relative with breast cancer to the risk profile of atypical hyperplasia doubles the relative risk to 10-fold, which is similar to the risk conferred by lobular carcinoma in situ (LCIS).

Irradiation of the Breast Area at an Early Age

As the population of pediatric cancer survivors ages, evidence is emerging that therapeutic irradiation of the breast region during the first, second, and third decades of life increases the risk of breast cancer. The greatest risk is seen in individuals treated with radiation therapy before age 15, with some studies suggesting as great as a 35% increased risk of breast cancer in such individuals by age 40. This risk is important to note because screening practices may need to be instituted earlier in this population than would normally be recommended.

Table 2–3. Breast Lesions and Relative Risk for Invasive Breast Cancer

No Increased Risk	Slightly Increased Risk (1.5–2.0×)	Moderately Increased Risk (5×)	Markedly Increased Risk (10×)
Adenosis	Hyperplasia	Atypical hyperplasia	Lobular carcinoma
Apocrine	(moderate or	(ductal or lobular)	in situ
metaplasia	florid, solid or		Atypical hyperplasia
Cysts	papillary)		with family
Duct ectasia	Papillomatosis		history of breast
Fibroadenoma			cancer
Fibrosis			
Hyperplasia,			
mild			
Mastitis			
Squamous			
metaplasia			

Source: Howell, 1995.

Personal History of Malignancy

It is well established that a personal history of breast cancer increases the risk of a subsequent breast cancer. In addition, a personal history of endometrial, ovarian, or colorectal cancer increases the relative risk as much as 2-fold.

Lifestyle Factors

Epidemiologic studies have identified a number of lifestyle factors that may influence breast cancer risk.

Diet and nutrition are controversial factors. Dietary fat has received much attention as a possible risk factor for breast cancer because of the high correlation between national per capita fat consumption and the incidence of the disease. In addition, a number of experiments in laboratory animals have suggested a link between the amount and type of dietary lipids and the growth of mammary tumors. However, studies addressing this issue have produced conflicting results. Even greater uncertainty persists regarding dietary supplements, such as soy, which has been suggested to both increase and decrease breast cancer risk. Until long-term, prospective studies that include more accurate and reliable assessments of dietary intake and supplementation are conducted, no definitive statements can be made regarding diet and nutrition and breast cancer risk.

In a pooled analysis of 6 prospective cohort studies, a slight increase in breast cancer risk was seen in women reporting consumption of 1 or more alcoholic beverages per day, compared with nondrinkers. The risk appeared to increase linearly with each 10-gram-per-day increase in consumption, ranging from a relative risk of 1.09 (95% confidence interval [CI], 1.04–1.13) for 1 drink per day to 1.41 (95% CI, 1.18–1.69) for 2 to 5 drinks per day, compared with nondrinkers. It has been suggested that alcohol consumption increases breast cancer risk either by decreasing the metabolic clearance of estrogen or by increasing the secretion of estrogen.

Because excess weight and weight gain are modifiable risk factors, a significant amount of interest and study has focused on the relationship between weight and breast cancer risk. Several prospective and case-control studies found an association between obesity and breast cancer risk. However, in other studies, the relationship between body size and risk of breast cancer differed according to menopausal status. Postmenopausal obesity and weight gain have been suggested to be associated with an increase in breast cancer risk.

A variety of other risk factors have also been investigated to determine whether they increase the risk of breast cancer. Epidemiologic studies have demonstrated an increase in breast cancer incidence in women with a higher level of education or higher socioeconomic status. Current evidence suggests that cigarette smoking does not influence breast cancer risk except possibly in women who are slow acetylators of aromatic amines. In addition, silicone implants and abortion do not appear to be associated with increased risk. Breast-feeding appears to confer some protective effect against premenopausal breast cancer.

RISK ASSESSMENT

Several mathematical models have been developed to predict the risk of developing breast cancer. The 2 models most commonly used are the Claus model and the Gail model. The Claus model assesses familial risk of breast cancer, whereas the Gail model assesses populational risk using nongenetic factors. Specifics pertaining to the Claus model are reviewed in chapter 3.

Risk factors used in the Gail model include age, family history of first-degree relatives with breast cancer, age at first live birth (or nulliparity), history of breast biopsy and atypical hyperplasia, and age at menarche. Because the incidence of breast cancer differs by race, the current, modified version of the Gail model includes race-specific data. This modified version of the Gail model was used in the Breast Cancer Prevention Trial (BCPT). The model accurately predicted the number of invasive breast cancers in the placebo arm of the trial: overall, the model predicted 159 cases of invasive breast cancer in the BCPT, and 155 cases were observed, yielding an expected-to-observed ratio close to unity (1.03).

Since the announcement of the results of the BCPT and the validation of the modified Gail model, the National Cancer Institute (NCI) has developed and distributed a computer program for calculating the projected risk of developing breast cancer. This program is available at http://bcra.nci.nih.gov/brc and can be used to facilitate the calculation of a woman's breast cancer risk in the clinical setting. The program is the first multifactorial model that has been developed and made available for clinicians to use for estimating the risk for a specific cancer.

The program prompts the user to input information about each of the risk factors and provides a printout showing the projected breast cancer risk in the next 5 years and the projected lifetime risk. For comparative purposes, the printout also includes the 5-year risk and lifetime risk for a woman of the same age and race as the woman evaluated but who is in the average risk category for all risk factors.

Increased risk is defined as a 5-year calculated risk of 1.7% or greater. This is the average risk of a 60-year-old woman. This risk was chosen as the cut-off point for elevated risk because 60 years is the median age at which breast cancer is diagnosed in the United States.

It is important to understand the limitations of the modified Gail model. It is not applicable to women with a personal history of invasive breast cancer, DCIS, or LCIS. In calculating breast cancer risk, the Gail model makes no adjustment for a first-degree relative with premenopausal or bilateral breast cancer. In addition, genetic mutations are not considered in the calculation of breast cancer risk. As a result, risk may be significantly underestimated. For these reasons, the risk calculation cannot be taken out of the context of the patient's overall personal and family history.

However, even with these limitations, the modified Gail model provides valuable information and serves as a key starting point in the evaluation of breast cancer risk. With the exception of women meeting the criteria for genetic-risk evaluation and counseling (Table 2–4), all women 35 years of age and older who present to the M. D. Anderson Cancer Prevention Center for breast cancer screening have a risk assessment calculation performed using the modified Gail model. On the basis of the estimated risk, a unique, personal prevention program is developed. This prevention program includes recommendations for primary prevention strategies and screening appropriate to the individual's risk level.

Three variables in the modified Gail model change or may change over time: age, family history of first-degree relatives with breast cancer, and history of breast biopsy with or without atypical hyperplasia. Because incremental increases in age produce only slight increases in the 5-year breast cancer risk, recalculations to adjust for age are done only periodically unless the patient just missed the 1.7% cut-off defining increased breast cancer risk. However, any change in the other 2 variables—i.e., a new breast cancer in a first-degree relative or an interim breast biopsy— prompts recalculation because the associated increase in breast cancer risk can significantly alter the benefit-versus-risk ratio for tamoxifen therapy (for more information, see the section Tamoxifen later in this chapter).

PRIMARY PREVENTION

Currently, 3 approaches have been proven to decrease breast cancer risk: prophylactic mastectomy, prophylactic oophorectomy, and chemoprevention with tamoxifen. Prophylactic surgery should be considered only by women with a known or suspected genetic predisposition. In contrast, chemoprevention with tamoxifen may be considered by any woman with

Table 2–4. M. D. Anderson Cancer Center Criteria for Genetic Risk Evaluation

- More than 2 relatives with breast cancer diagnosed before 50 years of age or with ovarian cancer
- 1 relative with breast and ovarian cancer
- 1 relative with bilateral breast cancer less than age 50
- 1 male relative with breast cancer
- Ashkenazi Jewish descent and breast or ovarian cancer in the family

increased risk. Lifestyle modifications have not been proven to reduce the risk of developing breast cancer, but because they can lead to better health, counseling about lifestyle modifications is nevertheless an important element of primary cancer prevention.

Lifestyle Modification

Studies exploring whether modification of lifestyle factors can reduce breast cancer risk have yielded inconsistent and controversial findings. However, regardless of their impact on breast cancer risk, lifestyle modifications can lead to better health and are recommended for individuals at all risk levels. These modifications include consuming a low-fat diet, limiting alcohol intake, avoiding smoking, exercising, and maintaining ideal body weight.

Prophylactic Mastectomy

Prophylactic mastectomy (see chapter 7) is an aggressive surgical procedure with many physiological and psychological ramifications. For most women with an increased risk of developing breast cancer, the drawbacks of prophylactic mastectomy outweigh the benefits, and the procedure is therefore not appropriate. However, for women with a considerable risk of developing breast cancer—primarily women with a genetic predisposition but also, to a lesser extent, women with LCIS—prophylactic mastectomy remains a risk reduction strategy to be considered. This is especially true in light of the recent findings by Hartmann et al (1999) showing a 90% reduction in breast cancer incidence in women at moderate to high risk after bilateral prophylactic mastectomy. Prophylactic mastectomy should be undertaken only after extensive counseling so that the patient has a thorough understanding of her breast cancer risk and other available risk reduction strategies as well as the psychological issues associated with the procedure. In addition, because total mastectomy is the current procedure of choice, the availability of immediate breast reconstruction should be discussed during the counseling process. There is currently no role for subcutaneous mastectomy in the primary prevention of breast cancer.

It is an interesting paradox that prophylactic mastectomy is considered as a prevention strategy while women diagnosed with breast cancer are given the option of breast conservation therapy. Because of advances in breast cancer chemoprevention, most breast cancer prevention experts are shifting the emphasis away from prophylactic surgery toward chemoprevention, especially for patients with LCIS. In the current M. D. Anderson practice algorithm, patients with LCIS are seen in the Cancer Prevention Center for risk counseling and a review of the primary prevention strategies currently available, with an emphasis placed on chemoprevention. Patients with LCIS are referred to a surgeon only if they are seriously considering and desiring prophylactic mastectomy.

Prophylactic Oophorectomy

Oophorectomy in women younger than 35 years of age has been shown to reduce the risk of breast cancer by as much as 60%. However, surgically induced menopause at this age is associated with its own risks. In the postmenopausal period, osteoporosis escalates, and there is an increased risk of cardiovascular disease. In addition, women with premature menopause can have a variety of associated symptoms that must be managed. For these reasons, prophylactic oophorectomy is typically considered only for women with a genetic predisposition, in whom the potential benefits of this procedure are increased because of the substantial reduction not only in breast cancer risk but also in ovarian cancer risk.

Chemoprevention

With the publication of the findings of the landmark BCPT in 1998, chemoprevention of breast cancer has emerged as a risk reduction strategy for women at increased risk for the disease.

Tamoxifen

Tamoxifen citrate is a selective estrogen receptor modulator that competes with circulating estrogen for binding to the estrogen receptor. Depending on the tissue and species, tamoxifen acts as an estrogen agonist or an estrogen antagonist.

In humans, tamoxifen has estrogen antagonistic properties in breast tissue and thus inhibits the growth of estrogen-dependent breast tumors. However, tamoxifen has estrogen agonistic effects on the endometrium, bones, and lipids. Tamoxifen induces cellular proliferation in the endometrium, preserves bone mass in postmenopausal women, and lowers low-density lipoprotein cholesterol.

For more than 20 years, tamoxifen has been used in the treatment of breast cancer. Tamoxifen was chosen as a potential breast cancer chemopreventive agent because studies showed that tamoxifen given for 5 years reduced the incidence of recurrent breast cancer by 42% and reduced the incidence of contralateral breast cancer by 47%.

In 1992, the National Surgical Adjuvant Breast and Bowel Project, with the support of the NCI, launched the landmark BCPT, also known as the P-1 trial or the tamoxifen prevention trial, to investigate the value of tamoxifen in reducing the risk of primary invasive breast cancer in women at increased risk for the disease. A total of 13,388 women aged 35 years or older who were at increased risk for breast cancer were entered into the trial and randomly assigned to receive either tamoxifen 20 mg daily or placebo daily for 5 years. Increased risk was defined as a personal history of LCIS, a 5-year risk of developing breast cancer of at least 1.7% as calculated using the modified Gail model, or age 60 years or older.

As of July 31, 1998, a total of 368 cases of invasive and noninvasive breast cancer had been observed among the 13,175 women with evaluable end points. There were 175 cases of invasive breast cancer in the placebo group, compared with 89 cases in the tamoxifen group, representing a 49% risk reduction (relative risk, 0.51; 95% CI, 0.39–0.66, $P<0.0001$). The annual event rate for invasive breast cancer among women taking tamoxifen was 3.4 per 1000 women, compared with 6.8 per 1000 women taking placebo. As can be seen from Table 2–5, the risk reduction was seen for all age groups in the trial as well as all projected levels of risk. Women with a history of LCIS had a risk reduction of 56%, and women with a history of atypical hyperplasia had a dramatic 86% risk reduction. The incidence of estrogen receptor (ER)-positive tumors was reduced 69% in the tamoxifen group compared with the placebo group; however, the rate of ER-negative tumors was not significantly different between the 2 groups. The risk reduction for invasive breast cancer was seen within the first year of the trial, and the lower incidence of breast cancer was seen for each subsequent year of the trial throughout 6 years of follow-up.

An additional benefit of tamoxifen suggested in the BCPT was the reduction in the incidence of osteoporotic fractures. The incidence of osteoporotic fractures of the hip, spine, or distal radius was reduced 19% among women receiving tamoxifen (137 events in the placebo group vs 111 events in the tamoxifen group). Most notable was a 45% reduction in fractures of the hip (Table 2–5).

Tamoxifen has many benefits, but it is also associated with risks. A 2.5-fold increase in the risk of developing endometrial cancer was observed in the women who received tamoxifen compared with the women who received placebo (Table 2–5). The average annual rates of endometrial cancer were 0.9 per 1000 women in the placebo group and 2.3 per 1000 women in the tamoxifen group. All 36 cases of invasive endometrial cancer that occurred among women receiving tamoxifen in the BCPT were stage I according to the classification of the International Federation of Gynecology and Obstetrics and had excellent clinical prognoses. It is also important to note that the increase in endometrial cancer risk was significant only among women aged 50 years or older (Table 2–5).

Tamoxifen was also associated with an increase in the number of thromboembolic vascular events (Table 2–5). While only the increase in the rate of pulmonary embolism reached statistical significance, the increased event rates for stroke, transient ischemic attack, and deep-vein thrombosis among women 50 years of age and older who took tamoxifen are cause for concern.

A marginal increase in the rate of cataract development was observed among women who took tamoxifen in the BCPT. The number of cataract surgeries was also increased in the tamoxifen-treated group.

Bothersome hot flashes were reported by 46% of women in the tamoxifen group, compared with only 29% in the placebo group. Vaginal

Table 2–5. Average Annual Rates for Outcomes in the Breast Cancer Prevention Trial

Cancer Outcome	Rate per 1000 Women		Risk Ratio (95% CI)
	Tamoxifen	Placebo	
Invasive breast cancer	3.4	6.8	0.51 (0.39–0.66)
Noninvasive breast cancer	1.4	2.7	0.50 (0.33–0.77)
Invasive breast cancer by patient characteristic			
Age, years			
≤ 49	3.8	6.7	0.56 (0.37–0.85)
50–59	3.1	6.3	0.49 (0.29–0.81)
≥ 60	3.3	7.3	0.45 (0.27–0.74)
History of LCIS			
Yes	5.7	13.0	0.44 (0.16–1.06)
No	3.3	6.4	0.51 (0.39–0.68)
History of atypical hyperplasia			
Yes	1.4	10.1	0.14 (0.03–0.47)
No	3.6	6.4	0.56 (0.42–0.73)
Number of 1st-degree relatives with breast cancer			
0	3.0	6.4	0.46 (0.24–0.84)
1	3.0	6.0	0.51 (0.35–0.73)
2	4.8	8.7	0.55 (0.30–0.97)
≥3	7.0	13.7	0.51 (0.15–1.55)
Risk of breast cancer within 5 years (%)			
≤ 2	2.1	5.5	0.37 (0.18–0.72)
2.01–3.0	3.5	5.2	0.68 (0.41–1.11)
3.01–5.0	3.9	5.9	0.66 (0.39–1.09)
≥ 5.01	4.5	13.3	0.34 (0.19–0.58)
Invasive endometrial cancer			
Overall	2.3	0.9	2.53 (1.35–4.97)
Age ≤ 49 years	1.3	1.1	1.21 (0.41–3.60)
Age ≥ 50 years	3.0	0.8	4.01 (1.70–10.90)
Fractures			
Hip	0.5	0.8	0.55 (0.25–1.15)
Hip, spine, and lower radius combined	4.3	5.3	0.81 (0.63–1.05)
Thromboembolic events			
Stroke	1.4	0.9	1.59 (0.93–2.77)
Transient ischemic attack	0.7	1.0	0.76 (0.40–1.44)
Pulmonary embolism	0.7	0.2	3.01 (1.15–9.27)
Deep vein thrombosis	1.3	0.8	1.60 (0.91–2.86)

Adapted from Fisher et al, 1998.

discharge reported as moderately bothersome or worse was seen in 29% of the treatment group, compared with 13% of the control group. Weight gain and depression were not associated with tamoxifen therapy. In the BCPT, there was no difference between the placebo and tamoxifen groups in the frequency of reported weight gain. Also, there was no difference between the placebo and tamoxifen groups in the frequency or severity of reported cases of depression or in the values of the depression scale measured at each follow-up visit as part of the quality-of-life assessment.

Since the unblinding of the BCPT results in April 1998, the findings of 2 European trials of tamoxifen for prevention of breast cancer have been published in *The Lancet* (Powles et al, 1998; Veronesi et al, 1998). The findings from these 2 trials differed significantly from those of the BCPT in that no prevention benefit was seen (Table 2–6). Because the BCPT was a well-designed and well-conducted trial with statistically significant findings, the contradictory findings from the 2 European trials do not negate the BCPT results. However, there are important differences between the European trials and the BCPT that should be noted.

In the Italian Tamoxifen Prevention Study (Veronesi et al, 1998), 5408 healthy women aged 35 to 70 years were randomly assigned to receive tamoxifen 20 mg daily for 5 years or placebo daily for 5 years. Women were not eligible unless they had previously undergone hysterectomy; this requirement ensured that women would not be affected by the increase in endometrial cancer risk due to tamoxifen. As a result of this eligibility restriction, the women in this study had either low risk of developing breast cancer (women who had undergone hysterectomy with bilateral oophorectomy) or normal risk of developing breast cancer (women who had undergone hysterectomy without bilateral oophorectomy).

At a median follow-up of 46 months, the investigators found no significant difference in the incidence of breast cancer between the treatment groups except among women taking hormone replacement therapy

Table 2–6. Summary of Tamoxifen Prevention Trials

Trial	Sample Size	Risk of Breast Cancer	Woman-years of Follow-up	Breast Cancers/ 1000 Woman-years Placebo	Tamoxifen
NSABP P-1	13,388	High (modified Gail model)	52,401	6.8	3.4
Royal Marsden	2471	Based on family history	12,355	5.0	4.7
Italian	5408	Low to normal	20,731	2.3	2.1

Reprinted with permission from Vogel VG: Breast cancer prevention: trial results. In: *Breast Cancer Prevention: Incorporating New Data into Clinical Practice.* Discovery International, 2000.

(HRT). Overall, a total of 22 breast cancers were diagnosed in the placebo group, compared with 19 in the tamoxifen-treated group. Among women taking HRT, 8 breast cancers were found in the placebo group (n = 390), compared with 1 in the tamoxifen group (n = 362).

The Italian trial had significant problems with compliance—26% of the women discontinued their study drug in the first year. The data from the Italian trial are confounded by the low-risk population, the small numbers enrolled, and the compliance issue, which resulted in a low power of the study to detect a significant difference.

The Royal Marsden Hospital Tamoxifen Prevention Pilot Trial (Powles et al, 1998) enrolled 2471 women with a family history of breast cancer. Whereas the BCPT based risk predominantly on nongenetic factors, the Royal Marsden trial used family history as the only risk criterion. The Royal Marsden study population was younger (61% under age 50) than the BCPT population (40% under age 50). Unlike the situation in the BCPT, in the European trials, postmenopausal women were allowed to use concomitant HRT.

At the time of the BCPT unblinding, an interim analysis of the Royal Marsden trial was conducted. With a median follow-up of 70 months, there was no benefit of tamoxifen over placebo in terms of reducing the incidence of breast cancer (34 cases in the tamoxifen group vs 36 in the placebo group). There also was no evidence that HRT confounded any possible benefit of tamoxifen.

According to the investigators' calculations, the Royal Marsden trial had sufficient power to detect a significant difference between the 2 study arms. The fact that no difference was detected may have been due to the younger population, as there is a higher incidence of ER-negative breast cancers in young women. As has been demonstrated in the BCPT and in treatment trials, tamoxifen is most effective in ER-positive breast cancers and has no significant impact on ER-negative tumors.

While the results of the Italian and Royal Marsden tamoxifen trials differed from those of the BCPT, the differences are most likely due to differences in study populations and design. On the basis of the BCPT findings, the US Food and Drug Administration has approved tamoxifen for the reduction of breast cancer risk in healthy women at increased risk for the disease.

Raloxifene

Raloxifene is a second-generation selective estrogen receptor modulator. The use of raloxifene in reducing the risk of fractures in postmenopausal women with osteoporosis was studied in the Multiple Outcomes of Raloxifene Evaluation (MORE) trial. In this placebo-controlled, double-blind trial, 7704 postmenopausal women were randomly assigned to receive raloxifene 60 mg daily, raloxifene 120 mg daily, or placebo. Analysis of the data was performed at a median of 40 months. Because raloxifene was found to reduce the incidence of fractures and increase bone density, the US Food and Drug Administration approved raloxifene for the prevention of osteoporosis.

The development of breast cancer was a secondary end point of the MORE trial. At 28.9 months follow-up, 11 cases of breast cancer (0.21%) had been detected in the raloxifene-treated patients, compared with 21 cases (0.82%) in the placebo group. This 74% reduction in the incidence of breast cancer with raloxifene (relative risk, 0.26; 95% CI, 0.13–0.52) was seen at both the 60-mg and 120-mg doses. Similar to the findings with tamoxifen, an increased incidence in venous thromboembolic events was seen in the raloxifene group (relative risk, 3.1; 95% CI, 1.5–6.2). In contrast to the findings with tamoxifen, raloxifene was not associated with an increase in the incidence of endometrial cancer (relative risk, 0.8; 95% CI, 0.2–2.7). However, the follow-up was too short to permit definitive judgement about this relationship, especially given that it took nearly a decade for the effects of tamoxifen on the endometrium to be fully understood.

In interpreting the findings of the MORE trial, some important characteristics of the study design should be understood. Women were not selected for the MORE trial on the basis of their breast cancer risk. Breast cancer risk was not determined prospectively, and this characteristic was not included in the stratification of the participants into the treatment arms. Given the known characteristics of the participants of this trial, specifically their personal history of osteoporosis, it could be argued that they are at decreased risk for both breast and endometrial cancer. As a result, the lack of demonstrated risk for endometrial cancer should be interpreted with caution.

The intriguing findings from the MORE study are the basis of the Study of Tamoxifen and Raloxifene (STAR) for the Prevention of Breast Cancer. Opened in May 1999, STAR will enroll 22,000 postmenopausal women at increased risk for breast cancer. Women will be randomly assigned to receive either tamoxifen 20 mg daily or raloxifene 60 mg daily for 5 years. The primary end point of this trial is the incidence of invasive breast cancer. Secondary end points are the incidences of DCIS and LCIS, endometrial cancer, bone fractures, and ischemic heart disease. In addition, the toxicity and side effects associated with each therapy will be compared.

Because raloxifene has not been proven to reduce breast cancer risk, raloxifene should not be used for breast cancer chemoprevention at this time outside of a clinical trial.

Counseling before Initiation of Therapy

Women who are found to be at increased risk for developing breast cancer—i.e., women with a personal history of LCIS, a genetic predisposition, or a 5-year risk of 1.7% or greater according to the modified Gail model—should be counseled regarding the benefits and risks of tamoxifen therapy.

However, women with a 5-year predicted breast cancer risk of less than 1.7% should not be considered for tamoxifen therapy at this time. Tamoxifen has not been demonstrated to have beneficial effects in individuals with this level of risk, and at best, any benefit is likely to be small and not sufficient to outweigh the risks of tamoxifen therapy. As previously noted, risk should be reassessed periodically, especially if any significant change occurs in breast cancer risk factors.

Tamoxifen has one of the most extensively documented benefit/risk profiles of any drug. The benefits and risks of the use of tamoxifen for breast cancer prevention were well delineated in the BCPT (Table 2–5). For any given woman, the potential benefits of tamoxifen therapy include reduced risks of invasive breast cancer, noninvasive breast cancer, and fractures of the hip, spine, and distal radius. These benefits were noted in women of all age groups in the BCPT. The potential risks of tamoxifen therapy include increased risks of endometrial cancer, thromboembolic vascular events (pulmonary embolism, deep vein thrombosis, and stroke), and cataracts. In the BCPT, the increase in these risks was seen only in women 50 years of age and older.

For any individual woman at increased risk for breast cancer, an attempt must be made to determine a net effect of tamoxifen therapy, either positive or negative. This net effect is primarily a function of the woman's predicted breast cancer risk, age, and hysterectomy status.

Tamoxifen therapy confers a 49% reduction in the incidence of invasive breast cancer and a 50% reduction in the incidence of noninvasive breast cancer. The magnitude of benefit of tamoxifen therapy in terms of breast cancer risk increases as a direct function of increasing 5-year predicted breast cancer risk (Table 2–7). In other words, a woman with a risk of 7% will experience greater benefit than will a woman with a risk of 1.0%. The expected risks of the other events potentially affected by tamoxifen are based only on age and race. For any given race, the magnitude of the expected effect (be it beneficial or harmful) will increase as a direct function of increasing age (Table 2–8). For example, a 60-year-old white woman has a higher risk for a vascular event than does a 40-year-old

Table 2–7. Magnitude of Breast Cancer Benefit

	Cases per 10,000 over 5 Years	
5-Year Risk (%)	Expected	Prevented
1.0	100	49
3.0	300	147
5.0	500	245
7.0	700	343

Reprinted with permission from Costantino JP, Vogel VG: Evaluating women for prevention prescription: risk assessment and counseling. In: *Breast Cancer Prevention: Incorporating New Data into Clinical Practice*. Discovery International, 2000.

Table 2–8. Annual Incidence Rates per 1000 Women for Other Events Associated with Tamoxifen Therapy

Event	Rates for Women of Ages			
	40–49 y	*50–59 y*	*60–69 y*	*70–79 y*
White Women				
Stroke	0.45	1.10	3.25	7.50
Pulmonary embolism	0.15	0.50	0.88	1.93
Deep vein thrombosis	0.49	0.55	0.98	1.61
Endometrial cancer	0.21	0.81	1.44	1.63
Hip fracture	0.04	1.02	2.42	7.44
Black Women				
Stroke	1.26	3.19	7.48	9.00
Pulmonary embolism	0.46	1.50	2.02	3.09
Deep vein thrombosis	1.52	1.65	2.25	2.58
Endometrial cancer	0.83	0.35	0.89	0.88
Hip fracture	0.03	0.55	0.92	2.83

Adapted from Gail et al, 1999.

white woman. It is important to note that there are some substantial differences by race. For example, depending on the age category, the baseline rates of vascular events among black women are between 1.5 and 2.5 times higher than the rates among white women.

When all the factors that affect the benefits and risks of tamoxifen are considered, it is possible to identify several groups of women in whom the positive effects of tamoxifen will most likely outweigh any negative effects:

1. Women with a very high risk of breast cancer (i.e., a personal history of LCIS or atypical hyperplasia or a 5-year predicted breast cancer risk of 6.5% or more).
2. Women under the age of 50 with a 5-year predicted risk of 1.7% or more.
3. Women 50 years of age or older with a 5-year predicted risk of 1.7% or more who have had a hysterectomy and either are at low risk for vascular events (nonsmoker, not obese, not diabetic, not hypertensive, and physically active) or are currently taking estrogen replacement therapy. (The risk of vascular events is the same with tamoxifen as with estrogen replacement therapy; thus, a change from estrogen to tamoxifen would not increase the risk of vascular events.)

Some women may still be considered for tamoxifen therapy even if the risk/benefit assessment indicates a negative net effect. Consideration should be given to the personal perspectives and desires of the woman. Each individual woman will have her own perception of how the various beneficial and detrimental effects should be weighed. Many individuals who are at increased risk for breast cancer are willing to incur the potential risks of therapy in exchange for the potential reduction in breast cancer risk. The health care provider should keep in mind that a woman's decision to take a drug for prevention is a personal decision. Except in extreme cases, once a woman fully understands the risks associated with tamoxifen therapy, no woman should be denied the opportunity to potentially reduce her risk of breast cancer if she has a strong desire to do so.

It is important that women with a known or suspected genetic predisposition for breast cancer be informed that the benefits of tamoxifen therapy in women with a genetic predisposition are uncertain. Individuals with genetic mutations are known to have a higher probability of ER-negative breast cancers, and tamoxifen has been shown to have no impact on the incidence of ER-negative breast cancers. Subset analyses of the BCPT participants are being conducted to determine the benefit of tamoxifen for women with a known or suspected genetic mutation. At present, such women may still be considered for tamoxifen therapy, but they should be aware that our knowledge of tamoxifen's benefits in their particular subgroup is limited. In addition to counseling about chemoprevention, women with a known or suspected genetic predisposition should receive counseling about prophylactic surgical options (mastectomy and oophorectomy)

Management of Women Taking Tamoxifen

The current recommended regimen for tamoxifen for chemoprevention of breast cancer is 20 mg once daily for 5 years. Women on tamoxifen therapy should have follow-up visits every 6 months. Each visit should include a clinical breast examination (CBE) and symptom assessment. Women receiving tamoxifen should also undergo annual screening mammography and—in women with an intact uterus—annual gynecologic examinations.

Symptom assessment should include inquiries about thromboembolic or gynecologic symptoms. Women taking tamoxifen should be educated about such symptoms and the need to promptly report any abnormal vaginal bleeding or symptoms of thromboembolic events (unilateral lower-extremity edema or acute onset of dyspnea or neurological symptoms). Any abnormal vaginal bleeding should be evaluated with transvaginal sonography, endometrial biopsy, or other procedures as the clinical situation dictates. There is currently no indication for routine endometrial screening, either by transvaginal sonography or endometrial biopsy, of asymptomatic women taking tamoxifen.

The common side effects of tamoxifen therapy have been well defined. Hot flashes are the most common reaction associated with therapy; the incidence of hot flashes is approximately 20% to 30% higher in patients taking tamoxifen than in those taking placebo. Symptomatic reactions are more common among women near the age of menopause and women who have just discontinued estrogen replacement therapy, but hot flashes can occur in women of any age.

Menopausal symptoms such as hot flashes can usually be managed with reassurance because the symptoms diminish with time in most patients. Some patients report symptomatic relief with vitamin E 400 to 800 IU daily or with evening primrose oil 1 to 2 tablets twice a day. If this conservative therapy is not effective, there are several prescription medications that may be of benefit. Paroxetine (Paxil) 10 to 20 mg daily and venlafaxine (Effexor) 25 mg 3 times a day have both been shown in randomized, controlled trials to reduce the incidence of hot flashes. Other agents that may be of benefit include Bellergal-S 1 tablet daily or twice a day and clonidine 0.1 to 0.2 mg daily or twice a day or by transdermal delivery. Each of these therapies should be tried for a minimum of 4 to 6 weeks before being abandoned in favor of another agent. If hot flashes become unresponsive to these approaches, tamoxifen may be discontinued for 4 to 6 weeks and then restarted; often symptoms do not reemerge when tamoxifen is restarted after a "drug holiday." When a drug holiday is implemented, it is important to instruct the patient that the plan is for tamoxifen to be restarted; this way both the patient and the health care provider are working under the same expectations. For some postmenopausal patients, the drug holiday may serve to demonstrate that the hot flashes are not a result of the tamoxifen therapy but rather are a consequence of an estrogen-deprived state.

Some patients taking tamoxifen experience vaginal dryness that can be managed with nonhormonal remedies available over the counter (e.g., Astroglide, Lubrin, Vagisil, Replens). Estrogen creams should be avoided because of the sustained systemic absorption seen with such preparations. However, Estring, a slow-release estrogen vaginal ring inserted every 3 months, is acceptable because systemic levels of estradiol are in the normal postmenopausal range after the first 24 hours of use.

Some patients taking tamoxifen experience a clear, nonodorous, nonirritating vaginal discharge. It is unusual for the discharge to occur in more than scant quantities. Once other causes of vaginal discharge have been eliminated, the patient can be reassured that this discharge is associated with the tamoxifen therapy and is harmless. This discharge is relatively rare and will frequently resolve spontaneously over time.

As previously noted, weight gain and depression are not associated with tamoxifen therapy. If other symptoms occur for which the etiology is not clear, therapy can be temporarily interrupted and restarted after a drug holiday.

Screening

The Cancer Prevention Center's approach to breast cancer screening is illustrated in panel 1 of appendix 2 at the end of this chapter. The cornerstones of screening are CBE, screening mammography, and breast self-examination (BSE), and specific recommendations depend on the woman's personal risk of breast cancer. Although a survival benefit from BSE has not yet been proven, BSE is encouraged for all individuals because it may reveal interval cancers between screenings.

Before screening is initiated, any severe comorbid conditions that limit life expectancy or therapeutic intervention should be considered. Screening may not be appropriate in women with a life expectancy of less than 10 years or in women in whom therapeutic intervention is not planned.

Individuals are stratified on the basis of their history of thoracic radiation therapy, history of proliferative breast disease, and genetic predisposition. Women who do not fall into one of these risk categories undergo routine screening, which consists of CBE every 1 to 3 years between the ages of 20 and 39 years and annually beginning at 40 years of age and annual screening mammography beginning at 40 years of age. If the predicted 5-year breast cancer risk is 1.7% or greater, annual CBE and mammography may be started at age 35, and risk reduction strategies should be considered.

Women who received thoracic radiation therapy during the second or early part of the third decade of life are at increased risk for developing breast cancer. The increase in incidence begins approximately 10 years after radiation therapy. For this reason, in women who received thoracic radiation therapy at a young age, CBE is recommended annually for women younger than 30 years of age and every 6 months for women 30 years of age or older. These women should also consider annual mammography beginning 10 years after radiation therapy but not earlier than age 30. Guidelines for women with a known or suspected genetic predisposition are similar to guidelines for women with a history of thoracic radiation therapy except that annual screening mammography is initiated 5 to 10 years prior to the earliest index case in the family and women should be encouraged to consider risk reduction strategies. Women with atypical hyperplasia or LCIS should have annual CBE and mammograms from the time of diagnosis and should consider risk reduction strategies.

Regardless of the level of breast cancer risk and the primary prevention strategies considered, risk-based breast cancer screening recommendations should be reinforced.

Diagnostic Evaluation of Breast Abnormalities

During the course of breast cancer screening, clinical and mammographic abnormalities will be identified that require further evaluation. Clinical abnormalities can be divided into 4 categories: dominant mass, asymmetric thickening or nodularity, nipple discharge, and skin changes. Guidelines have been developed to direct the diagnostic evaluation of both mammographic and clinical abnormalities.

Mammographic Abnormality with Normal Findings on Clinical Breast Examination

If the findings on mammography are abnormal, a diagnostic work-up is necessary to definitively evaluate the abnormality (see appendix 2, panel 2). The American College of Radiology (ACR) has established the Breast Imaging Reporting and Data System (BI-RADS) to standardize mammography reports (for more information, see chapter 4). The ACR category 0 refers to mammograms for which some combination of additional mammographic views, sonography, and comparison with prior films is necessary to determine the final ACR category. In the screening setting, women with mammographic findings classified as ACR category 1 (normal) or 2 (benign finding) may return to routine screening. Mammographic findings classified as ACR category 3, 4, or 5 warrant additional diagnostic management.

Mammographic findings classified as ACR category 4 (suspicious) or 5 (highly suggestive of malignancy) require tissue diagnosis for definitive assessment. The tissue diagnosis may be accomplished with the use of fine-needle aspiration, core needle biopsy, or excisional biopsy. Establishing concordance between the pathologic findings on fine-needle aspiration or core needle biopsy and the findings on diagnostic imaging is integral in determining that the area of concern has been adequately assessed. Benign pathologic findings would not be concordant with a highly suspicious mammogram. If findings are concordant, women with benign results may be followed with diagnostic mammography in 6 to 12 months, and women with malignant results require an oncologic referral. Findings of atypical hyperplasia or radial scar warrant surgical excision to determine whether the lesion is benign or malignant. However, if the pathology and diagnostic imaging findings are discordant, reimaging or rebiopsy may be indicated to achieve concordance.

Women with findings classified as ACR category 3 (probably benign) may reasonably be managed with close surveillance with diagnostic mammograms every 6 months for 1 to 2 years. Stable lesions may permit the patient to return to routine screening; however, lesions that change over the course of surveillance require further evaluation by tissue diagnosis as just outlined. If the patient is noncompliant or highly anxious, further evaluation by tissue diagnosis may be indicated.

Dominant Mass

The diagnostic evaluation of a dominant mass is based on the woman's age (see appendix 2, panel 3). In women 30 years of age or older, the mass should be investigated with mammography and sonography. In women under the age of 30, breast cancers are rare, and the sensitivity of mammography and risks associated with mammography are of concern. In women in this age group, observation, direct needle biopsy, and breast sonography are options for the initial diagnostic evaluation of the palpable finding.

Clinical suspicion plays a critical role in the approach to women under the age of 30 who present with a dominant mass. If the risk or likelihood of malignancy is determined to be low on the basis of history and physical examination, observation of the mass for 1 or 2 menstrual cycles may be the initial approach. The patient should be reevaluated after the appropriate interval to ascertain whether the mass has resolved. Persistence of the mass necessitates further evaluation with either direct needle biopsy or breast sonography.

Direct needle biopsy, usually by fine-needle aspiration, will yield either fluid, which suggests a cyst, or a cellular aspirate. When fine-needle aspiration yields a cellular aspirate and pathologic evaluation of the aspirate suggests a fibroadenoma, a 6-month follow-up CBE is done to assess the stability of the mass. Alternatively, the lesion may be surgically excised to confirm the benign findings. Nondiagnostic or indeterminate specimens necessitate reaspiration or biopsy under ultrasound guidance. If the level of suspicion has increased, a mammogram may be indicated prior to rebiopsy. If direct needle biopsy reveals cancer, regardless of whether the biopsy yielded fluid or a cellular aspirate, a mammogram should be obtained before the patient is referred for oncologic management if a mammogram has not already been obtained.

When fine-needle aspiration yields fluid with benign cytologic features and results in resolution of the mass, the mass is most likely a cyst; however, a CBE should be performed in 2 to 3 months to ascertain that the mass has not recurred. If the mass persists after fluid is aspirated, the mass should be further investigated with mammography and sonography to rule out a suspicious intracystic mass.

Finally, a dominant mass in a woman under the age of 30 may be evaluated with breast sonography. This is managed in the same way as a dominant mass in a woman 30 years of age or older with the exception that a mammogram is obtained prior to the sonogram for the older age group. Sonography will reveal whether the mass is solid or cystic. Fine-needle aspiration is indicated if the sonographic findings are indeterminate for a cyst or if there is uncertainty regarding concordance between the sonographic findings and the mammographic abnormality. In addition, the cyst may be aspirated if the patient is symptomatic or the cyst limits future mammographic interpretation. If sonography reveals a solid lesion with the characteristics of a fibroadenoma, the lesion can be reevaluated in 6 months with CBE and the appropriate breast imaging study to assess stability, or the lesion can be evaluated pathologically with either needle biopsy or excision. Solid lesions that are indeterminate or suspicious on sonography should be biopsied, preferably under ultrasound guidance. If an intracystic mass is identified sonographically, surgical excision is recommended.

In interpreting the results of the biopsy, it is important to determine whether the pathologic diagnosis is concordant with the findings on CBE and the diagnostic imaging studies. Discordant results should prompt reevaluation of the clinical examination and imaging studies as well as the pathologic diagnosis. Repeat biopsy, either ultrasound-guided needle biopsy or excisional biopsy, may be necessary. Any biopsy that is indeterminate or yields atypia necessitates excision to ascertain the correct diagnosis.

Asymmetric Thickening or Nodularity

An area of asymmetric thickening or nodularity is less distinct than a dominant mass, and for many health care providers it carries a slightly less ominous connotation. All cases of asymmetric thickening or nodularity should be assessed with sonography (see appendix 2, panel 4). Mammography is considered a necessary part of the diagnostic evaluation only for women 30 years of age or older. Women under the age of 30 years should have mammography only if it is clinically indicated—e.g., in the case of abnormal findings on sonography.

If the findings on mammography and sonography are negative, additional diagnostic evaluation can be limited to a follow-up CBE in 8 to 12 weeks to assess stability. In the case of stable findings on CBE, the patient can return to routine screening; in the case of progression of the area of thickening or nodularity, the lesion would most appropriately be further evaluated according to the guidelines for evaluation of a dominant mass.

Women with abnormal mammographic findings (ACR category 3, 4, or 5) should undergo diagnostic evaluation as previously described (see the section Mammographic Abnormality with Normal Findings on Clinical Breast Examination).

Nipple Discharge

It is important to characterize nipple discharge so that an appropriate diagnostic evaluation can be conducted (see appendix 2, panel 5). Discharge that is nonspontaneous and from multiple ducts should not raise suspicion of breast cancer. For women aged 40 and over, a diagnostic mammogram should be done as would be recommended for any 40-year-old woman. Women with mammographic findings classified as ACR category 0, 3, 4, or 5 should be managed according to the guidelines for evaluation of mammographic abnormalities with normal findings on clinical breast examination. Women with this type of nipple discharge should be instructed to stop compression of the breast and the elicitation of the nipple discharge. They should also be advised to report if the discharge becomes spontaneous. Women with bilateral, milky discharge should have pregnancy ruled out and undergo an endocrine evaluation.

The most worrisome discharge is spontaneous, unilateral discharge from a single duct, typically serous, sanguinous, or serosanguinous in nature. A diagnostic mammogram is the initial step in the diagnostic evaluation of this type of discharge. Lesions classified as ACR category 4 or 5 should be evaluated according to the guidelines for evaluation of mammographic abnormalities with normal findings on clinical breast examination. Unless breast conservation therapy is planned, a diagnosis of cancer in the breast under evaluation will usually end the diagnostic evaluation. If breast conservation therapy is planned, no malignancy is diagnosed, or the mammogram is ACR category 1, 2, or 3, then ductography should be performed as the prelude to a duct excision. Duct excision not only allows a pathologic diagnosis of the etiology of the nipple discharge but also allows for resolution of the discharge. Although nipple discharge is rarely a symptom of cancer, it is important to rule this out as well as to manage the patient's symptoms.

Skin Changes

Although seemingly innocuous, skin changes of the breast require careful evaluation (see appendix 2, panel 6). Not uncommonly, patients are seen in the Cancer Prevention Center for evaluation of an isolated skin change of the breast that turns out to be a symptom of breast cancer. These patients have frequently been reassured by their outside health care provider that the skin findings are of no consequence. Special attention should be given to any breast skin change in a woman over the age of 40. The primary considerations are inflammatory breast cancer—with the usual skin changes of erythema and peau d'orange (skin thickening)—and Paget's disease, symptoms of which can include scaling, eczema, or nipple excoriation. Mammographic and/or sonographic evaluation is undertaken as indicated by age and other breast findings. Abnormalities found on diagnostic imaging should be evaluated according to the guidelines for evaluation of mammographic abnormalities with normal findings on CBE. If inflammatory breast cancer is a consideration and mammographic findings are benign, further evaluation with a skin punch biopsy or blind core needle biopsy of breast parenchyma is warranted. Benign findings on biopsy should prompt reassessment and possible rebiopsy depending on the level of suspicion.

CONCLUSION

The paradigm for breast cancer prevention has changed dramatically in the past several years. Whereas the focus was once on breast cancer screen

KEY PRACTICE POINTS

- Unless a genetic predisposition is suspected, the initial step of breast cancer prevention is risk assessment using the NCI Breast Cancer Risk Assessment Tool.

- Risk-based breast cancer screening recommendations should be reinforced regardless of the level of breast cancer risk.

- Women at increased risk for breast cancer should receive information and counseling about the risks and benefits of tamoxifen therapy. In addition, women with a known or suspected genetic predisposition should receive counseling about the options of prophylactic surgery.

- Clinical and mammographic breast abnormalities can be systematically evaluated. In the diagnostic work-up, concordance between the final radiographic and/or pathologic results and the initial clinical findings and level of suspicion is essential.

ing with the triad of BSE, CBE, and mammography, now the paradigm has expanded to include breast cancer risk assessment and primary prevention strategies. Women who present for breast cancer screening should have a risk assessment performed to ascertain the risk level and appropriate recommendations for primary prevention strategies. Regardless of the risk level or primary prevention strategy employed, the benefits of breast cancer screening should be reinforced.

Any clinical or mammographic breast abnormality should be subjected to diagnostic evaluation. A key component of this evaluation is concordance between the results of diagnostic evaluation and the initial clinical findings and level of suspicion. Discordant results should prompt reevaluation.

The mission of M. D. Anderson's Cancer Prevention Center is to provide research-based cancer risk assessment and risk reduction counseling as well as primary and secondary cancer prevention services for individuals with a cancer concern. Women with average or increased risk for breast cancer can be referred by their outside physician or can self-refer to any of the programs offered. With the comprehensive breast cancer prevention program serving as the template upon which programs for other cancer sites are being developed, the Cancer Prevention Center is setting the pace in clinical cancer prevention services and research.

Suggested Readings

American Cancer Society. *Breast Cancer Facts & Figures, 1999–2000.* Atlanta: American Cancer Society, 1999.

Armstrong K, Eisen A, Weber B. Assessing the risk of breast cancer. *N Engl J Med* 2000;342:564–571.

Cummings SR, Eckert S, Krueger KA, et al. The effect of raloxifene on risk of breast cancer in postmenopausal women: results from the MORE randomized trial. Multiple Outcomes of Raloxifene Evaluation. *JAMA* 1999;281:2189–2197.

Day R, Ganz PA, Costantino JP, Cronin WM, Wickerham DL, Fisher B. Health-related quality of life and tamoxifen in breast cancer prevention: a report from the National Surgical Adjuvant Breast and Bowel Project P-1 Study. *J Clin Oncol* 1999;17:2659–2669.

Fisher B, Costantino JP, Wickerham DL, et al. Tamoxifen for prevention of breast cancer: report of the National Surgical Adjuvant Breast and Bowel Project P-1 Study. *J Natl Cancer Inst* 1998;90:1371–1388.

Gail MH, Costantino JP, Bryant J, et al. Weighing the risks and benefits of tamoxifen treatment for preventing breast cancer. *J Natl Cancer Inst* 1999;91:1829–1846.

Hartmann LC, Schaid DJ, Woods JE, et al. Efficacy of bilateral prophylactic mastectomy in women with a family history of breast cancer. *N Engl J Med* 1999;340:77–84.

Howell LP. The pathway to cancer. In: O'Grady LF, Lindfors KK, Howell PL, Rippon MB, eds. *A Practical Approach to Breast Disease.* Boston: Little, Brown and Co.; 1995:23–29.

Marchant DJ. Risk factors. In: Marchant DJ, ed. *Breast Disease.* Philadelphia: W.B. Saunders Co.; 1997:115–133.

National Cancer Institute. CancerNet Web site. Available at: http://www.cancernet.nci.nih.gov. Accessed September 2000.

Powles T, Eeles R, Ashley S, et al. Interim analysis of the incidence of breast cancer in the Royal Marsden Hospital tamoxifen randomised chemoprevention trial. *Lancet* 1998;352:98–101.

Schairer C, Lubin J, Troisi R, Sturgeon S, Brinton L, Hoover R. Menopausal estrogen and estrogen-progestin replacement therapy and breast cancer risk. *JAMA* 2000;283:485–491.

Veronesi U, Maisonneuve P, Costa A, et al. Prevention of breast cancer with tamoxifen: preliminary findings from the Italian randomised trial among hysterectomised women. Italian Tamoxifen Prevention Study. *Lancet* 1998;352:93–97.

Vogel VG. Breast cancer prevention: a review of current evidence. *CA Cancer J Clin* 2000;50:156–170.

Vogel VG. Prevention of breast cancer. In: Singletary SE, Robb GL, eds. *Advanced Therapy of Breast Disease.* Hamilton: B. C. Decker; 2000:27–35.

Appendix 2: M. D. Anderson Cancer Center Breast Screening and Diagnostic Guidelines

Panel 1: Screening

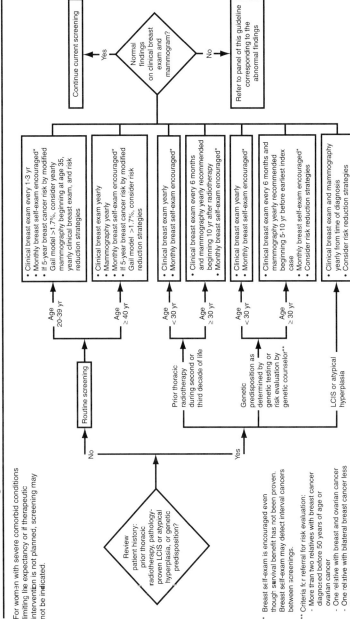

For woman with severe comorbid conditions limiting life expectancy or if therapeutic intervention is not planned, screening may not be indicated.

Review patient history: prior thoracic radiotherapy, pathology-proven LCIS or atypical hyperplasia, or genetic predisposition?

No → Routine screening

Yes →

Prior thoracic radiotherapy during second or third decade of life

Genetic predisposition as determined by genetic testing or risk evaluation by genetic counselor**

LCIS or atypical hyperplasia

Age 20-39 yr
- Clinical breast exam every 1-3 yr
- Monthly breast self-exam encouraged*
- If 5-year breast cancer risk by modified Gail model >1.7%, consider yearly mammography beginning at age 35, yearly clinical breast exam, and risk reduction strategies

Age ≥ 40 yr
- Clinical breast exam yearly
- Mammography yearly
- Monthly breast self-exam encouraged*
- If 5-year breast cancer risk by modified Gail model >1.7%, consider risk reduction strategies

Age < 30 yr
- Clinical breast exam yearly
- Monthly breast self-exam encouraged*

Age ≥ 30 yr
- Clinical breast exam every 6 months and mammography yearly recommended beginning 10 yr after radiotherapy
- Monthly breast self-exam encouraged*

Age < 30 yr
- Clinical breast exam yearly
- Monthly breast self-exam encouraged*

Age ≥ 30 yr
- Clinical breast exam every 6 months and mammography yearly recommended beginning 5-10 yr before earliest index case
- Monthly breast self-exam encouraged*
- Consider risk reduction strategies

- Clinical breast exam and mammography yearly from time of diagnosis
- Consider risk reduction strategies

Normal findings on clinical breast exam and mammogram?

Yes → Continue current screening

No → Refer to panel of this guideline corresponding to the abnormal findings

* Breast self-exam is encouraged even though survival benefit has not been proven. Breast self-exam may detect interval cancers between screenings.

** Criteria for referral for risk evaluation:
- More than two relatives with breast cancer diagnosed before 50 years of age or ovarian cancer
- One relative with breast and ovarian cancer
- One relative with bilateral breast cancer less than age 50
- One male relative with breast cancer
- Ashkenazi Jewish descent and breast or ovarian cancer in the family

Panel 2: Mammographic Abnormality

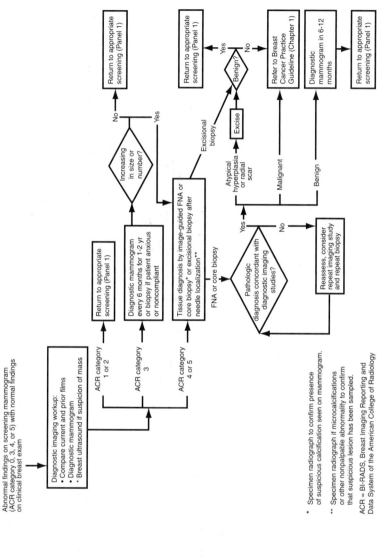

Abnormal findings on screening mammogram
(ACR category 0, 3, 4, or 5) with normal findings
on clinical breast exam

Diagnostic imaging workup:
• Compare current and prior films
• Diagnostic mammogram
• Breast ultrasound if suspicion of mass

ACR category 1 or 2 → Return to appropriate screening (Panel 1)

ACR category 3 → Diagnostic mammogram every 6 months for 1-2 yr or biopsy if patient anxious or noncompliant → Increasing in size or number?
  - No → Return to appropriate screening (Panel 1)
  - Yes →

ACR category 4 or 5 → Tissue diagnosis by image-guided FNA or core biopsy* or excisional biopsy after needle localization**

Excisional biopsy → Benign?
  - Yes → Return to appropriate screening (Panel 1)
  - No → Refer to Breast Cancer Practice Guideline (Chapter 1)

FNA or core biopsy → Pathologic diagnosis concordant with diagnostic imaging studies?
  - Yes → Atypical hyperplasia or radial scar → Excise → Benign?
    - Yes → Return to appropriate screening (Panel 1)
    - No → Refer to Breast Cancer Practice Guideline (Chapter 1)
  - Yes → Malignant → Refer to Breast Cancer Practice Guideline (Chapter 1)
  - Yes → Benign → Diagnostic mammogram in 6-12 months → Return to appropriate screening (Panel 1)
  - No → Reassess, consider repeat imaging study and repeat biopsy

*   Specimen radiograph to confirm presence
    of suspicious calcification seen on mammogram.

** Specimen radiograph if microcalcifications
    or other nonpalpable abnormality to confirm
    that suspicious lesion has been sampled.

ACR = BI-RADS, Breast Imaging Reporting and
Data System of the American College of Radiology

Panel 3: Dominant Mass

Abnormal findings on clinical breast exam: dominant mass

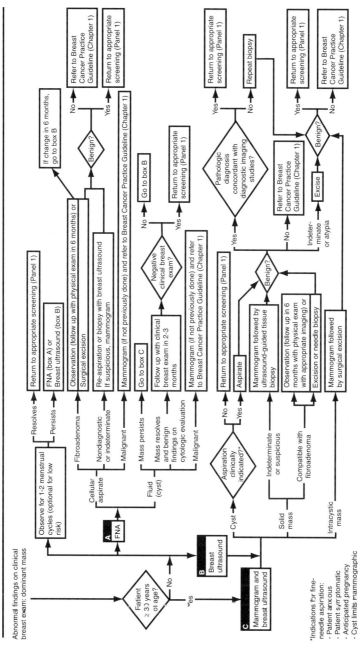

Panel 4: Asymmetric Thickening or Nodularity

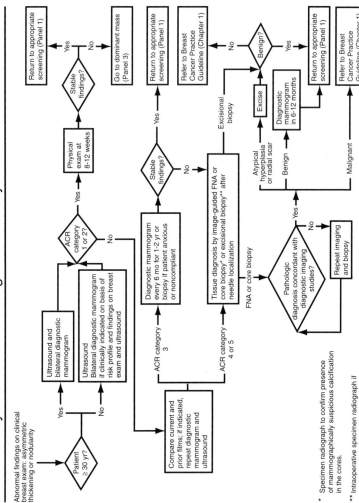

Abnormal findings on clinical breast exam: asymmetric thickening or nodularity

* Specimen radiograph to confirm presence of mammographically suspicious calcification in the cores.

** Intraoperative specimen radiograph if microcalcifications or occult mass.

ACR = BI-RADS, Breast Imaging Reporting and Data System of the American College of Radiology

Panel 5: Nipple Discharge

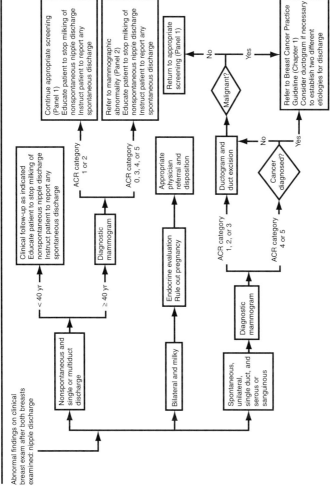

Abnormal findings on clinical breast exam after both breasts examined: nipple discharge

Nonspontaneous and single or multiduct discharge

< 40 yr → Clinical follow-up as indicated
Educate patient to stop milking of nonspontaneous nipple discharge
Instruct patient to report any spontaneous discharge

≥ 40 yr → Diagnostic mammogram

ACR category 1 or 2 → Continue appropriate screening (Panel 1)
Educate patient to stop milking of nonspontaneous nipple discharge
Instruct patient to report any spontaneous discharge

ACR category 0, 3, 4, or 5 → Refer to mammographic abnormality (Panel 2)
Educate patient to stop milking of nonspontaneous nipple discharge
Instruct patient to report any spontaneous discharge

Bilateral and milky → Endocrine evaluation
Rule out pregnancy → Appropriate physician referral and disposition

Spontaneous, unilateral, single duct, and serous or sanguinous → Diagnostic mammogram

ACR category 1, 2, or 3 → Ductogram and duct excision

ACR category 4 or 5 → Cancer diagnosed?

Cancer diagnosed? — Yes → Refer to Breast Cancer Practice Guideline (Chapter 1)
Consider ductogram if necessary to establish two different etiologies for discharge

Cancer diagnosed? — No → Malignant?

Malignant? — No → Return to appropriate screening (Panel 1)

Malignant? — Yes → Refer to Breast Cancer Practice Guideline (Chapter 1)
Consider ductogram if necessary to establish two different etiologies for discharge

ACR = BI-RADS, Breast Imaging Reporting and Data System of the American College of Radiology

Panel 6: Skin Changes

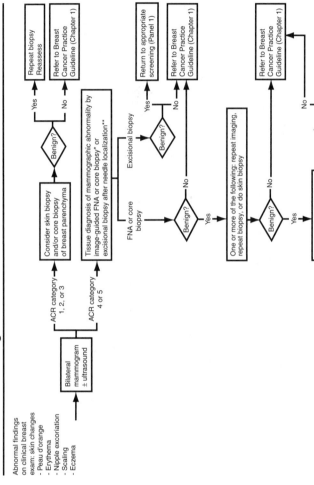

Abnormal findings
on clinical breast
exam: skin changes
- Peau d'orange
- Erythema
- Nipple excoriation
- Scaling
- Eczema

Bilateral mammogram ± ultrasound

ACR category 1, 2, or 3 → Consider skin biopsy and/or core biopsy of breast parenchyma → Benign? — Yes → Repeat biopsy Reassess
                                                                                      — No → Refer to Breast Cancer Practice Guideline (Chapter 1)

ACR category 4 or 5 → Tissue diagnosis of mammographic abnormality by image-guided FNA or core biopsy* or excisional biopsy after needle localization**

Excisional biopsy → Benign? — Yes → Return to appropriate screening (Panel 1)
                             — No → Refer to Breast Cancer Practice Guideline (Chapter 1)

FNA or core biopsy → Benign? — No → Refer to Breast Cancer Practice Guideline (Chapter 1)
                              — Yes → One or more of the following: repeat imaging, repeat biopsy, or do skin biopsy → Benign? — No → Refer to Breast Cancer Practice Guideline (Chapter 1)
                              — Yes → Reassess clinical and radiographic findings and consider excisional biopsy → Benign? — No → Refer to Breast Cancer Practice Guideline (Chapter 1)
                                                                                                                                — Yes → Return to appropriate screening (Panel 1)

* Specimen radiograph to confirm presence
   of suspicious calcification seen on mammogram.

** Specimen radiograph if microcalcifications
   or other nonpalpable abnormality to confirm
   that suspicious lesion has been sampled.

ACR = BI-RADS, Breast Imaging Reporting and
Data System of the American College of Radiology

3 GENETIC PREDISPOSITION TO BREAST CANCER

Gordon B. Mills and Paula Trahan Rieger

CHAPTER OVERVIEW

In the past decade, the tools required to more clearly define a woman's risk for development of breast cancer have begun to emerge. Our understanding of cancer at a molecular level and our understanding of how certain genetic mutations contribute to the development of cancer have facilitated this work. Advances in medical technology and discoveries stemming from the Human Genome Project now provide the means to test individuals for the presence of genetic mutations associated with some known hereditary cancer syndromes. Although many ethical, legal, and psychosocial issues associated with testing remain unresolved, genetic testing is having and will continue to have a significant impact on cancer care. Physicians in the community will have vital roles in educating individuals about the availability of cancer genetic testing, making referrals for cancer genetic counseling, and providing follow-up care.

INTRODUCTION

Since the 18th century, it has been observed that certain types of cancers tend to cluster within some families at a higher rate than could be attributed to chance. This observation led many researchers to believe that such cancers were "hereditary." Today we know that approximately 5% to 10% of all tumors arise in individuals who inherit a genetic mutation that predisposes them to the development of cancer, including breast cancer.

Several developments in recent years have broadened our understanding of cancer biology and of the role of genetics in the development of cancer. One such development is the Human Genome Project. Through this research effort, the genes associated with hereditary cancer syndromes are rapidly being delineated. Currently, more than 50 cancer predisposition genes have been identified. Being able to recognize the characteristics that signal the presence of a hereditary cancer syndrome in a family and to initiate appropriate risk management referrals for family members has become an important component in the care of women who are at high risk for developing breast and ovarian cancers.

This chapter focuses on how current knowledge of the role of genetics in cancer development is being applied in the field of breast cancer risk management. Included are discussions of some of the hereditary cancer syndromes and the associated genes that predispose individuals to the development of breast cancer, the processes involved in cancer genetic counseling and cancer genetic testing, and risk management strategies for women found to have a genetic predisposition for breast and ovarian cancers.

CANCER PREDISPOSITION GENES

Underlying the development of cancer are changes in gene structure or function caused by genetic mutations or epigenetic alterations in the expression of the genes that control cell growth and differentiation, DNA repair, and cell death. The majority of cancers are sporadic, resulting from a series of genetic or epigenetic changes in somatic or body cells. The mutated, highly penetrant, rare cancer predisposition genes associated with hereditary cancer syndromes are carried in germ cells and thus have the potential to be passed from generation to generation and to confer an inheritable predisposition for cancer development. This means that a person who inherits a mutated gene known to cause cancer has an increased likelihood of developing cancer, although for cancer to develop, other genetic mutations must also occur. Cultural, lifestyle, and environmental factors are also thought to play a role in the development of cancer. Thus, although cancer predisposition genes increase the likelihood that cancer will develop, cancer is not an inevitable outcome. It is important that this concept be fully conveyed in cancer genetic counseling and stressed as an essential underpinning for cancer prevention.

Cancer predisposition genes are generally transmitted in an autosomal dominant pattern with incomplete penetrance. Despite the autosomal dominant pattern of cancer presentation at the organism level, most inherited gene mutations are recessive at the cellular level, requiring loss of the normal copy of a gene for expressivity. Although loss of the normal copy of a gene is rare at the cellular level, loss of the normal copy of a gene is most likely a frequent occurrence at the level of the human body, with its billions of cells. Thus, individuals who harbor a mutated cancer predisposition gene are in essence "born with a strike against them" because at birth, every cell in their body already has a genetic change, and these altered genes confer an increased risk for the development of cancer.

Cancer predisposition genes are also transmitted vertically, which means that successive generations are affected. Depending on the type of cancer, male and female family members are generally affected at an equal rate. In classic autosomal dominant inheritance, every affected person in a pedigree has an affected parent. However, for several reasons, this may not be the case among kindreds in families with a hereditary cancer syndrome. One reason is that, within a family, individuals may inherit a gene that predisposes them to the development of cancer, yet they may not develop cancer. Another reason is that the gene that causes a specific type of cancer may not be expressed equally in male and female family members. For example, men cannot develop ovarian cancer and generally do not develop breast cancer as a consequence of *BRCA1* mutations; however, men may carry the altered gene associated with hereditary breast and ovarian cancers (*BRCA1*). For these reasons, in families with a hereditary cancer syndrome, generations may be "skipped" or not affected by cancer. However, history of breast cancer, ovarian cancer, or both among the paternal kindred is as important in the assessment of an individual's risk for cancer as is the history of these diseases among maternal relatives.

Some of the cancer predisposition genes known to be associated with hereditary breast cancer syndromes are BRCA1, BRCA2, MMAC/PTEN, and *p53*. As well, a hypothetical group of genes as yet undiscovered, including the BRCA3 gene, may also increase susceptibility to breast and other cancers. Figure 3–1 shows a pedigree of a family with high-risk characteristics and a known mutation in a cancer predisposition gene.

HEREDITARY CANCER SYNDROMES

A hereditary cancer syndrome is the presence, in several generations of a family, of multiple cases of cancer that are associated with a mutated gene in the germline. The genes specific to each syndrome have not yet been identified. In most hereditary cancer syndromes, an individual inherits an abnormality in a tumor suppressor gene that triggers a loss of function and leads to multiple other genetic changes. Many of the tumor suppressor genes involved in hereditary cancer syndromes contribute to genetic stability by either mediating DNA repair or detecting abnormalities in genomic structure leading to cell cycle arrest and repair or to apoptosis and clearance of aberrant cells. However, in other syndromes, individuals inherit a mutation that results in a gain of function and the development of an activated oncogene. In this case, the inheritance of the abnormality confers an increased proliferative or survival advantage.

Several characteristics are common in families with a hereditary cancer syndrome:

- The occurrence, within a single lineage (i.e., maternal relatives or paternal relatives), of multiple cases of cancer, especially cancers of the same type (e.g., breast cancer, colorectal cancer, or melanoma) or cancers related to a specific abnormality (e.g., breast and ovarian cancer in carriers of BRCA1 or BRCA2 abnormalities, bowel and endometrium cancers in carriers of hereditary nonpolyposis colon cancer [HNPCC] complex abnormalities, and leukemia and sarcoma in carriers of *p53* abnormalities)
- A diagnosis of cancer at an earlier age than is seen in the general population (e.g., a diagnosis of breast cancer before age 50 years)
- The occurrence of multiple cancers in a family member (e.g., a person with both breast and ovarian cancer)
- The presence of rare cancers, such as retinoblastomas or brain tumors
- Cancer in paired organs (e.g., both breasts or both kidneys)
- Nonmalignant manifestations of a hereditary cancer syndrome (e.g., hamartomas of the skin and mucous membranes and palmar pits, as seen in Cowden disease)

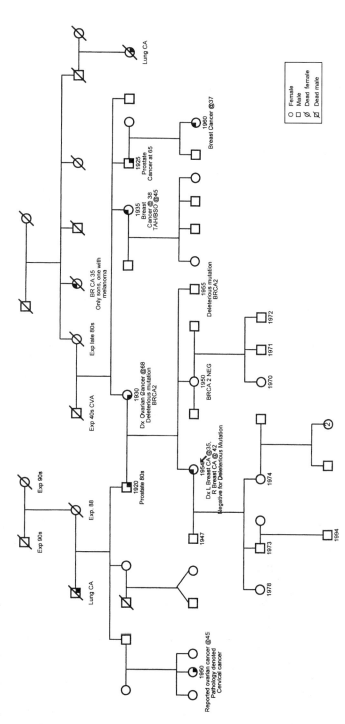

Figure 3–1. This figure depicts the history (pedigree) of a family with a known alteration in *BRCA2*, a gene that predisposes individuals to the development of breast and ovarian cancers. Several characteristics often seen in families with a predisposition for breast cancer are depicted on this pedigree. A strong family history of breast and ovarian cancer is seen on the maternal side, with several cases of early-onset breast cancer and ovarian cancer. In this family, the proband (patient with the arrow) tested negative for the *BRCA2* mutation, even though she had an early-onset breast cancer. Her brother, born in 1955, has inherited the known mutation. This pedigree also demonstrates a cancer on the paternal side that was reported to be ovarian cancer but proven by pathology report to be cervical cancer. Also, the proband's maternal grandmother would be an obligate carrier who never had breast or ovarian cancer. @, at; BR, breast; CA, cancer; CVA, cardiovascular accident; Dx, diagnosed; Exp, expired; L, left; NEG, negative; R, right; TAH/BSO, total abdominal hysterectomy and bilateral salpingo-oophorectomy.

When any of these characteristics is present, alone or in combinations, the possibility of a hereditary cancer syndrome should be considered. These criteria should serve as "flags" to identify individuals who should be referred for intensive cancer genetic counseling.

Following is a brief review of the hereditary cancer syndromes associated with breast and ovarian cancer that are most commonly seen in clinical practice.

BRCA1 and *BRCA2* Syndromes

The *BRCA1* gene, which was identified in 1994, is located on chromosome 17q and appears to account for 30% to 35% of breast cancers in families with a high incidence of early-onset breast and ovarian cancers. The *BRCA2* gene, identified in 1995, is located on chromosome 13q and appears to account for about 25% of breast cancers in families with early-onset breast cancer. It is believed that *BRCA1* and *BRCA2* mutations account for the majority of familial ovarian cancers.

The mechanisms by which mutations in *BRCA1* or *BRCA2* contribute to the development of breast cancer are not yet fully elucidated. These genes are components of the *BRCA1*-associated genome surveillance complex, which has been implicated in the detection or repair of abnormal or damaged DNA. Other members of this complex include:

- BRCA2
- RAD51
- The retinoblastoma gene product
- p53
- BARD1
- The *BRCA1*-associated protein (BAP1)
- Histone deacetylases
- RNA polymerase II
- myc
- ATM (a member of the phosphatidylinositol kinase superfamily, which is mutated in ataxia telangiectasia)
- BLM recQ helicase, which is mutated in Bloom syndrome
- RAD50-MRE11-NBS1 protein complex
- Replication factor C
- *MSH2*, *MSH6*, and *MLH1* mismatch repair genes and their products

In addition, *BRCA1* regulates the expression of multiple proteins, including p21, p53, GADD45, and GADD153, most of which are implicated in the detection or repair of abnormal or damaged DNA. However, the association of *BRCA1* with BAP1, which is a de-ubiquitinating enzyme, also implicates *BRCA1* in protein stability.

The *BRCA1* gene is most clearly implicated in transcription-coupled DNA repair—that is, the repair of double-stranded DNA breaks. It also appears to contribute to the passage of cells through the G_2-M checkpoint and to centrosome duplication. The association of BRCA1 with the ATM, BLM, and RAD50-MRE11-NBS1 proteins also implicates the gene in repair of radiation-induced DNA damage. Replication factor C, which loads proliferating cell nuclear antigen onto DNA, may play a role in cell cycle transit. The association of BRCA1 with the MSH2, MSH6, and MLH1 mismatch repair genes and their products, which are aberrant in patients with HNPCC, may contribute to a predisposition to the development of ovarian cancer in families with BRCA1 and BRCA2 mutations as well as families with HNPCC. However, this association fails to explain the high frequency of breast cancer in families with BRCA1 and BRCA2 mutations but not in families with HNPCC.

Thus, BRCA1 appears to be a critical caretaker gene that is required to maintain genomic integrity during DNA replication. This suggests that loss of BRCA1 function, and likely loss of BRCA2 function as well, may predispose families to cancer development by increasing the frequency of mutations in other important tumor suppressor genes.

The lifetime risk of developing breast cancer for members of BRCA1-linked families is relatively high (Table 3–1). In the general population, the cumulative incidence of breast cancer by age 50 is 2%, whereas in women with an alteration in BRCA1, the cumulative incidence of breast cancer by age 50 may be as high as 50%. Some mutations carry a lower penetrance; thus, lifetime risk for breast cancer in some families may range from 40% to as high as 80%. Women with breast cancer and an abnormality in BRCA1 have up to a 65% chance of developing a contra-

Table 3–1. Lifetime Risk and Increase in Risk for Development of Breast and Ovarian Cancers in Carriers of the BRCA1 Mutation

Cancer Type/Penetrance	Lifetime Risk (%)	Increase in Risk*
Breast cancer		
High	80	17-fold
Medium	60	5-fold
Low	40	3-fold
Contralateral breast cancer		
High	65	6-fold
Medium	43	4-fold
Low	24	3-fold
Ovarian cancer		
High	40	20-fold
Medium	16	8-fold
Low	6	3-fold

* Increase in risk compared with the general population (individuals who do not carry the BRCA1 mutation).

Table 3–2. **Increase in Risk for Development of Breast and Other Cancers in Carriers of the** *BRCA2* **Mutation**

Cancer Type	Increase in Risk*
Breast	3-fold
Contralateral breast	5-fold
Ovarian	8-fold
Prostate	5-fold
Prostate before age 65	7-fold
Pancreatic	4-fold
Gallbladder and bile duct	5-fold
Stomach	3-fold
Melanoma	3-fold

* Increase in risk compared with the general population (individuals who do not carry the *BRCA2* mutation).
Source: Breast Cancer Linkage Consortium, 1999.

lateral breast cancer. In the general population, the lifetime risk for ovarian cancer is in the range of 1% to 2%; however, in women with an alteration in *BRCA1*, the lifetime risk for ovarian cancer may range from 6% to 40%. There may also be a small but significantly increased risk for prostate cancer in men and for colon cancer in men and women who have *BRCA1* mutations.

The lifetime risk of developing breast cancer for women in families with *BRCA2* mutations is approximately 30% (a 3-fold increase in risk compared with women in the general population), and these women have a 5-fold increased risk of developing a contralateral breast cancer (Table 3–2). Individuals with an inherited abnormality in *BRCA2* also have an increased risk of developing ovarian cancer, prostate cancer (5-fold, with a 7-fold increase before age 65), pancreatic cancer, gallbladder and bile duct cancer, stomach cancer, and melanoma. Why *BRCA2* predisposes individuals to these yet not other cancers remains unknown. The estimated lifetime risk of breast cancer for men who carry *BRCA2* mutations is roughly 6%. The trend of breast cancer development in families with the *BRCA2* mutation shows a lesser skew to younger age than is seen in families with the *BRCA1* mutation.

BRCA1 and *BRCA2* are rarely mutated in sporadic breast cancers, although there may be abnormalities in expression or function of *BRCA1* and *BRCA2* in sporadic breast cancers. This trend suggests that patients with breast cancer as a consequence of inherited abnormalities in *BRCA1* or *BRCA2* could have a different prognosis than women with sporadic breast cancers. Indeed, tumors that arise in patients with abnormalities in *BRCA1* tend to exhibit increased grade, increased mitotic index, and increased frequency of *p53* mutations as well as decreased frequency of estrogen and progesterone receptor positivity compared with sporadic breast cancers. These characteristics would be expected to contribute to a poor prognosis. However, reports in the literature of studies of more than 400 patients tested for abnormalities in *BRCA1* indicate that the prognosis of patients with breast cancer who have such abnormalities is only slightly worse, if worse at all, than that of patients with breast cancer who do not have these abnormalities (Phillips et al, 1999). Interestingly, there is a markedly reduced incidence of ductal carcinoma in situ and lobular carcinoma in situ in families with abnormalities in *BRCA1* mutations. Whether this represents a different natural history wherein tumors do not pass through an in situ phase or a shortening of the interval that tumors spend at the in situ phase is not known. No obvious difference has been reported in nodal status, tumor size, or positivity for the *erb*B-2/*neu* oncogene based on *BRCA1* or *BRCA2* mutation status. As well, in the approximately 130 *BRCA2*-positive tumors that have been reported, there have been no obvious differences in pathological markers or patient outcome compared with sporadic breast cancers (Phillips et al, 1999).

Cowden Disease

Cowden disease is a rare syndrome that accounts for only a few cases of hereditary breast cancers. Cowden disease is one of a large number of genetic syndromes associated with dermatoses. It is characterized by mucocutaneous lesions, trichilemmomas, acral keratoses, papillomatous papules, mucosal lesions, macroencephaly, and Lhermitte-Duclos disease. Some individuals may exhibit fibroids, lipomas, fibromas, hamartomas, or thyroid adenomas. Individuals with this syndrome exhibit a high frequency of breast and gastrointestinal cancers and thyroid disease.

Cowden disease is caused by abnormalities in the *MMAC/PTEN* gene, which was cloned by Dr. Peter Steck at M. D. Anderson Cancer Center. The *MMAC/PTEN* gene, a tumor suppressor gene located at 10q23, encodes a unique phosphatase with the ability to dephosphorylate proteins and lipids. *MMAC/PTEN* terminates transmembrane signaling, decreasing transit through the G_1 phase of the cell cycle and predisposing cells to death through anoikis and apoptosis. (Anoikis occurs when a cell loses contact with surrounding cells. The ability to bypass anoikis is a critical component in the metastatic cascade. The majority of tumor cells that enter the circulation die by anoikis.) Breast cancers occur in 25% to 50% of carriers of a *MMAC/PTEN* mutation. These women tend to be young and to have bilateral disease. Unlike the *BRCA1* and *BRCA2* genes, the *MMAC/PTEN* gene is frequently mutated in sporadic tumors, including tumors of the brain, endometrium, and prostate.

Li-Fraumeni Syndrome

The Li-Fraumeni syndrome is rare, accounting for only 1% of all inherited breast cancers. The most common components of the Li-Fraumeni syndrome are childhood leukemias and lymphomas, brain tumors, and sarcomas. Premenopausal breast cancer is a relatively uncommon component of this syndrome. Li-Fraumeni cancers occur in very young women; therefore, in families with this syndrome, screening should be initiated at age 20 to 25 years.

The Li-Fraumeni syndrome is caused by mutations in the *p53* gene. The *p53* gene plays a critical role in regulating cell cycle transit and apoptosis, particularly in response to DNA damage. As has been noted, *p53* interacts with *BRCA1*, suggesting that both genes may function in a complex that surveys genomic stability. Mutations in *p53* are the most common genetic abnormality in sporadic tumors, which indicates the importance of this tumor suppressor gene.

Founder Effects

Founder effects are the unusual prevalence of specific genotypes in a population. Founder effects occur when specific mutations are found in a greater than expected frequency in a population or in people of a certain heritage. Founder effects frequently occur as a result of geographical migration, a limited number of ancestors, and catastrophes. Founder effect mutations in the *BRCA1* and *BRCA2* genes are most commonly seen in people of Ashkenazi Jewish, Dutch, French-Canadian, Icelandic, or Sephardic Jewish (from Iraq) descent. Indeed, although the frequency of mutations in the *BRCA1* and *BRCA2* genes is approximately 0.1% in the general population, the frequency of mutations in the *BRCA1* and *BRCA2* genes in people in these ethnic groups is between 1.0% and 5.0%. Thus, an individual's heritage may provide an important clue about his or her genetic predisposition for cancer and about a specific site for DNA analysis. This is why it is important to consider a person's ethnic origin during assessment of cancer risk.

Cancer Genetic Counseling

The goals of cancer genetic counseling are to educate the at-risk or affected individual about the role of genetics in the transmission of cancer; to assess the individual for the possible presence of a hereditary cancer syndrome in his or her family; to explain the positive and negative implications of cancer genetic testing; to recommend a risk management plan; and to provide support to help the individual cope with psychosocial issues that may arise during the process. Cancer genetic counseling should always be provided before cancer genetic testing to ensure that the individual has adequate information when deciding whether to proceed with testing.

Cancer genetic counseling is a comprehensive program. At M. D. Anderson, the steps involved in cancer genetic counseling are as follows:

- Collecting data that will provide an in-depth review of the individual's medical history, the individual's family history (a minimum of 3 complete generations is required), and occurrences of cancer within the family
- Evaluating the individual's knowledge of hereditary cancer syndromes and cancer genetics, self-perception of risk of developing cancer, and motivation for seeking genetic counseling and testing
- Assessing risk
- Determining the likelihood that an affected family member would test positive for an alteration in a cancer predisposition gene
- Explaining the testing process and the benefits, risks, limitations, costs, and potential outcomes of testing
- Assessing the individual's psychosocial status and support systems to determine his or her ability to cope with test results
- Determining whether the individual wants to know the results of the genetic test once test results are received
- Recommending a risk management program (e.g., surveillance, chemoprevention, or prophylactic surgery) and referring the individual to a specialist who can perform the service

A key component in assessing an individual's risk for development of cancer is evaluating the family history, particularly the history of cancers that have occurred in the family. Studies have shown that self-reports of family history are often inaccurate, especially with respect to gynecological cancers such as cervical, endometrial, and ovarian cancers. The best source for this information is pathology records or death certificates. Accessing this information can be time-consuming, but the health care team can help the patient obtain the necessary records. A sample authorization for disclosure of medical records is shown in appendix 3A at the end of this chapter.

A thorough explanation of genetic testing is also important. Information about cancer genetic testing abounds in the lay media and on the Internet. Thus, individuals frequently seek cancer genetic testing with unrealistic expectations of the purpose and implications of testing. Counselors must explain what type of test will be given (e.g., protein truncation or full gene sequencing), how the test will be performed, which family member is the best candidate for testing and why, potential test results, and what certain test results might mean.

Another key component in cancer genetic counseling is the risk management recommendation. The nondirective provision of information has been the standard of practice in genetic counseling. The goal of this approach is to provide the individual with the information needed to make decisions about his or her care but not to make recommendations. In the cancer setting, however, clear medically warranted recommendations can be made about ways to manage cancer risk. For example, effective surgical options exist for treating individuals at increased risk for developing colorectal cancer, and the health care team is obligated to recommend these options. Nevertheless, the ultimate goal of cancer genetic counseling is the provision of balanced and complete information so that an individual can make an informed decision concerning his or her health. It is important for the members of the health care team to be aware of their own biases and philosophies about testing and to take care that their opinions do not in any way influence the individual's decisions.

At many centers that provide cancer genetic counseling, it is standard procedure to send the individual a post-counseling follow-up letter that summarizes the family history; the individual's potential risk for development of cancer; the benefits, risks, and limitations of testing; and recommendations for risk management (see appendix 3B at the end of this chapter).

At M. D. Anderson, cancer genetic counseling is facilitated by a multidisciplinary team that includes oncologists, advanced-practice oncology nurses, genetic counselors, and medical geneticists. The oncologists and advanced-practice oncology nurses bring expertise in screening, prophylactic therapy, cancer treatment, and psychosocial support. The genetic counselors and medical geneticists bring expertise in the assessment of family genetic history, hereditary cancer syndromes, inheritance patterns, and issues related to genetic testing.

Cancer genetic counseling is accomplished in a series of sessions. The first visit usually covers 1.5 to 2 hours; however, it takes another 6 to 8 hours to prepare and validate the pedigree; to present the pedigree at a disposition conference; to provide referrals for screening, prevention, and prophylaxis; and to write the post-counseling follow-up letter. In order to obtain the necessary information, several visits may be required. At many centers, including M. D. Anderson, test results are delivered face to face so that psychosocial and educational issues can be evaluated at that time.

CANCER GENETIC TESTING

Cancer genetic testing is the process of testing an individual to determine the presence of alterations of specific genes that predispose him or her to the development of certain cancers. This section discusses several issues regarding cancer genetic testing, including testing procedures, interpretation of results, psychosocial response to testing, risk management, and confidentiality.

Testing Procedures

Cancer genetic testing is commercially available for a number of cancers; however, controversy persists over whether testing should be offered outside the research setting and without the benefit of cancer genetic counseling. Some groups contend that cancer genetic testing should always be conducted within the context of clinical research because there are still many unanswered questions regarding genetic testing for hereditary cancer syndromes and regarding the management of individuals who are at increased risk for developing cancer; these questions can be more easily addressed in the clinical trial setting. An example of a study designed to answer a question about cancer genetic testing is one that would identify additional genetic mutations associated with hereditary cancer syndromes.

As has been explained, the goal of cancer genetic counseling is to provide the individual with information that he or she can use to make decisions about genetic testing. Many feel that performing cancer genetic testing within the context of a clinical trial will ensure that individuals receive adequate information because written informed consent is required for participation in clinical trials. Numerous position statements have been published about cancer genetic counseling and cancer genetic testing, and the majority agree about the necessity of informed consent. The Task Force on Genetic Testing strongly advocates for written informed consent and emphasizes that respect for personal autonomy is paramount.

Interpretation of Results

It is the individual's choice whether to be informed of the genetic test results. At M. D. Anderson, our standard of care is to discuss the genetic test results in a meeting with the person tested.

The results of each genetic test and the implications of the results must be reviewed in detail. If a deleterious mutation (a positive test result) is found, it must be clearly communicated to the individual that this denotes a "predisposition" for the development of cancer, not a diagnosis or even a prediction of cancer development. Information related to penetrance, the likelihood that an individual will develop cancer, must be reviewed. Likewise, when there is a known mutation in a family but the individual tests negative for that mutation, it is important for the individual to realize that he or she still has the general-population risk for developing cancer.

Some test results provide no information for an individual or the family about an inherited predisposition for cancer. When no known mutation is detected in a family, a negative result on a cancer genetic test can be difficult to interpret. Negative test results may be obtained if an abnormality is missed (i.e., a false-negative result) because the mutation was located in a region of the gene that was not tested (e.g., a promoter, enhancer, or intronic region); because an undiscovered gene is responsible for the aggregation of cancers seen in the family; or because the aggregation of cancers may be the result of pure chance. Test results are considered inconclusive when there is insufficient information to determine whether the sequence changes are deleterious or simply a harmless genetic polymorphism within the population. In the latter instance, it is difficult to assess cancer risk. In some cases, depending on the family history of cancer, the individual could still be considered at high risk.

The *BRCA1* and *BRCA2* genes are both extremely large. Therefore, they require full-length sequencing including the intron-exon boundaries and the putative promoter region. Even under these circumstances, however, there is a significant rate of false-negative results. False-negative results are not errors in sequencing; rather, they appear to represent mutations in important areas of the genes that have not yet been identified. Thus, in an individual who is considered at high risk for breast cancer on the basis of family cancer history, a negative test result has little or no impact on the likelihood of a mutation in *BRCA1* or *BRCA2* or possibly another gene in the family. As has been noted, there are a number of founder effect mutations in *BRCA1* and *BRCA2* genes in individuals of certain ethnic backgrounds. Individuals should first be tested for these abnormalities; if they are not found, the pedigree should be reassessed. If the individual is still considered at high risk, full-length sequencing would be an appropriate follow-up test. When a mutation is found, testing can be offered to all family members. Information from multiple tests will distinguish mutation carriers who warrant intensive management from individuals who do not carry abnormalities and thus have only a general-population risk. Failure to identify a deleterious mutation or a mutation of unknown significance does not provide useful information for other family members.

To provide the most information for a family, it is best to first test an affected individual (e.g., one who already has cancer). However, although this person is a member of a family with a known genetic mutation, his or her own cancer may be a sporadic tumor (see Figure 3–1). Many centers will only test affected individuals. This may not always be possible, however, because all affected individuals may have died or those still living may not wish to be tested. Therefore, testing an unaffected individual is acceptable; however, it is important to emphasize the limitations of this approach and how results will ultimately be interpreted with respect to other family members. A positive test result for a known deleterious mutation provides beneficial information for the entire family; however, depending on the specific hereditary cancer syndrome, a negative test result (no evidence of a mutation) provides information only for the individual being tested.

Psychosocial Response to Testing

Genetic testing to determine susceptibility to cancer carries with it unique psychosocial implications of which the health care team must be aware. Assessing the psychological impact of test results is an important research area.

Studies have only recently begun to evaluate why people seek genetic testing and how they decide whether to have test results disclosed to them. The majority of the published studies on psychosocial issues associated with cancer genetic counseling and testing have evaluated high-risk families that participated in the original research studies designed to identify cancer predisposition genes.

To prevent or manage an emotional response to the disclosure of an unfavorable genetic status, the health care team providing cancer genetic counseling must explain the benefits, risks, and limitations of the test before testing is done and again before results are disclosed. The health care team must evaluate family dynamics and the individual's cultural and health care beliefs, reinforce the individual's existing coping skills and teach new ones, provide nondirective counseling to help the individual make decisions about his or her care, and identify individuals who may need a psychological referral.

For women from high-risk families, it can be a catastrophic experience to see a parent or close relative die of cancer at a young age, and the experience can alter the woman's view of life. It is crucial that individuals be empowered to make decisions that are appropriate to their individual risks, perceptions, and life experiences. As well, the health care team must be cautious not to allow their own value judgements to influence their interactions with the individual.

Confidentiality

There are many concerns about misuse of information derived from test results and the negative sequelae that may result from release of test results, such as discrimination with respect to employment and approval for health, life, disability, and mortgage insurance coverage.

In 1995, at a workshop jointly sponsored by the Ethical, Legal, and Social Implications Working Group and the National Action Plan on Breast Cancer (a public-private partnership created to eliminate breast cancer), issues related to genetic discrimination and health insurance were discussed, and recommendations were formulated to protect individuals against discrimination based on genetic inheritance. Several states have enacted legislation prohibiting discrimination by health insurers and, in some cases, employers. The Kennedy-Kassebaum Bill, passed in 1996, includes safeguards to protect consumers against discrimination based on genetic information; however, the effectiveness of this bill has not been tested in the courts. It is anticipated that in the future, additional federal and state bills will be enacted to address these concerns. To date, few if any cases of overt discrimination related to cancer genetic testing have been documented. Nevertheless, an individual's fears of discrimination have a direct impact on his or her willingness to seek genetic counseling and testing.

Consideration must be given to how results are documented, communicated, and managed to ensure confidentiality. Many institutions do not place results obtained from cancer genetic testing in the patient's medical record; in addition, they may require signed consent from the individual before test results are released to or discussed with family members, insurers, or other health care professionals.

RECENT DEVELOPMENTS WITH IMPLICATIONS FOR CANCER GENETIC TESTING

Several recent developments resulting from clinical trials or the establishment of guidelines by national organizations and individual investigators have important implications for cancer genetic testing.

Guidelines for Cancer Risk Assessment and Cancer Genetic Testing

The National Comprehensive Cancer Network (NCCN), a not-for-profit, tax-exempt corporation, is an alliance of 18 of the leading cancer centers in the United States. In addition to providing superior cancer care, the NCCN member institutions continuously improve this care through the implementation of oncology practice guidelines and through performance measurement.

In 1997, the NCCN published an article that identified 6 aspects of cancer genetic testing that could potentially be encompassed within practice guidelines: the process of informed consent, the need for counseling on nonmedical issues, a process for ensuring the use of current information to guide medical decision making, training for those providing counseling, mandatory follow-up, and the value of participating in research. The practice guidelines for genetics were presented at the annual NCCN conference in February 1999 and published in November 1999 (Daly, 1999).

The American Society of Clinical Oncology has also established guidelines for consideration in the conduct of cancer genetic testing (ASCO, 1996).

Cancer Risk Assessment Models

Models have been developed for use in assessing risk for some cancers. The Gail model, based on information gathered from the Breast Cancer Detection and Demonstration Project, was used to determine eligibility for the Breast Cancer Prevention Trial and is reviewed in chapter 2. Tabular data compiled by Claus et al (1994) using information from the Cancer and Steroid Hormone study are especially useful for evaluating family breast cancer history because they take into account the age of affected relatives at the onset of cancer. Analysis of this information enabled the researchers to construct tables that can be used to predict a woman's cumulative lifetime risk of developing breast cancer. The risk estimates are based on the age of affected relatives at the time of cancer diagnosis. The histories of various family members and combinations of family members can be evaluated (e.g., mother, mother and sister, and mother and maternal aunt); however, the relatives evaluated must have breast cancer and must be from the same lineage (i.e., maternal or paternal). In general, the Claus model is used to estimate risk in families at moderate risk for developing cancer—for example, families in which several cases of breast cancer are present yet the age of onset is later and the cases are not reflective of a hereditary breast or ovarian cancer syndrome.

Although the Gail and Claus models are useful, they have limitations. The data collected using these models have been obtained primarily from white women; thus, the models may not be applicable to women of other races. As well, both models were developed prior to the discovery of the genes associated with hereditary cancer syndromes; thus, the models tend to underestimate the risks for individuals from families with hereditary breast cancer and to overestimate the risks for others.

Several models now enable clinicians to predict the probability that an individual may test positive for a mutation in either *BRCA1* or *BRCA2*. Frank et al (1998) developed a statistical model using data from 238 women who had undergone sequence analysis of the *BRCA1* and *BRCA2* genes. For consideration in this study, women had to have been diagnosed with breast cancer before age 50 or to have had an ovarian cancer at any age and at least 1 first- or second-degree relative with either diagnosis. Results of testing were correlated with personal and family history of malignancy to yield tables predicting whether a family with a specific set of characteristics (e.g., a proband with breast cancer before age 40 and a relative with ovarian cancer) would test positive. These tables do not separate women of Ashkenazi Jewish heritage (who are known to have a higher prevalence of *BRCA1* and *BRCA2* mutations) from women of European and other heritages.

Parmigiani et al (1998) developed and applied a mathematical model for calculating the probability that a woman with a family history of breast cancer, ovarian cancer, or both might carry a mutation in *BRCA1* or *BRCA2*. This model has been named the BRCAPRO model, and it is currently being validated. The probability is based on family history of breast and ovarian cancers in first- and second-degree relatives. The cancer probabilities are obtained from Bayes' theorem using family history as the evidence and using mutation prevalence as the prior distribution. There is some evidence that other, undiscovered cancer predisposition genes may account for breast cancer in these families; this is a potential limitation of the BRCAPRO model. This model is useful for determining the probability that a woman may be a carrier for a mutation in either *BRCA1* or *BRCA2*; however, these data must also be balanced with clinical evaluation and expertise. In families with a small number of breast cancer cases, BRCAPRO may provide spurious predictions of risk. Characteristics found to be predictive of testing positive for a mutation in *BRCA1* or *BRCA2* in families with 3 to 5 cases of breast or ovarian cancer include a case of ovarian cancer, bilateral breast cancer, or breast cancer diagnosed before age 40 (Table 3–3).

These cancer risk assessment models were developed for use with families with a large number of breast and ovarian cancers and are probably most representative of families with a high-penetrance genetic mutation. In many cases, either because of nuclear families (families in which only a small number of women are available for testing) or as the result of migration, estrangement, adoption, or the Holocaust, family history information is limited. In these cases, the health care team must derive the best possible estimate of risk. In some instances, the team must inform the individual that a risk assessment cannot be made; these families will be considered to have an indeterminate cancer risk. Table 3–4 outlines criteria published by the NCCN that would signify the potential presence of a hereditary breast or ovarian cancer syndrome or both in a family. Families that meet these criteria would be appropriate candidates for further evaluation and cancer genetic counseling.

BREAST CANCER AND OVARIAN CANCER PREVENTION STRATEGIES

As more is understood about the nature of carcinogenesis, the ability to intervene at the earliest stages of tumor development is becoming a

Table 3–3. Factors Predictive of Testing Positive for a *BRCA1* or *BRCA2* Mutation in Families with 3 to 5 Cases of Breast or Ovarian Cancer

Family Cancer History Factors	Likelihood of Testing Positive (%)
Breast and ovarian cancer history	
One ovarian and 2 breast	57
Breast cancer only	
Bilateral breast cancer	36
None in women younger than 40	14
One or more in women younger than 40	48
No bilateral breast cancer	7
None in women younger than 30	0
One or more in women younger than 40	14
Breast cancer before age 40	30
No breast cancer before age 40	6

Source: Ligtenberg et al, 1999.

Table 3–4. Criteria Suggestive of Hereditary Breast or Ovarian Cancer Syndrome that Warrants Further Professional Evaluation

1. Member of known *BRCA1/BRCA2* kindred

2. Personal history of breast cancer + one or more of the following:
   a. Diagnosed age ≤ 40 yr, with or without family history
   b. Diagnosed age ≤ 50 yr or bilateral, with ≥ 1 close blood relative with breast cancer *or* ≥ 1 close blood relative with ovarian cancer
   c. Diagnosed at any age, with ≥ 2 close blood relatives with ovarian cancer at any age, *or* breast cancer, especially if ≥ 1 woman is diagnosed before age 50 yr or has bilateral disease
   d. Close male blood relative has breast cancer
   e. If of Ashkenazi Jewish descent and diagnosed age ≤ 50 yr, no additional family history required *or* at any age if history of breast and/or ovarian cancer in close blood relative

3. Personal history of ovarian cancer + one or more of the following:
   a. ≥ 1 close blood relative with ovarian cancer
   b. ≥ 1 close female blood relative with breast cancer at age ≤ 50 yr *or* bilateral breast cancer
   c. ≥ 2 close blood relatives with breast cancer
   d. ≥ 1 close male blood relative with breast cancer
   e. If of Ashkenazi Jewish descent, no additional family history is required

4. Personal history of male breast cancer + one or more of the following:
   a. ≥ 1 close male blood relative with breast cancer
   b. ≥ 1 close female blood relative with breast or ovarian cancer
   c. If of Ashkenazi Jewish descent, no additional family history is required

5. Family history only—one or more of the following:
   a. ≥ 1 close blood relative with breast cancer age ≤ 40 yr or bilateral breast cancer
   b. ≥ 2 close blood relatives with ovarian cancer
   c. ≥ 2 close blood relatives with breast cancer, especially if ≥ 1 is age ≤ 50 yr
   d. ≥ 1 close blood relative with breast cancer, ≥ 1 with ovarian cancer, any age
   e. If of Ashkenazi Jewish descent, 1 close relative with breast or ovarian cancer

greater possibility. Recognizing that dysplastic lesions are biologically significant in the preinvasive stage and understanding the intrinsic biological mechanisms that may prevent these lesions from becoming invasive and metastatic may lead to the design of more effective prevention measures. Currently, there are 3 basic strategies for prevention of breast and ovarian cancers: chemoprevention, prophylactic surgery, and screening and detection.

Chemoprevention

The term chemoprevention, which is defined as the use of natural or synthetic chemical agents to reverse, suppress, or prevent carcinogenic progression to invasive cancer, was coined by Michael Sporn in 1976. Today, several drugs are being investigated for their efficacy in chemoprevention. Among them are tamoxifen, oral contraceptives, and retinoids.

Tamoxifen

A meta-analysis of trials evaluating the effectiveness of tamoxifen in decreasing the incidence of contralateral breast cancer was published by the Early Breast Cancer Trialists' Collaborative Group in 1992. These data led to the concept that the drug might play a role in breast cancer prevention. To test this hypothesis, the National Surgical Adjuvant Breast and Bowel Project initiated the Breast Cancer Prevention Trial in 1992. Women at increased risk for breast cancer were randomly assigned to receive placebo or tamoxifen 20 mg per day for 5 years. The Gail model, based on a multivariate logistic regression model using combinations of risk factors, was used to estimate the probability of occurrence of breast cancer over time. Tamoxifen reduced the risk of invasive breast cancer in these women by 49%. The cumulative incidences of breast cancer through 69 months of follow-up were 43.4 cases per 1000 women in the placebo group and 22.0 cases per 1000 women in the tamoxifen group. Tamoxifen reduced the risk of noninvasive breast cancer by 50% and reduced the occurrence of estrogen receptor–positive tumors by 69%; however, no difference was seen in the occurrence of estrogen receptor–negative tumors. Because breast cancer in individuals with abnormalities in *BRCA1* tends to be estrogen receptor negative, it is not clear whether tamoxifen will decrease breast cancer development in women with abnormalities in *BRCA1*. A subset of patients in the Breast Cancer Prevention Trial are being reanalyzed because of proven abnormalities in either *BRCA1* or *BRCA2*, and definitive data on the efficacy of tamoxifen in these women are expected in the second half of 2001.

Oral Contraceptives

Oral contraceptives have been proven to provide protection against ovarian cancer in the general population. Indeed, oral contraceptives provide definitive proof of the concept that a major life-threatening cancer can be prevented by a simple, relatively nontoxic approach.

Narod and colleagues enrolled 207 women with hereditary ovarian cancer and 161 of their sisters as controls in a case-control study (Narod et al, 1998). Lifetime history of oral contraceptive use was obtained by interview or by written questionnaire and was compared between patients and controls after adjustment for year of birth and parity. The results demonstrated that risk for developing ovarian cancer decreased with increasing duration of oral contraceptive use, with an approximate 2-fold decrease in the incidence of ovarian cancer in women with proven abnormalities in *BRCA1* or *BRCA2*. Follow-up prospective trials are needed; however, oral contraceptives represent a reasonable temporizing step in women who have not completed their families. There may be a slight increase in the incidence of breast cancer in women with abnormalities in *BRCA1* and *BRCA2* who receive exogenous estrogens; however, ovarian cancer is much more difficult to detect than breast cancer and thus much more lethal, making the use of oral contraceptives a reasonable prevention approach for this cancer type.

Retinoids

Retinoids are under investigation as a preventive therapy for a number of cancers, including breast and ovarian cancers, because they have been shown to inhibit cellular proliferation and to induce cellular differentiation.

Fenretinide, a synthetic retinoic acid derivative, was selected for use in breast cancer prevention studies because of its low toxicity profile and its prevention efficacy in preclinical studies. A randomized trial of fenretinide conducted in Milan, Italy, demonstrated a potential decrease in the occurrence of second breast malignancies in premenopausal women. There was no major activity in other population groups. This agent is now being assessed in combination with tamoxifen in a phase II breast cancer prevention trial.

Chemoprevention trials with oral contraceptives plus retinoids will be important in determining whether these drugs are effective in selected populations, such as women who are carriers of a genetic change that predisposes them to the development of breast or ovarian cancer.

Prophylactic Surgery

Many individuals faced with a high lifetime risk of developing breast cancer consider prophylactic surgery as a means to manage their risk. However, minimal data exist on the effectiveness of this intervention. For some hereditary conditions, such as familial adenomatous polyposis and hereditary medullary thyroid cancer, prophylactic surgery is accepted practice. However, for other types of cancer, such as hereditary breast and ovarian cancers, prophylactic surgery is more controversial. Although it is often assumed that prophylactic mastectomy will greatly decrease the risk of breast cancer, realistically, not all breast tissue can be removed. The precise degree of risk reduction associated with prophylactic mastectomy or oophorectomy has not yet been determined for individuals who carry a mutation that predisposes them to breast or ovarian cancer. Therefore, individuals who choose prophylactic mastectomy must realize that some risk remains.

Hartmann et al (1999) published results from a retrospective study of all women with a family history of breast cancer who underwent bilateral prophylactic mastectomy at the Mayo Clinic between 1960 and 1993. The women were divided into a high-risk group (n = 214) and a moderate-risk group (n = 425) on the basis of family history of cancer. A control group of the sisters of the high-risk probands and the Gail model were used to predict the number of breast cancers expected in the 2 groups in the absence of prophylactic mastectomy. The median length of follow-up was 14 years. The median age at prophylactic mastectomy was 42 years. According to the Gail model, 37.4 breast cancers were expected in the moderate-risk group; however, only 4 breast cancers occurred in this group, for an 89.5% reduction in risk ($P < .001$).

Hartmann and colleagues also compared the number of breast cancers among the 214 high-risk probands with the number among their 403 sisters who had not undergone prophylactic mastectomy. Of these sisters, 38.7% (156) had been given a diagnosis of breast cancer (115 cases were diagnosed before the respective proband's prophylactic mastectomy and 38 were diagnosed afterward; the time of the diagnosis was unknown in 3 cases). By contrast, breast cancer was diagnosed in 1.4% (3 of 214) of the probands. Thus, prophylactic mastectomy was associated with a reduction of at least 90% in the incidence of breast cancer. The authors concluded that in women with a high risk of breast cancer based on family history of breast cancer, prophylactic mastectomy can significantly reduce the incidence of breast cancer. A limitation of this study was that cancer genetic testing was not done; thus, it is unknown whether the women in this high-risk group were carriers of mutations in either BRCA1 or BRCA2.

In April 2000, Hartmann et al published an update of this study. At that time, they had completed analysis of BRCA1 and BRCA2 for germline mutations for 110 high-risk families, and they identified 16 women with inherited mutations in either BRCA1 or BRCA2. At the time of the study, at a median follow-up of 16.1 years since prophylactic mastectomy, none of these women had developed breast cancer. The investigators concluded that bilateral prophylactic mastectomy results in a significant reduction in the risk of developing breast cancer in women carrying abnormalities in BRCA1 or BRCA2.

Several other studies have attempted to evaluate the outcome of prophylactic mastectomy in women at high risk for breast cancer. Remarkably, in 2 large studies, 1 each at Memorial Sloan-Kettering Cancer Center and M. D. Anderson, more than 95% of patients were extremely pleased with the outcome of prophylactic mastectomy. The only significant indicators that would place women in the 5% group (those not satisfied with the outcome of the prophylactic mastectomy) were whether the patient decided on her own to undergo the mastectomy or based her decision on her physician's recommendation and whether there were complications, such as infection, associated with either the original or subsequent surgery.

Screening and Detection

Another option for breast cancer prevention is aggressive cancer screening beginning at an earlier age and at more frequent intervals. A task force of the Cancer Genetics Studies Consortium, a group of researchers investigating the psychosocial implications of cancer susceptibility testing, has published follow-up recommendations for individuals at high risk of developing cancer. However, it is important to note that the efficacy of mammography, Sestamibi scans, ultrasonography, and magnetic resonance imaging in the high-risk population is not known. Indeed, the efficacy of mammography is much lower in premenopausal women, with higher false-negative and false-positive rates. Clinical trials are needed to determine the most appropriate surveillance measures for individuals carrying mutated cancer predisposition genes and to develop more sensitive screening tests. Screening is discussed in detail in chapter 2.

Currently, there is no standard of care for the management of individuals who carry alterations in either *BRCA1* or *BRCA2*. Table 3–5 outlines the NCCN recommendations for preventive care of women and men who are members of families with the hereditary breast or ovarian cancer syndrome.

Comparison of Outcomes of Prevention Strategies

A number of models have been used to evaluate the effects of prophylactic surgery on patient outcomes. The predicted outcomes are limited by the lack of definitive data but are useful for discussions with patients. For example, in a 30-year-old carrier of the *BRCA1* mutation, tamoxifen, raloxifene, and prophylactic oophorectomy are each predicted to decrease the chance of developing breast cancer approximately 2-fold, translating into a 0.4- to 2.8-year increase in life span (Table 3–6). Prophylactic mastectomy is predicted to result in a 10-fold decrease in the chance of developing cancer and a 2.7- to 3.7-year increase in life span. A combination of prophylactic oophorectomy and mastectomy may result in a 3.8- to 4.6-year increase in life span. These outcomes are very similar to the outcomes of prevention therapies in women who have already developed breast cancer. In this patient group, prophylactic mastectomy is predicted to re-

Table 3–5. Management of Hereditary Breast and Ovarian Cancer Syndrome

Women	Men
• Training in breast self-exam and regular monthly practice starting at age 18 yr	• Consider annual mammogram for *BRCA2* mutation carriers
• Clinical breast exam, annual or semi-annual, starting at age 25 yr	• Clinical breast exam for *BRCA2* carriers
• Annual mammogram starting at age 25 yr	• Breast self-exam training and regular monthly practice for *BRCA2* carriers
• Consider prophylactic mastectomy on case-by-base basis. Counsel regarding degree of protection and reconstruction options	• Refer to other NCCN guidelines for other cancer screening
• Transvaginal ultrasound + CA-125 + pelvic exam, annually or semi-annually, starting at age 25–35 yr and done concurrently	• Education regarding signs and symptoms of cancer
• Counsel regarding prophylactic oophorectomy on case-by-case basis, including discussion of reproductive desires, extent of cancer risk, degree of protection, and management of menopausal symptoms	
• Consider chemoprevention options (category 1, see NCCN Breast Cancer Risk Reduction Guidelines)	
• Education regarding signs and symptoms of cancer	
• Consider participation in investigational breast imaging studies when available	

sult in a 0.6- to 2.1-year increase in life span, and chemoprevention and oophorectomy each result in a 2-fold decrease in the risk of developing breast cancer (Table 3–7).

Potential cost benefits in terms of years of life saved are another important consideration when breast cancer prevention strategies are compared. A recent study has suggested that the cost per year of life saved for an Ashkenazi Jewish woman would range from $20,000 for screening plus mastectomy and oophorectomy to $30,000 for screening plus mastectomy, compared with $134,000 for screening alone. These numbers

Table 3–6. Effect of Breast Cancer Prevention Strategies in a 30-Year-Old
BRCA1 Mutation Carrier

Treatment	Decrease in Chance of Developing Breast Cancer	Years of Life Saved
Tamoxifen	2-fold	1.0–2.1
Raloxifene	2-fold	1.3–2.8
Prophylactic oophorectomy	2-fold	0.4–1.2
Prophylactic mastectomy	10-fold	2.7–3.7
Prophylactic mastectomy and oophorectomy	15-fold	3.8–4.6

Source: Grann et al, 2000.

Table 3–7. Effect of Breast Cancer Prevention Strategies in Women with
Breast Cancer and _BRCA1_ or _BRCA2_ Mutations

Treatment	Decrease in Chance of Developing Cancer	Years of Life Saved
Breast cancer		
Tamoxifen	2-fold	0.4–1.3
Prophylactic oophorectomy	2-fold	0.2–1.8
Prophylactic mastectomy	10-fold	0.6–2.1
Ovarian cancer		
Oral contraceptives	2-fold	Not known
Prophylactic oophorectomy	2-fold	0.2–1.8

Source: Schrag et al, 2000.

compare very favorably with treatment of hypertension or a 3-artery cardiac bypass.

IMPLICATIONS FOR THE ONCOLOGIST

Our understanding of cancer at a molecular level and of the role of certain genetic mutations in the development of cancer has enabled us to more clearly define genetic predisposition for breast and ovarian cancers and, thus, the risk for women in families with hereditary breast and ovarian cancer syndromes. With this new knowledge, we can begin to improve prevention techniques to reduce the risk for these women. Cancer genetic counseling and cancer genetic testing are complex and labor-intensive processes. Many centers, including M. D. Anderson, utilize a multidisciplinary approach in conducting these processes. Although cancer genetic counseling and cancer genetic testing are typically conducted at specialized centers, community physicians must be fully aware of the full scope of services associated with genetic testing so they can make appropriate referrals for the individual.

KEY PRACTICE POINTS

- Approximately 5% to 10% of all tumors arise in individuals who inherit a genetic abnormality that predisposes them to the development of cancer, including breast cancer.

- Cancer is not an inevitable outcome of an inherited predisposition; other genetic mutations must occur for cancer to develop.

- Characteristics seen in hereditary cancer syndromes include clustering of like cancers, the occurrence of cancers before the age of 50, and multiple cancers in one person. Paternal heritage is as important as maternal heritage.

- Founder effect mutations in breast cancer predisposition genes are known to occur in people of Ashkenazi Jewish, Dutch, Icelandic, French-Canadian, and Sephardic Jewish heritage.

- Cancer genetic counseling is a vital preparative step that helps to ensure that the individual fully understands the issues related to cancer genetic testing.

- Options for management of increased risk for breast cancer include more frequent and earlier screening, chemoprevention, and prophylactic mastectomies.

Suggested Readings

American Society of Clinical Oncology. Statement of the American Society of Clinical Oncology: genetic testing for cancer susceptibility. *J Clin Oncol* 1996;14:1730–1736.

Blackwood MA, Weber BL. BRCA1 and BRCA2: from molecular genetics to clinical medicine. *J Clin Oncol* 1998;16:1969–1977.

Breast Cancer Linkage Consortium. Cancer risks in BRCA2 mutation carriers. *J Natl Cancer Inst* 1999;91:1310–1316.

Claus EB, Risch N, Thompson WD. Autosomal dominant inheritance of early-onset breast cancer. Implications for risk prediction. *Cancer* 1994;73:643–651.

Cummings S, Olopade OI. Predisposition testing for breast cancer. *Oncology* 1998;12:1227–1242.

Daly M. NCCN proceedings: genetics/familial high-risk cancer screening. *Oncology* 1999;13:161–183.

Early Breast Cancer Trialists' Collaborative Group. Systemic treatment of early breast cancer by hormonal, cytotoxic, or immune therapy. *Lancet* 1992;339:1–15.

Eng C. Genetics of Cowden syndrome: through the looking glass of oncology. *Int J Oncol* 1998;12:701–710.

Frank TS, Manley SA, Olopade OI, et al. Sequence analysis of BRCA1 and BRCA2: correlation of mutations with family history and ovarian cancer risk. *J Clin Oncol* 1998;16:2417–2425.

Grann VR, Jacobson JS, Whang W, et al. Prevention with tamoxifen or other hormones versus prophylactic surgery in BRCA1/2-positive women: a decision analysis. *Cancer J Sci Am* 2000;6:13–20.

Hartmann LC, Schaid D, Sellers T. Bilateral prophylactic mastectomy (PM) in BRCA1/2 mutation carriers. *Proceedings of the American Association for Cancer Research* 2000;41 (abstract 1417).

Hartmann LC, Schaid DJ, Woods JE, et al. Efficacy of bilateral prophylactic mastectomy in women with a family history of breast cancer. *N Engl J Med* 1999;340:77–84.

Li FP. Cancer control in susceptible groups: opportunities and challenges. *J Clin Oncol* 1999;17:719–725.

Ligtenberg MJ, Hogervorst FB, Willems HW, et al. Characteristics of small breast and/or ovarian cancer families with germline mutations in BRCA1 and BRCA2. *Br J Cancer* 1999;79:1475–1478.

Lindor NM, Greene MH. The concise handbook of family cancer syndromes. Mayo Familial Cancer Program. *J Natl Cancer Inst* 1998;90:1039–1071.

Lynch HT, Casey MJ, Lynch J, et al. Genetics and ovarian carcinoma. *Semin Oncol* 1998;25:265–280.

Mills GB, Rieger PT, Watt MA, Graham CC, Pentz RB. Genetic predisposition to cancer. In: Pollock R, ed. *Manual of Clinical Oncology*. New York: Springer-Verlag; 1998:63–97.

Narod SA, Risch H, Moslehi R, et al. Oral contraceptives and the risk of hereditary ovarian cancer. Hereditary Ovarian Cancer Clinical Study Group. *N Engl J Med* 1998;339:424–428.

Parmigiani G, Berry D, Aguilar O. Determining carrier probabilities for breast cancer-susceptibility genes BRCA1 and BRCA2. *Am J Hum Genet* 1998;62:145–158.

Phillips KA, Andrulis IL, Goodwin PJ. Breast carcinomas arising in carriers of mutations in BRCA1 or BRCA2: are they prognostically different? *J Clin Oncol* 1999;17:3653–3663.

Rieger PT, Pentz RB. Genetic testing and informed consent. *Semin Oncol Nurs* 1999;15:104–115.

Schrag D, Kuntz KM, Garber JE, Weeks JC. Life expectancy gains from cancer prevention strategies for women with breast cancer and BRCA1 or BRCA2 mutations. *JAMA* 2000;283:617–624.

Varley JM, Evans DG, Birch JM. Li-Fraumeni syndrome—a molecular and clinical review. *Br J Cancer* 1997;76:1–14.

Weitzel JN. Genetic cancer risk assessment. Putting it all together. *Cancer* 1999;86(suppl 11):2483–2492.

Appendix 3A:
Authorization for
Disclosure of Medical
Records

THE UNIVERSITY OF TEXAS
MD ANDERSON
CANCER CENTER

Risk Assessment Clinic
(713) 745–8040
(713) 745–8046 fax
Box 51

AUTHORIZATION FOR DISCLOSURE OF MEDICAL RECORD INFORMATION

I hereby authorize my health care providers to release information concerning my medical history to the Risk Assessment Clinic at The University of Texas M. D. Anderson Cancer Center. This authorization applies to my past and future visits at your hospital/clinic and will be beneficial in the assessment of my cancer risk.

Patient Name: _____   Date of Birth: _____

Address: _____   Telephone: _____

_____   Patient Number: _____

Covering the period(s) of health care: From: _____ To: _____
(date)   (date)

A. Information to be disclosed:

☐ Complete health record(s)   ☐ Pelvic exam (pelvic exam/Pap smear reports)
☐ Primary medical evaluation   ☐ Mammogram/ultrasound (report)
☐ X-ray reports   ☐ Pathology reports related to cancer diagnosis
☐ Laboratory tests   ☐ Radiology reports
☐ Consultation reports   ☐ Admission records & discharge summary
☐ Other: _____

_____

_____

B. Please fax or mail the requested medical records to:

The University of Texas M. D. Anderson Cancer Center   Fax: (713) 745–8046
Paula Rieger, RN/Risk Assessment Clinic   Phone: (713) 745–8040
1515 Holcombe—Box 51
Houston, Texas 77030

C. I HEREBY RELEASE YOU FROM LIABILITY FOR FOLLOWING THIS AUTHORIZATION AND REQUEST.

_____   _____
Name (please print)   Signature

_____
Relationship to Patient (deceased)

REGARDING M. D. ANDERSON PATIENT:

_____   _____
(Name)   (MDACC Number)

TEXAS MEDICAL CENTER
1515 HOLCOMBE BOULEVARD • HOUSTON, TEXAS 77030 • (713) 792–2121
A Comprehensive Cancer Center Designated by the National Cancer Institute

Appendix 3B: Follow-up Letter Sent after Cancer Genetic Counseling

May 5, 2000

Dear Ms. James:

It was a pleasure meeting with you again on May 1, 2000, at the M. D. Anderson Cancer Center Risk Assessment Clinic. This letter outlines our assessment of your family history and of the risk of there being a mutated (altered) gene in your family that predisposes individuals to the development of breast, ovarian, or other cancers.

Summation of Family History of Cancer

Breast and Ovarian Cancer

To summarize once again, based on the information you provided, there are 4 women with known breast cancers in your family history: (1) yourself, diagnosed at age 35 and again in the opposite breast at age 45; (2) a maternal aunt diagnosed at age 38; (3) a maternal cousin diagnosed at age 37; and (4) a maternal great-aunt diagnosed at age 35. These breast cancers were all diagnosed before menopause (premenopausal).

One woman, your mother, had an ovarian cancer, which was diagnosed at age 68.

You have a personal history of biopsy of a mass in the left breast, which was positive for an infiltrating intraductal carcinoma. Lymph node dissection showed that 3 were positive. You were treated with a modified radical mastectomy of the left breast, post-operative radiation therapy, and adjuvant chemotherapy. You had no evidence of disease until 1996, when you were diagnosed with a second breast cancer. This cancer was detected early and was treated with a segmental mastectomy.

Other Cancers

On the maternal side of your family, a cousin had a lung cancer at an unknown age.

On the paternal side of your family, your father had a prostate cancer in his 80s. You reported that a paternal cousin had an ovarian cancer at age 45; however, pathology reports proved this to be a cervical cancer.

Verification of Cancer Occurrence

Pathology reports of the known cancer diagnoses in your family would help us verify the occurrence of cancers in your family and would enable us to refine our estimates of cancer risk in your family. The validity of our assessment is based on the extent and the accuracy of the information you have provided. We have provided you with the appropriate pathology request forms. We must reiterate once again that it is especially prudent to obtain pathological documentation to verify any diagnosis of ovarian cancer. We have found, through experience, that ovarian cancer is often confused with cancers of other internal organs or with other female cancers. In addition, the presence of ovarian cancer in a family is significant in that it can significantly alter the assessment of the presence of a hereditary cancer syndrome in a family.

Probability of the Presence of an Altered Breast Cancer Gene in Your Family

Breast cancer is a common cancer in women, and it is seen frequently in the population. Thus, in a large family, it is not uncommon that 1 or several women will have breast cancer. Certain characteristics are seen in families with hereditary cancer syndromes: (1) a clustering of specific cancers—for example, breast and ovarian cancer—more than would be expected to occur by chance alone; (2) earlier age at onset of cancer than is seen in the general population; and (3) evidence of cancer in each generation of the family. Women may also tend to have bilateral breast cancers.

In your family, there are several cases of early-onset breast cancer and an ovarian cancer. We would estimate that there is a greater than 50% probability that an alteration in either the *BRCA1* or *BRCA2* gene might be found in your family if cancer genetic testing were done on an affected family member (one who has developed a breast or ovarian cancer). You reported that your mother has undergone testing using full sequencing of the *BRCA1* and *BRCA2* genes and that an alteration was found in the *BRCA2* gene. Your mother's first-degree relatives can now be tested for this alteration if they so choose. Each would have a 50% probability of having inherited the *BRCA2* alteration.

We do not yet completely understand the process that takes place in the development of breast cancer. We do know that alterations, or mutations, in either the *BRCA1* or *BRCA2* genes increase an individual's chance of developing breast cancer.

Overview of the Frequency of and Risks Associated with Inheritance of *BRCA1* and *BRCA2* Alterations

It is estimated that, for the general population, the probability of having an alteration in either *BRCA1* or *BRCA2* is approximately 1 in 800. For those of Ashkenazi Jewish descent, the probability of an alteration in either of these genes is estimated to be 1 in 50. As we discussed, alterations in these genes are inherited in a dominant pattern. Each of us carries 2 copies of a gene, and an alteration in 1 copy is sufficient to increase cancer risk. Only 1 copy of a gene is transmitted to our offspring. So, for each gene, there is a 50% chance that the copy that is transmitted to our offspring will be the normal copy and, likewise, a 50% chance that the transmitted copy will be the altered copy. Thus, even if we carry an altered gene, each of our offspring has only a 50% chance of inheriting the altered copy.

Although the precise risk is uncertain, our best data at this time indicate that women with abnormalities in the *BRCA1* gene carry the following lifetime risk of developing cancer: up to a 40% to 60% lifetime risk for breast cancer, with an increased risk of bilateral disease, and a 20% to 40% lifetime risk for ovarian cancer. These cancers tend to develop at an earlier age than in the general population. There is also an increased risk of developing a cancer in the second breast if one has already developed a breast cancer. There may be a slightly increased risk for the development of colorectal cancer and, for men, prostate cancer.

Abnormalities in the *BRCA2* gene in women are thought to confer a similar lifetime risk of developing breast cancer (30%–50%) and a moderate risk of developing ovarian cancer (approximately 10%–30%), although data about this gene are more limited. Alterations in the *BRCA2* gene also increase the risk of breast cancer in males, with an approximate 6% lifetime risk by age 70. Research is beginning to identify other cancers that may also be associated with alterations in *BRCA2*, and it appears that families in which this gene is present have an increased incidence of prostate cancer, pancreatic cancer, gallbladder and bile duct cancer, stomach cancer, and malignant melanoma.

In the future, we will continue to look for other cancers that are associated with alterations in the *BRCA1* and *BRCA2* genes.

The Benefits, Risks, and Limitations of Cancer Genetic Testing

Currently, there are only a few cancer susceptibility genes for which cancer genetic testing is available, and as we discussed in your clinic visit, these tests have limitations. The tests are new, and new information about them is becoming available as more people undergo testing. With the current technology, it takes a minimum of 4 to 6 weeks to obtain cancer genetic test results. The cost of full sequencing of the *BRCA1* and *BRCA2* genes is approximately $2500. Many insurers are beginning to cover the cost of testing. By testing an affected person, the likelihood of detecting an alteration, if it is present, is increased. In your family, your mother has already tested positive. Hence, the cost of testing for other first-degree relatives, who may choose this option, would be approximately $300.

Although a positive test result can tell you whether you carry the alteration, it cannot tell you when or if cancer will develop. The effect of environmental and other factors on cancer development is not known. Some 40% to 60% of patients who carry alterations in these cancer susceptibility genes may *never* develop cancer. Screening guidelines and prevention measures for those at high risk of developing cancer are currently being outlined. There are no measures that are known to completely prevent cancer or to guarantee early detection. The knowledge of carrying an altered cancer susceptibility gene may cause some people to feel anxious, whereas such knowledge may cause others to feel more in control.

It is important to understand that a negative test *does not* mean the individual has no cancer risk. A negative test result in a family in which no genetic alteration has been identified and in which no affected family member is available for testing provides little information about family members' risk for cancer. The detection system may miss certain true alterations in an estimated 10% to 30% of cases. There may also be alterations in other genes that have yet to be discovered. It is possible that the cancers in your family occurred by chance, but it is still very important to follow cancer screening guidelines. In your family, a known deleterious mutation has been found. A first-degree relative who tests negative would carry the same risk as the general population for developing a breast or ovarian cancer.

As we discussed, there are many ethical, legal, and social issues associated with cancer genetic testing. Insurance companies may deny you or members of your family insurance coverage if the results are positive or if they are aware that you have been tested. It is even remotely possible that they could use your family history data as evidence of increased risk and alter your coverage based only on that information. If your insurance provider will not pay for the testing or if you choose to pay out of pocket, the cost can be high. Recent genetic nondiscrimination legislation passed at both the state- and federal-government levels is beginning to address this issue and to provide protection for those who are currently insured. M. D. Anderson continues to work with the Texas legislature to formulate and enact genetic nondiscrimination laws that will, hopefully, correct these problems. A bill was passed and became effective September 1, 1997, that prohibits discrimination in determination of eligibility for employment, occupational licenses, and coverage under certain health benefit plans based on the use of certain cancer genetic tests.

Every attempt is made to keep all information regarding your risk for cancer confidential. Information derived through counseling and testing is not included in your medical record at M. D. Anderson, but there is no absolute guarantee that insurers cannot access this information. However, your written authorization would be required before any information is released. If a potential employer is aware that a candidate for employment has an increased risk for cancer, employment might be denied.

The decision to undergo cancer genetic testing is yours, as is the decision whether to receive the results of testing. When making these decisions, remember that cancer genetic testing might reveal information that is important to other family members—for example, information regarding adoption or paternity (fatherhood). Some of your family members may want to be tested and know their results, whereas others may not. It is important that you discuss these issues with your health care team and your family before deciding to undergo cancer genetic testing.

Cancer Prevention and Counseling

There is currently no known treatment to definitively prevent the development of breast or ovarian cancer in individuals who have a greater risk for developing these diseases compared with that of the general population. However, many strategies are currently being studied, and data exist to support the efficacy of several of these strategies in decreasing the risk for developing a breast or ovarian cancer. Current options for managing increased risk include prophylactic surgery with continued annual screening, chemoprevention, and increased screening measures.

Prophylactic Surgery and Continued Annual Screening

- Prophylactic hysterectomy/oophorectomy
  This procedure may decrease the risk for developing an ovarian cancer but will not eliminate it entirely. New evidence published in August 1999 by Weber and colleagues in the *Journal of the National Cancer Institute* indicates that women carrying an alteration in the *BRCA1* gene can decrease their risk for developing breast cancer by up to 70% by having a bilateral prophylactic oophorectomy.
- Prophylactic mastectomy
  This procedure may decrease the risk for developing a breast cancer but will not eliminate it entirely. You have had a modified radical mastectomy of the left breast and a segmental mastectomy of the right breast. At this time, we do not know the precise degree of protection that these prophylactic surgeries will provide. A study published by Hartmann in 1999 reviewed data from the Mayo Clinic and showed a substantial reduction in the risk for breast cancer following prophylactic mastectomy, even in women who had a family history of breast cancer. This study included a retrospective evaluation of women with a family history of breast cancer who had bilateral prophylactic mastectomy at the Mayo Clinic between 1960 and 1993. Two hundred fourteen women met study-specific criteria for high risk, and 3 of them had developed breast cancer. There was an approximate 90% reduction in breast cancer risk in the group overall.

  This study did not evaluate women who were known carriers of either *BRCA1* or *BRCA2* mutations. In April of 2000, Hartmann and colleagues provided an update of this study. Thus far, they have completed germline *BRCA1* and *BRCA2* analyses in 110 families at high risk for cancer. They have identified 16 women who have inherited mutations in either *BRCA1* or *BRCA2* to date, and none of these women have developed breast cancer. These patients have been followed for a median 16.1 years since prophylactic mastectomy. Hartmann and colleagues concluded that bilateral prophylactic mastectomy yields a significant reduction in risk for cancer.

Chemoprevention

Results from the Breast Cancer Prevention Trial completed in 1998 suggested that tamoxifen may decrease the frequency of breast cancer in women at high risk for the disease. The degree of protection this approach provides for individuals with a genetic abnormality is currently not clear. Furthermore, research by Narod and colleagues has indicated that the birth control pill may decrease the risk for ovarian cancer in women who carry alterations in the *BRCA1* and *BRCA2* genes. Thus, the birth control pill and tamoxifen may decrease the incidence of ovarian and breast cancer, respectively, in individuals at risk for these diseases. It is important, however, that women weigh the risks and benefits of taking a drug such as tamoxifen.

In 1999, a trial was initiated by the National Cancer Institute that will compare the effects of tamoxifen and raloxifene in decreasing the risk for breast cancer in postmenopausal women at increased risk for this disease. Accrual for this important trial has begun at M. D. Anderson and at other centers across the United States. If you have family members who are interested in more information about this trial, please have them call 713-792-8064 or 1-800-4CANCER (1-800-422-6237) from outside the Houston area.

Screening

The following recommendations for cancer screening have been modified for your level of risk.

- Breast Cancer
  - Mammography—We would defer to the recommendations of your oncologist.
  - Clinical breast exam—We would defer to the recommendations of your oncologist.
  - Monthly breast self examination.

- Cervical Cancer
  Annual Pap smear and pelvic examination beginning at age of initiation of sexual activity.

- Ovarian Cancer
  - Annual transvaginal ultrasound
  - Annual CA-125 level

For women who are known carriers of an alteration in either *BRCA1* or *BRCA2*, a panel of experts have published guidelines (published by Burke and colleagues) that recommend screening for ovarian cancer on an annual or semiannual basis. For women considered to be at increased risk for ovarian cancer, based on personal or family history, the National Cancer Institute has recommended that screening measures for the detection of ovarian cancer be instituted when a woman carries of 5% or higher lifetime risk of developing ovarian cancer. We estimate that you would fall above this number; thus, special screening is recommended.

Dr. Diane Bodurka Bevers conducts a special ovarian cancer screening program here at M. D. Anderson. We have requested an appointment for you to undergo ovarian cancer screening through this program at your follow-up visit with us. You may call them directly at 713-792-6810 for further information or to cancel the appointment, if you so choose.

- Colorectal Cancer
  The American Cancer Society recommends that, beginning at age 50, both men and women should follow this testing schedule for colorectal cancer:
  - Flexible sigmoidoscopy and digital rectal examination every 5 years if there are no abnormal findings, and annual fecal occult blood testing, or
  - Double contrast barium enema and digital rectal examination every 10 years if there are no abnormal findings, or
  - Full colonoscopy and digital rectal examination every 10 years if there are no abnormal findings

- Skin Cancer
  - Monthly skin self exam
  - Beginning at 40, annual professional examination for individuals at increased risk (e.g., people with fair skin, a family or personal history of skin cancer, history of significant sun exposure)

These screening options do not guarantee that a cancer will be found at an early, curable stage. Clinical trials across the country are currently being conducted to determine the most appropriate screening tests and guidelines for individuals at high risk for cancer. Please stay in touch with us regarding new information on clinical trials that may become available. You may wish to consider participating in clinical trials here at M. D. Anderson that are designed to answer these questions.

M. D. Anderson offers a variety of specialized cancer prevention and screening services through our Prevention Center, including full cancer screening examinations for both men and women that build upon the long-standing expertise of this institution in cancer screening.

Counseling

We recommend that your first-degree relatives also seek cancer genetic counseling at a clinic such as ours to discuss their risk for cancer related to personal and family history. We would be pleased to counsel them if they so desire.

We advise you to consider continuing risk assessment counseling every 6 months to 1 year to evaluate new information and how that information might impact your personal risk for developing breast or ovarian cancer.

Recommended Surveillance Plan

We recommend the following cancer surveillance plan for you:

- Screening
  We have scheduled an appointment for you for ovarian cancer screening.
- Testing
  Following discussion regarding available cancer genetic testing options, you chose to have a genetic test done that will determine whether you have inherited the alteration in the *BRCA2* gene that is known to be present in your family. As we discussed, our standard of care is that test results be given in person. We will not mail the results or give them to you over the telephone. Once we receive your test results, we will contact you to schedule a follow-up visit where we will disclose the results of the test to you.
- Change in family history
  Please notify us of any changes in your family history (particularly with respect to cancer status).

We hope this information will be of help to you as you make decisions about your health. If you have any further questions or concerns, please feel free to call us.

Sincerely,

Gordon B. Mills, M.D., Ph.D.
Chairman, Department of Molecular Therapeutics
Ad-interim Medical Director
Human Clinical Cancer Genetics
Ransom Horne Jr. Professorship for Cancer Research
The University of Texas M. D. Anderson Cancer Center
1515 Holcombe Blvd., Box 317
Houston, TX 77030
713-792-7770

Paula Trahan Rieger, MSN, RN, CS, AOCN®, FAAN
Nurse Practitioner, Human Clinical Cancer Genetics Program
The University of Texas M. D. Anderson Cancer Center
1515 Holcombe Blvd., Box 336
Houston, TX 77030
713-745-8040

4 Mammography, Magnetic Resonance Imaging of the Breast, and Radionuclide Imaging of the Breast

Gary J. Whitman, Anne Chmielewski Kushwaha,
Barbara S. Monsees, and Carol B. Stelling

CHAPTER OVERVIEW

Breast imaging plays an important role in screening for breast cancer, classifying and sampling nonpalpable breast abnormalities, and defining the extent of breast tumors. Randomized clinical trials and meta-analyses have demonstrated decreased mortality rates in women who undergo mammographic screening compared with unscreened controls. In the past decade, there have been notable improvements in mammographic image quality and positioning. In breast conservation therapy, mammography is used to define the extent of malignancy before definitive segmentectomy and to monitor the breast after surgery and radiation therapy. Percutaneous biopsy techniques have been developed to facilitate safe, accurate tissue acquisition. The use of stereotactic and ultrasound-guided biopsies has resulted in a decrease in the number of surgical biopsies performed. Mammography can also be used to guide needle localizations, most of which, in our practice, are performed to help guide the excision of known cancers. Whereas technetium Tc 99m sestamibi imaging has been reasonably accurate in the evaluation of palpable lesions, sestamibi imaging is thought to be limited in the evaluation of nonpalpable lesions. Magnetic resonance imaging shows promise for detecting breast cancers and defining the extent of disease. Magnetic resonance imaging–guided needle localization and core needle biopsy techniques are being developed, and these techniques should allow for the increased utilization of magnetic resonance imaging in the staging of breast cancers. Digital imaging systems offer opportunities for postprocessing and reconfiguring of the original data. Digital mammography should result in improved image quality, a lower call-back rate, and, perhaps, a decreased radiation dose.

Introduction

Over the past decade, major advances have occurred in breast imaging. Mammographic positioning and film quality have improved significantly, and advances in stereotactic biopsy techniques have allowed for safe, accurate biopsy of nonpalpable lesions. These technological advances have occurred at the same time as an expansion in the role of breast imagers as consultants in the diagnosis and management of breast lesions. Mammographers play active roles in every phase of breast lesion detection and characterization, from screening mammography to diagnostic work-up views to biopsy. In women with breast cancer who are being considered for breast conservation therapy (BCT), mammography is critical in determining whether there is multicentric or multifocal disease that may preclude breast conservation. In this chapter, current mammographic practices are reviewed, magnetic resonance imaging (MRI) of the breast is discussed, and radionuclide techniques (technetium Tc 99m sestamibi imaging and the use of technetium Tc 99m sulfur colloid for lymph node mapping) are reviewed.

SCREENING MAMMOGRAPHY

Mammography, clinical breast examination, and breast self-examination are the cornerstones of breast cancer screening and early detection. In the United States, screening mammography is an established health service and widely accepted as a standard of care in cancer prevention. The screening program at the Julie and Ben Rogers Diagnostic Clinic is an important component of M. D. Anderson Cancer Center's missions of cancer screening and prevention.

Efficacy of Screening Mammography

Screening mammography recommendations have been a controversial subject among epidemiologists and breast cancer specialists around the world. Much of the controversy centers around the efficacy of screening mammography in women aged 40 to 49. The current United States recommendations for screening mammography are based on evidence gathered in 7 randomized controlled trials performed between 1963 and 1988 and several meta-analyses. These studies have shown that screening mammography in women aged 40 years and older has reduced cancer deaths by 29% to 45%.

In evaluating the results of the screening mammography trials, a few potential biases should be considered. Lead-time bias refers to the interval between disease detection and the usual manifestations of the disease. The estimated lead time in cancer detection with mammography is 18 months ± 6 months. Length-time bias refers to differences in the rate of growth of tumors. It is thought that interval cancers (those detected during the interval between regularly scheduled annual mammographic screening examinations) are the fastest-growing cancers and have a worse prognosis than cancers detected at regularly scheduled screening mammography. Self-selection bias refers to the fact that patients who volunteer for studies tend to have an increased health awareness compared with the general population. Overdiagnosis is the detection of lesions that have questionable malignant potential. In breast cancer screening, one example of possible overdiagnosis is small-cell ductal carcinoma in situ (DCIS). The natural history of small-cell DCIS is unknown. In general, small-cell DCIS and large-cell DCIS have been treated in a similar manner, and some reports have questioned the invasive potential of small-cell DCIS. Another potential bias in some of the screening trials is cross-contamination, whereby women assigned to the control groups could and did obtain mammograms outside the study confines. This practice may have diminished the observed benefits of mammography.

Some of the randomized controlled trials have been criticized for specific flaws. The Edinburgh trial has been criticized for its randomization techniques. The Canadian trials were criticized for selection bias, questionable randomization practices, and poor mammographic quality. In addition, in all of the randomized controlled studies, poor compliance, cross-contamination, too-lengthy screening intervals, and the limitations of mammographic techniques in the 1970s and 1980s may lead to underestimation of the effects of screening mammography.

Screening Mammography Recommendations

The M. D. Anderson recommendations for screening mammography are the same as those of the American Cancer Society and the American College of Radiology: annual mammography is recommended beginning at age 40. Initiation of screening mammography before age 40 is recommended for women who are known carriers of *BRCA1* or *BRCA2* gene mutations and women who have a first-degree relative with premenopausal breast cancer or evidence of a high hereditary risk for breast cancer. Women with *BRCA1* or *BRCA2* mutations are at increased risk for the development of breast cancer at a young age. Women with *BRCA1* mutations also have a high risk for developing ovarian cancer and colon cancer. Mutations in the *BRCA2* gene are associated with an increased risk of developing breast cancer (including breast cancer in men), endometrial cancer, prostate cancer, and other adenocarcinomas. In women with a high risk of breast cancer based on hereditary factors, mammographic screening is usually started 10 years before the age of the index patient at diagnosis but not before age 25 (i.e., a woman whose mother was diagnosed with breast cancer at age 43 would begin annual screening mammography at age 33).

Initiation of screening mammography prior to age 40 is also suggested for women who received radiation therapy to the chest before age 30. It is known that women who received radiation to the chest before age 30 are at increased risk for breast cancer because of possible radiation damage to the breast tissue at a genetically sensitive time in development. This increased risk appears to be dose and age related. The most common indication for irradiation of the chest today is treatment of Hodgkin's disease. Occasionally, young women with other malignancies, including thyroid carcinoma and sarcomas, undergo radiation therapy to the chest. In women who have undergone irradiation of the chest before age 30, mammographic screening should start 10 years after the completion of radiation therapy but not before age 25; thereafter, annual mammography is suggested.

Design of Screening Mammography Programs

The goal of a screening mammography program is to detect early cancers (Figure 4–1). The mammographer's emphasis should be on the detection of masses smaller than 1 cm and the identification of suspicious calcifications. If an abnormality is identified on a screening study, additional imaging (i.e., diagnostic mammography) is suggested. Call-back rates below 10% in a population undergoing regular, annual screening are

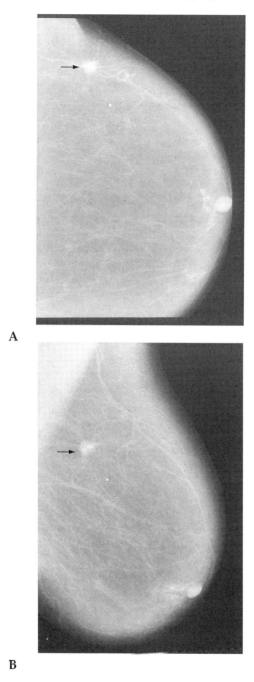

Figure 4–1. Craniocaudal (A) and mediolateral oblique (B) views of a high-density, irregular, spiculated mass (arrow) in the upper outer left breast identified on screening mammography. Surgical excision revealed tubular carcinoma.

suggested. Efforts are ongoing to bolster compliance, improve efficiency, and decrease overhead costs. Costs can be lowered by separating screening from diagnostic studies and batch-reading the screening studies. At M. D. Anderson, we have 2 separate mammography reading rooms. One room is for current diagnostic studies and on-line monitoring of work-ups. The second room, where screening mammograms are read, is a quieter room with 2 large mammography alternators. The screening studies are hung on the alternators, and reporting is performed with a computerized system. A computer-aided diagnosis device (ImageChecker, R2 Technology, Los Altos, CA) has been added to our screening program to serve as a "second reader."

Mammographic screening programs should detect 6 to 10 cancers per 1000 women on their first screen and 2 to 4 cancers per 1000 women on subsequent screens. Biopsy should be recommended in less than 2% of the first screens and in less than 1% of the subsequent screens. Six-month follow-up mammograms (to document the stability of probably benign findings for lesions classified as category 3 in the Breast Imaging Reporting and Data System [BI-RADS] of the American College of Radiology [Table 4–1]) should be recommended in approximately 4% to 5% of cases. The positive predictive value for patients undergoing biopsy should be 25% to 35%. Ductal carcinoma in situ should comprise 20% to 35% of the cancers detected. At least 40% of all invasive cancers detected should be less than 1 cm in diameter.

MAMMOGRAPHIC WORK-UPS

At M. D. Anderson, our mammography practice is divided into 2 components: screening studies and diagnostic studies. Screening mammography is performed on asymptomatic women without a personal history of breast cancer. Diagnostic mammography is performed on women with abnormal

Table 4–1. American College of Radiology's Breast Imaging Reporting and Data System (BI-RADS)

Category 0	Need additional imaging evaluation
Category 1	Negative
Category 2	Benign finding
Category 3	Probably benign finding—short interval follow-up suggested
Category 4	Suspicious abnormality—biopsy should be considered
Category 5	Highly suggestive of malignancy—appropriate action should be taken

American College of Radiology (ACR). Breast Imaging Reporting and Data System (BI-RADS™). Third Edition. Reston [VA]. American College of Radiology, 1998. No other representation of this material is authorized without express, written permission from the American College of Radiology.

findings on screening studies, women with signs or symptoms of breast cancer, women with a history of breast cancer (women treated with BCT and women treated with mastectomy), and women with breast implants.

The additional mammographic views obtained for diagnostic work-ups vary according to the specific problem being addressed and, to some degree, according to the radiologist supervising the study. In general, we approach diagnostic mammographic work-ups in the following manner:

1. For calcifications, magnification views are obtained in the cranio-caudal and the 90° lateral projections (Figure 4–2).
2. Masses are evaluated with spot compression views or magnification spot compression views and then sonography, as needed.
3. Palpable masses are imaged with tangential spot compression views and then sonography, as needed (Figure 4–3).
4. Comparison with prior mammograms is suggested for all diagnostic work-ups.

In addition to general guidelines for mammographic work-ups (Figures 4–4 and 4–5), we have established detailed guidelines for specific scenarios. In the case of multiple obscured nonpalpable masses without a dominant mass, if old studies are not available, most mammographers tend to recommend 6-month follow-up mammography to document stability of the findings. However, a recent study has shown that in cases of multiple obscured masses, annual mammography may be more appropriate than 6-month follow-up mammography. For analyzing and localizing densities seen only on the craniocaudal view, rolled views in the craniocaudal projection are helpful, especially if the mammographer is trying to determine whether the mammographic findings are real. If a region of increased density is seen only on the mediolateral oblique view, obtaining a mediolateral oblique view at the same angle as on the prior year's study can help in determining whether the region of increased density is due to a new lesion or to overlap of normal structures. Mammograms obtained after cyst aspirations or pneumocystography (mammography performed following injection of air into the cyst cavity after the cyst contents are aspirated) can be used to verify that a mass seen on mammography corresponds with a mass seen on sonography. Alternatively, a mammogram could be obtained after sonographically guided placement of a needle in the mass to establish mammographic-sonographic concordance.

In evaluating cases with calcifications, the mammographer should carefully analyze the morphology of the calcifications. Calcifications with typically benign characteristics (such as the popcorn-like, coarse calcifications of a fibroadenoma) require no further evaluation. Indeterminate or malignant-appearing calcifications should be evaluated with magnification imaging to facilitate appropriate categorization and determination of the extent of the calcifications. The breast imager should consider skin

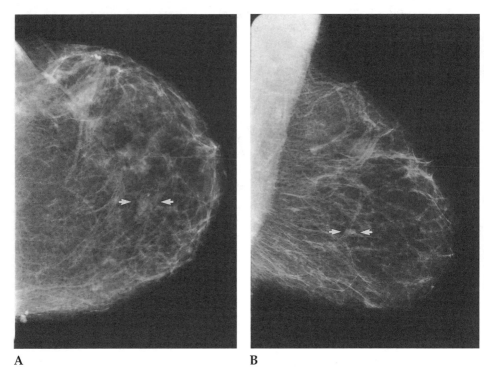

A   B

Figure 4–2. Screening mammograms were obtained in a 47-year-old woman. On the craniocaudal (A) and mediolateral oblique (B) views of the left breast, faint calcifications are seen, associated with a vague mass (arrows).

calcifications if the calcifications are seen on only 1 view or if the calcifications are identified close to a skin surface. Skin localization procedures, performed to determine whether the calcifications are located in the skin or in the breast parenchyma, can be performed in the mammographic unit with a fenestrated compression paddle.

At M. D. Anderson, diagnostic mammographic work-up cases are supervised by an interpreting physician. Each case is individualized to answer a specific question or to solve a specific problem. After the images have been reviewed and an assessment has been rendered, it is the radiologist's responsibility to communicate the results to the referring physician and the patient, especially in the case of worrisome or unanticipated findings.

ROLE OF MAMMOGRAPHY IN BREAST CONSERVATION THERAPY

Mammography plays an important role in BCT. Before breast-conserving surgery, mammography is used to evaluate the extent of the malignant

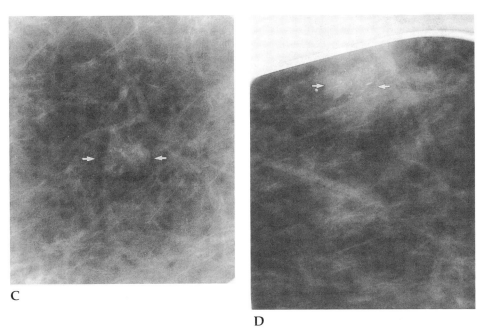

C

D

Figure 4–2. *(continued)*   On the craniocaudal magnification view (C), the calcifications are smudgy and the mass is lobular in shape (arrows). On the lateromedial
magnification view (D), the calcifications (arrows) layer in the dependent portion
of round structures. The findings are consistent with milk-of-calcium layering in
microcysts.

process and to screen the contralateral breast for an unsuspected cancer.
After surgery, mammography is used to identify residual tumor, especially in cases in which the original malignancy presented as microcalcifications. After radiation therapy, mammography is used to identify nonpalpable lesions and to help characterize palpable abnormalities.

Mammography before Breast-Conserving Surgery

Breast cancers may be detected by breast self-examination, clinical breast
examination performed by a health care professional, mammography, or
sonography. Once a probable malignancy has been identified, defining the
extent of disease may require mammography, sonography, and, in some
cases, MRI. When a lesion suspicious for cancer (BI-RADS category 4 or
5) is detected, the breast imager must define the lesion in terms of its size,
shape, and associated microcalcifications. The use of spot magnification
views is recommended to help identify microcalcifications, which may be
subtle and faint. Also, it is advisable to obtain a 90° lateral view to demonstrate the precise location of the lesion prior to stereotactic core needle

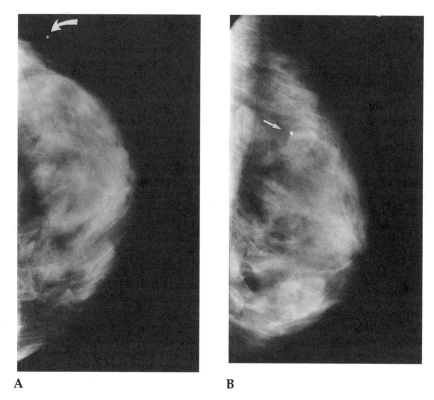

A   **B**

Figure 4–3. Clinical examination revealed a palpable abnormality in the upper outer left breast. The craniocaudal view (A) shows a metallic marker (arrow) that was placed on the skin in the region of the palpable abnormality. On the medio-lateral oblique view (B), a vague round density is seen in the region of the metallic marker (arrow).

biopsy (SCNB) or needle localization and surgical excision. Spot magnification views should be obtained between the malignant-appearing lesion and the nipple to define the anterior extent of the malignant process. In some patients, a spot magnification view of the subareolar region with the nipple in profile will demonstrate calcifications at the base of the nipple, raising the possibility of Paget's disease. At some facilities, nipple-areolar involvement precludes BCT, whereas at other centers, central segmentec-tomies are performed, in which the entire nipple-areolar complex is re-moved.

When analyzing mammograms from a patient with a known or sus-pected malignancy, the radiologist should insist on high-quality films. Op-timal compression and appropriate x-ray penetration are critical for im-aging the primary lesion as well as the entire breast. Identification of additional lesions on mammography can indicate multicentric (2 or more

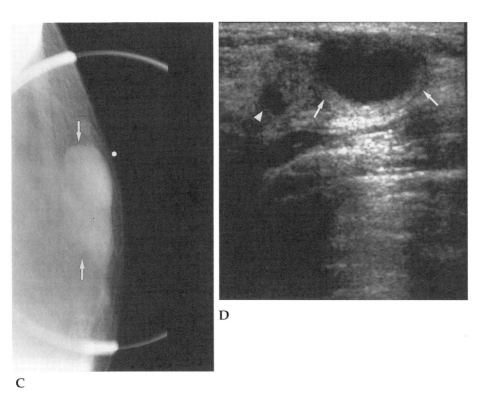

C

D

Figure 4–3. *(continued)* Magnified spot compression view (C), obtained tangential to the metallic marker, shows an oval mass (arrows). Sonogram (D) shows a thick-walled cyst (arrows) corresponding to the mammographic and sonographic findings and a smaller, adjacent cyst (arrowhead).

lesions in different quadrants) or multifocal (2 or more lesions in the same quadrant) disease and requires tailored work-ups with mammography and sonography.

In women with known breast cancer, there may be a synchronous cancer in the contralateral breast. It is important that the mammographer not be distracted from carefully analyzing the contralateral breast. At our center, women who come for evaluation often bring mammograms obtained at outside facilities. If copy films are provided, the original films should be requested or the entire study should be repeated. All images should be reviewed, including special mammographic views and sonograms.

Mammography after Breast-Conserving Surgery

In evaluating the breast after a segmental resection that revealed malignancy, the radiologist's task is to identify evidence of residual tumor. The

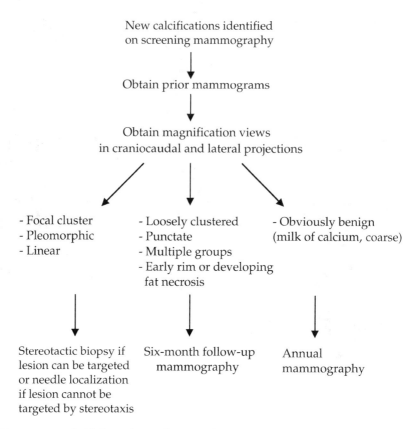

New calcifications identified
on screening mammography

Obtain prior mammograms

Obtain magnification views
in craniocaudal and lateral projections

- Focal cluster
- Pleomorphic
- Linear

- Loosely clustered
- Punctate
- Multiple groups
- Early rim or developing
  fat necrosis

- Obviously benign
(milk of calcium, coarse)

Stereotactic biopsy if
lesion can be targeted
or needle localization
if lesion cannot be
targeted by stereotaxis

Six-month follow-up
mammography

Annual
mammography

Figure 4–4.   Guidelines for evaluation of new calcifications identified on screening mammography.

radiologist should carefully analyze the mammograms, looking for suspicious microcalcifications and suspicious masses. Large postoperative hematomas and seromas can make visualization of the surgical site difficult. High-kVp technique can be helpful in thick, noncompressible breasts with postoperative fluid collections. Occasionally, a postoperative seroma is aspirated to allow for improved imaging of the surgical site. Reexcision should be performed if there is mammographic evidence of residual tumor or if there were positive margins at surgery.

Follow-up Mammography after Completion of Breast Conservation Therapy

The appropriate timing of follow-up mammography after BCT is debatable; the optimal regimen has not been scientifically established. In some practices, the treated breast is imaged 3 to 6 months after the completion

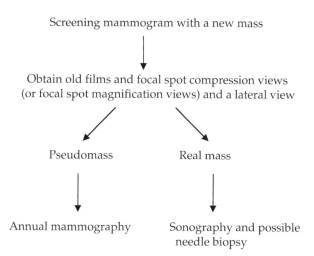

Figure 4–5. Guidelines for evaluation of a new mass identified on screening mammography.

of radiation therapy; at other facilities, the treated breast is imaged at 6-month intervals; and at other centers, mammography is performed yearly after the completion of radiation therapy. At M. D. Anderson, the treated breast and the contralateral breast are imaged 6 months after the completion of radiation therapy, and annual bilateral mammography is performed thereafter. Subtle clinical or mammographic changes in the conservatively treated breast should be carefully evaluated. Also, abnormalities in the contralateral breast should be analyzed in a meticulous manner because women with a history of malignancy in one breast are at high risk for developing cancer in the contralateral breast.

Typical changes on mammography after BCT include localized findings at the surgical site (Figure 4–6) as well as more diffuse changes due to radiation therapy. Postoperative fluid collections (hematomas and seromas) usually appear as round or oval, dense, fairly well marginated masses, and they may demonstrate fat-fluid levels on the lateral view. As these fluid collections resolve, they may develop spiculated margins. The surgical bed usually demonstrates architectural distortion, which resolves over time. Some scars may appear as spiculated masses at the postoperative site. The center of the scar will frequently show entrapped fat, and scars usually demonstrate a changing appearance on different views. It is often helpful to obtain tangential views in women who have undergone BCT to visualize the postoperative site separately from the skin changes.

In women who have undergone BCT, calcifications frequently develop in or adjacent to the surgical site. Benign calcifications include dystrophic calcifications, calcifications due to fat necrosis, and suture calcifications.

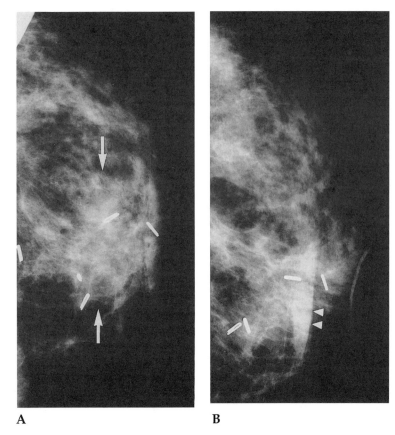

A   **B**

Figure 4–6. After BCT, the left craniocaudal view (A) shows postoperative architectural distortion (arrows). The laterally exaggerated craniocaudal view (B) demonstrates a changed appearance at the surgical site, consistent with architectural distortion, and associated skin thickening (arrowheads).

As they begin to appear, calcifications near the surgical site are often small and faint, making it difficult to differentiate recurrent tumor from developing benign calcifications. After radiation therapy, there is edema of the treated breast, and high-kVp techniques may be needed because the breast is less compressible. Skin thickening, trabecular thickening, and increased parenchymal density usually remain for 2 to 3 years after BCT and resolve slowly over time.

Local recurrence in the treated breast occurs at a rate of about 1% per year. Mammographic signs of tumor recurrence include a new mass (Figure 4–7), suspicious microcalcifications, enlargement or thickening of the scar, and an increase in breast edema. Recurrence prior to 18 months after completion of BCT is rare. In the first 6 years after BCT, recurrence is more likely to occur in the same quadrant as the original tumor. In the follow-up evaluation of women who have undergone BCT, sonography and MRI are employed as adjuncts to clinical examination and mammography.

MAMMOGRAPHY IN WOMEN WITH OTHER MALIGNANCIES

Mammography can detect primary cancers that are not breast cancer, such as primary and secondary lymphoma and metastases from other malignancies (Figure 4–8). Primary breast lymphoma is defined as extranodal lymphoma in a patient with no history of lymphoma in the past and no evidence of known lymphoma at other sites. Secondary breast lymphoma, which is more common than primary breast lymphoma, is defined as involvement of the breast tissue in a patient who has systemic or nodal involvement elsewhere. Primary breast lymphoma usually presents as a mass with circumscribed or partially circumscribed margins. Enlarged axillary lymph nodes may be identified on mammography in patients with lymphoma or leukemia.

Metastases to the breast are rare. Metastases are usually solitary, ill-defined masses in the periphery of the breast. Metastases may be multiple, and occasionally, metastatic disease may simulate inflammatory breast carcinoma. The tumors most likely to metastasize to the breast, in addition to contralateral primary breast tumors, are malignant melanoma (Figure 4–9) and cancers of the lung, ovary, kidney, gastrointestinal tract, thyroid, and cervix. Metastases to the breast from other cancers have been reported (Figure 4–10).

At M. D. Anderson, mammography is used occasionally to monitor treatment response in patients with known metastatic disease. The decision to order a mammogram for a patient with a nonbreast primary cancer is made on an individual basis, and the decision to perform imaging should depend on the patient's overall prognosis.

GALACTOGRAPHY

Galactography, also known as ductography, is a contrast examination of the ductal system of the breast. Galactography is used to detect and localize intraductal growths suspected because of spontaneous discharge from the nipple and to aid in localization of known lesions prior to surgical excision. Preoperative galactography on the day of surgery has resulted in decreased operating and anesthesia time.

Spontaneous nipple discharge is defined as persistent, nonlactational discharge that occurs without nipple manipulation or manual expression and comes from a single duct orifice. Often the patient notices a spot of wetness on her night clothing or on her bra. The discharge may be watery,

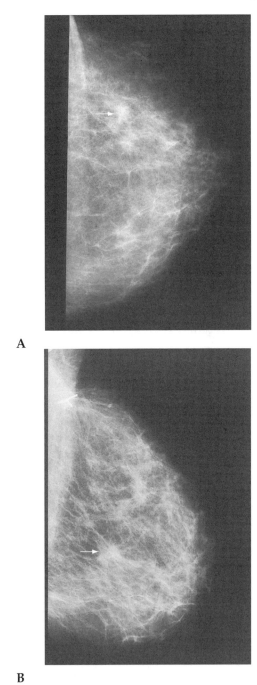

A

B

Figure 4–7. Craniocaudal (A) and mediolateral oblique (B) views demonstrate a new, irregular, spiculated mass (arrow) in the upper outer aspect of the treated left breast.

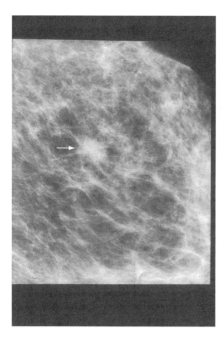

C

Figure 4–7. *(continued)* Magnified mediolateral view (C) demonstrates the mass (arrow) with associated pleomorphic calcifications. Stereotactic biopsy revealed invasive ductal carcinoma, and a mastectomy was subsequently performed.

clear, serous, serosanguinous, or bloody. Green or cloudy discharge is usually nonspontaneous and originates from multiple duct openings, indicating a benign cause, such as duct ectasia.

Before a woman is referred for galactography, a careful physical examination and a detailed history should be performed to rule out benign causes of galactorrhea. Physical examination often reveals discharge from multiple duct openings in the symptomatic or the contralateral breast. In addition to characterizing the number of discharging ducts, the color of the discharge, and the spontaneity of the discharge, the physical examination of the breast should involve a systematic search for a pressure point. There may be a palpable mass or a dilated duct beneath the nipple. Such findings would tend to point to an intraductal growth causing ductal distention. Most intraductal growths are caused by solitary intraductal papillomas. The differential diagnosis, however, includes ductal carcinoma. Multiple papillomas are uncommon, but they are risk markers for subsequent development of breast cancer. The diagnosis of multiple peripheral papillomas cannot be made on the basis of imaging alone. Only histopathologic evaluation can confirm the diagnosis.

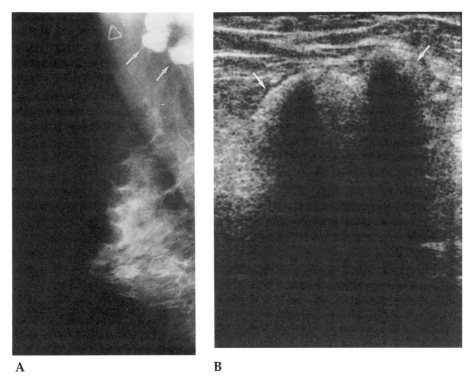

A   B

Figure 4–8. The right mediolateral oblique view (A) demonstrates calcified masses (arrows) in the region of the palpable abnormality (triangle) in a woman with a history of ovarian carcinoma. Sonogram (B) shows calcified axillary lymph nodes (arrows) with marked shadowing, representing metastatic disease.

If spontaneous nipple discharge from a single duct opening is confirmed, then a breast imaging consultation is appropriate. For women younger than 30 years of age, sonography is performed to search for a distended duct. Antegrade or retrograde ductography can then be performed to document an intraductal growth, its size and location, and the distance from the nipple. For women 30 years of age or older, a diagnostic mammogram is indicated. Focal spot compression views are often performed behind the nipple to search for a mass or a clue to the cause of the discharge. Rarely, mammography may show typical casting calcifications indicating DCIS. Often the mammogram is normal because the intraductal growth is too small to be identified without galactography. Cytologic evaluation of the nipple discharge is not considered a reliable diagnostic test, and cytologic evaluation is not routinely performed in our practice. Cytologic evaluation of nipple discharge to determine whether malignancy is present is associated with a relatively high false-negative rate.

Galactography is performed using a small, blunt-tipped, 30- or 31-gauge cannula (a sialography catheter with an end hole or a specialized catheter designed for galactography). The woman must have expressible discharge on the day of the ductogram to show which of the 15 to 25 nipple ducts is the one with the discharge. Relative contraindications to galactography include acute mastitis and purulent drainage. Cannulating the duct opening may be tedious, but the procedure is not difficult, and it should not be painful to the patient. The duct is filled with ionic contrast material (usually 0.5 to 1.0 cc) in a retrograde manner until there is a sensation of fullness or slight burning. Mammographic images are then obtained in the craniocaudal and the mediolateral projections. Magnification views are often obtained, especially when small intraductal filling defects are identified.

If an intraductal growth is located, the surgeon may request a repeat ductogram with injection of ionic contrast material plus methylene blue (to facilitate the duct excision) on the morning of the scheduled surgical excision. For intraductal growths several centimeters deep to the nipple, placement of a localization needle or wire adjacent to the intraductal growth may help to ensure excision of the appropriate region.

Most intraductal masses identified on galactography are benign, solitary papillomas. Malignancy is diagnosed in less than 10% of cases. Factors that are often associated with malignancy include watery discharge, male gender, older age, suspicious mammographic findings, positive cytologic findings, and irregular duct walls on the ductograms.

STEREOTACTIC CORE NEEDLE BIOPSY

At M. D. Anderson, our current approach is to perform a percutaneous biopsy with stereotactic or sonographic guidance to obtain histopathologic information before a definitive, 1-step surgical procedure is performed (Figure 4–11). Obtaining histopathologic information with percutaneous techniques allows treatment options to be discussed with the patient and her family before surgery. A definitive preoperative diagnosis of malignancy increases the chances of obtaining adequate margins with a single surgical procedure, and this approach can avoid the costs and morbidity associated with multiple surgical procedures.

At our institution, percutaneous techniques are regularly used to diagnose small, node negative cancers identified by mammography. Nonpalpable breast masses are biopsied under sonographic guidance with either fine-needle aspiration or core needle technique. Suspicious calcifications and masses not identified on sonography are sampled with SCNB techniques. The introduction of SCNB techniques has allowed for a reduction in the number of surgical biopsies. Stereotactic core needle biopsy

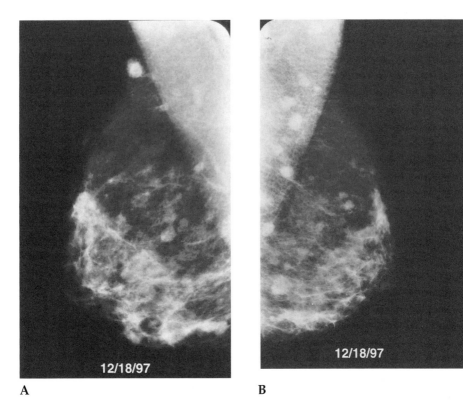

A   B

Figure 4–9. Right (A) and left (B) mediolateral oblique views show multiple bilateral masses consistent with metastatic disease in a patient with known melanoma.

is less expensive than surgical biopsy, is associated with less morbidity, and results in minimal or no scarring. Stereotactic core needle biopsy is safe, quick, and efficacious.

Stereotactic core needle biopsy should not be scheduled until a careful, detailed mammographic work-up is completed. Stereotactic core needle biopsy should be considered for suspicious lesions (BI-RADS category 4) and highly suspicious lesions (BI-RADS category 5) but should not be used instead of follow-up mammography for lesions that are probably benign (BI-RADS category 3). In addition, SCNB may be performed in cases of multiple lesions to rule out multicentric or multifocal disease and to facilitate surgical planning.

Stereotactic core needle biopsy may be performed with add-on attachments to upright mammography units or with prone biopsy tables. At M. D. Anderson, nearly all SCNBs are performed on a dedicated prone biopsy table; the use of upright add-on devices is reserved for women with neck or back problems and women who are unable to lie in the prone

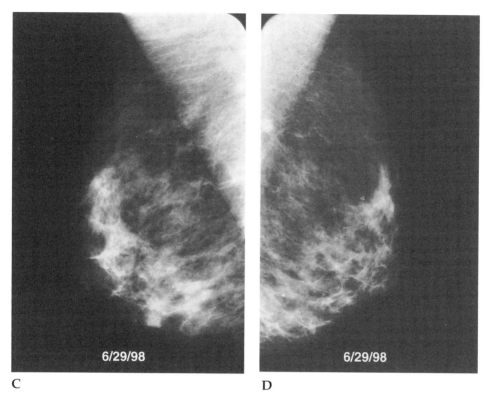

C   D

Figure 4–9. *(continued)*   The patient was treated with chemotherapy, and right (C) and left (D) mediolateral oblique views obtained 6 months later show a marked decrease in the number of masses and the size of the masses, consistent with a response to chemotherapy.

position. Stereotactic systems enable targeting of a single point (with x, y, and z coordinates, determined by a computerized calculation). If the lesion cannot be targeted with stereotaxis (i.e., if the mass is vague or the calcifications are faint), then SCNB should not be performed, and needle localization and surgical excision should be considered. Lesions near the chest wall, superficial lesions, and periareolar lesions may be difficult to biopsy with SCNB techniques. If the breast compresses to less than 3 cm, the case may not be well suited for SCNB. With some stereotactic units, the maximal compressed breast thickness that can be accommodated is 10 cm. In our practice, if we are unsure of the visibility of the target or if we think that the compressed breast thickness may be suboptimal, we perform a stereotactic scout examination. During the stereotactic scout examination, the woman lies prone on the table, the lesion is targeted, and measurements, including the compressed breast thickness, are obtained to determine if SCNB is feasible.

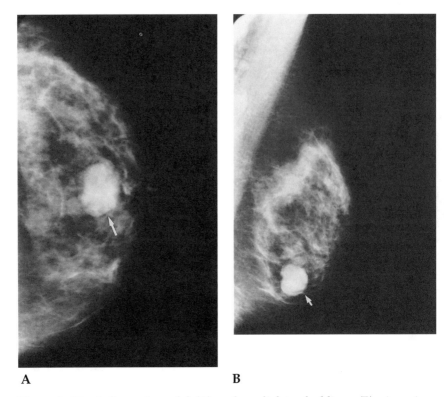

A   **B**

Figure 4–10. Left craniocaudal (A) and mediolateral oblique (B) views in a woman with a history of cloacogenic carcinoma show a high-density mass (arrow) in the 6 o'clock position, corresponding to a palpable abnormality.

Stereotactic core needle biopsy is associated with few complications. Hematomas requiring percutaneous or surgical drainage are rare. However, small hematomas and mild bruising may occur. Infection is rare, and pain is usually minimal. Prior to the SCNB, we administer lidocaine mixed with sodium bicarbonate for local anesthesia. Additional local anesthesia may be administered through the biopsy device as needed during the procedure. Tumor seeding in the biopsy needle track is not considered a significant risk.

At our center, we use directional vacuum-assisted biopsy instruments for all SCNBs. These instruments consist of 11- or 14-gauge biopsy devices connected to a vacuum chamber that draws tissue into a cutting notch. In our practice, nearly all SCNBs are performed with an 11-gauge vacuum-assisted biopsy instrument (Mammotome, Ethicon Endo-Surgery, Cincinnati, OH). In selected cases (i.e., in thin breasts and in superficial lesions), a 14-gauge vacuum-assisted biopsy device is used. Vacuum-assisted biopsy units can sample calcifications in a larger area and more contiguously than

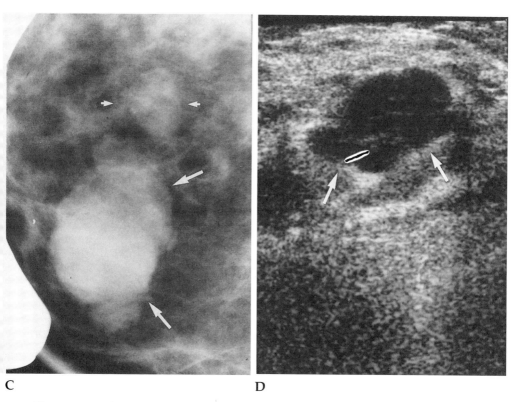

C   D

Figure 4–10. *(continued)*   Lateromedial spot magnification view (C) demonstrates the lobular mass at 6 o'clock (large arrows) and an adjacent satellite lesion (small arrows). Sonogram (D) shows a hypoechoic lobular mass (arrows) with internal echoes and some through-transmission. Biopsy demonstrated metastatic disease.

can an automated gun. Directional vacuum-assisted SCNB has become a standard procedure for biopsy of microcalcifications. Directional vacuum-assisted biopsy devices have allowed for more accurate histopathologic diagnoses, especially in differentiating DCIS from atypical ductal hyperplasia. Surgical excision is recommended when SCNB reveals invasive carcinoma, DCIS, or atypical ductal hyperplasia. A diagnosis of atypical ductal hyperplasia by vacuum-assisted SCNB requires surgical excision because 15% of cases of atypical ductal hyperplasia will be found at surgery to have associated DCIS or invasive ductal carcinoma. In 15% of patients in whom DCIS is diagnosed by SCNB performed with a vacuum-assisted device, invasive ductal carcinoma will be identified on surgical excision.

An important component of SCNB is mammographic-pathologic concordance. For example, if the targeted lesion is an irregular mass with spiculated margins (BI-RADS category 5) and the final histopathologic diag-

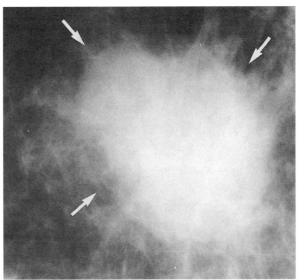

A

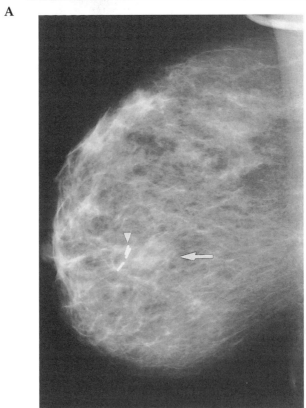

B

Figure 4–11. Screening mammography in a 47-year-old woman revealed a mass in the 2 o'clock position of the right breast. A straight-on scout view (A) obtained prior to SCNB shows a large lobular mass with indistinct margins (arrows). Stereo-tactic core needle biopsy demonstrated invasive ductal carcinoma. The patient was then treated with chemotherapy. A mediolateral oblique view (B) obtained 3 months after SCNB shows that the tumor (arrow) has shrunk. Three metal markers (arrow-head) were placed at the anterior aspect of the tumor.

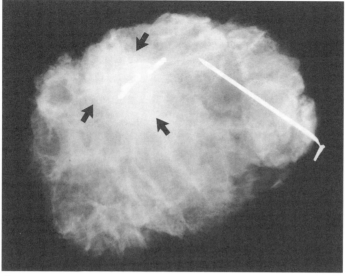

C

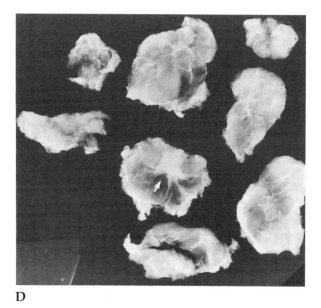

D

Figure 4 11. *(continued)*   Following needle localization, specimen radiograph (C) shows the residual tumor (arrows) and the metal markers. Radiographs of the sliced specimen (D) demonstrate an irregular mass with spiculated margins (arrow) in the middle slice of the second column. Pathologic examination revealed invasive ductal carcinoma, and there were no metastatic axillary lymph nodes (20 axillary lymph nodes were removed).

nosis is benign, then repeat biopsy (with SCNB or by surgical excision) should be performed. The sensitivity of SCNB ranges from 71% when a 20-gauge cutting needle is used to 99% when a 14-gauge cutting needle is used. If the lesion identified on mammography is thought to represent a radial scar, excisional biopsy should be considered, especially if the lesion is large (greater than 2 cm in diameter). Accurate histopathologic diagnosis of a radial scar may require complete removal of the entire lesion, and radial scars may be associated with mammographically occult malignancies.

Vacuum-assisted biopsy instruments allow for the placement of small (3 mm) stainless steel clips (MicroMark, Ethicon Endo-Surgery, Cincinnati, OH) at the biopsy site. These clips are deployed through vacuum-assisted biopsy instruments and serve as markers in cases in which the entire lesion is removed at the time of biopsy. Also, the stainless steel clips are helpful in documenting the site of the biopsy, helping to focus mammographic follow-up, and marking the location of lesions that may disappear or shrink with preoperative chemotherapy.

MAMMOGRAPHICALLY GUIDED NEEDLE LOCALIZATION

Screening mammography permits the detection of small, clinically occult, nonpalpable cancers. The identification of small nonpalpable lesions by mammography has necessitated the development of needle localization techniques to guide surgical excision. The goal of needle localization procedures is to transfix the lesion with the localizing device or to place the localizing device alongside the lesion. Needle localizations are usually performed with mammographic or sonographic guidance. Needle localization procedures can also be performed with computed tomography, and techniques are evolving to allow for needle localization with MRI guidance. In our practice, we perform most needle localizations with mammographic guidance.

Over the past decade, diagnostic excisional biopsies have become less common because of the introduction of percutaneous biopsy techniques (SCNB and ultrasound-guided biopsies), by which a histopathologic diagnosis can be established before surgery. In the current practice milieu, the most common indication for needle localization is to help guide definitive resection (with negative margins) of a known cancer.

A complete mammographic work-up must be performed before needle localization to determine the number of lesions and the extent of the mammographic abnormality. In the mammographic suite, needle localizations are usually performed with a fenestrated alphanumeric compression device. Some procedures may be performed with a freehand technique. A number of needles and hookwires have been developed for mammographic needle localizations. The localizing device is placed through or adjacent to the mammographic abnormality, enabling the surgeon to remove the targeted abnormality and a small amount of adjacent normal tissue. In general, needle localization can be performed accurately, and in most cases, the needle or wire can be positioned within 5 mm of the targeted abnormality.

For needle localization procedures, the breast is positioned in a standard mammographic unit, and compression is employed. In nearly all cases the patient is seated; however, with some procedures performed with a caudal-to-cranial approach, the patient is standing. Needle localizations are performed parallel to the chest wall. The skin surface closest to the mammographic abnormality is chosen as the entry point. For example, if the mammographic abnormality is close to the top of the breast, a craniocaudal approach is used. If the lesion is located in the medial aspect of the breast, a mediolateral approach is used.

The recent introduction of small-field-of-view digital detectors has eliminated the need for film processing and increased the efficiency of needle localizations. With digital detectors, an image appears on a screen almost immediately after an exposure is taken. Thus, the amount of time that the woman's breast is in compression is decreased, as is the overall procedure time.

Once the mammographic abnormality is identified within the fenestrated compression device, the skin is cleaned in the usual sterile manner with povidone-iodine and alcohol. Thereafter, lidocaine mixed with sodium bicarbonate is administered to anesthetize the skin and the subcutaneous tissues. After appropriate needle positioning is verified on the first projection, the breast is taken out of compression, and then needle position is verified with an orthogonal view. The needle may then be retracted slightly to allow for the distal tip to be situated approximately 1 cm beyond the distal aspect of the lesion. Then a hookwire may be placed through the localizing needle. The outer needle may be withdrawn, or the outer needle may remain in place. Thereafter, the localizing device may be gently taped to the skin. Alternatively, the localizing device may be secured to the skin with a bandage and tape. Also, a small cup may be placed over the needle to protect it.

The films confirming proper positioning of the localizing needle are reviewed and labeled for the surgeon, and a diagram showing the needle and the targeted lesion is prepared. The patient is then escorted to the surgical holding area with the films and the diagram. After surgical removal of the targeted abnormality, specimen radiography is performed to verify the presence of the lesion within the specimen and to document that the localizing device has been removed (Figure 4 11). While the patient is still under anesthesia, we routinely obtain a radiograph of the entire specimen without compression. Then the specimen is sliced in the pathology laboratory, and radiographs of the serial slices are obtained. Once the radiologist views the specimen radiographs, information regarding removal of the targeted lesion is relayed to the surgeon and the surgical pathologist. The information from specimen radiography may be particularly helpful in evaluating margins in cases of known or suspected cancers. Close or involved margins may necessitate the removal of additional tissue.

Lymph Node Mapping

The status of the axillary lymph nodes is an important prognostic indicator in patients with breast cancer. Conventional axillary lymph node dissection is associated with sampling error and potential morbidity. Sentinel lymph node mapping has recently been applied to axillary lymph node staging in patients with breast cancer in an effort to increase the accuracy and reduce the morbidity of surgical evaluation of the regional lymph nodes. The fundamental concept underlying sentinel node mapping is that the lymphatic effluent of a tumor drains initially to a sentinel node (or to a few sentinel nodes) before other nodes in the group receive tumoral drainage. The status of the sentinel node(s), determined through careful evaluation, is thought to be an accurate indicator of regional nodal involvement. If the sentinel node is found to be negative (no evidence of metastatic disease), then the other lymph nodes in that nodal group are likely to be negative as well, and a more extensive lymph node dissection is not needed.

Technetium Tc 99m sulfur colloid (usually filtered) is the most commonly used radiopharmaceutical in lymph node mapping. The usual dose is 0.5 mCi, and the radiopharmaceutical is usually administered in 3 to 6 mL of saline. A higher dose (2.5 mCi) is injected if lymphoscintigraphy is performed on the day before surgery. The higher dose allows for imaging in the nuclear medicine area on the first day and intraoperative lymph node mapping on the second day, without the need for a second injection of the radiopharmaceutical. Various injection techniques have been reported, including intratumoral, peritumoral, periareolar, and subdermal injections.

At our institution, lymph node mapping is usually performed with peritumoral injections. In the case of a palpable abnormality, injection of the radiopharmaceutical is guided by palpation. In the case of a nonpalpable lesion, injection of the radiopharmaceutical may be guided by either sonography or mammography. When mammographic guidance is utilized, 1 or 2 needles are placed through or adjacent to the mammographic abnormality. The needles are secured in place, and the patient is then escorted to the nuclear medicine area, where the radiopharmaceutical is administered. Four separate injections are usually performed around the lesion. After lymphoscintigraphy, the patient may be sent to the operating room for lymph node mapping and surgical excision.

In the operating room, the surgeon usually injects isosulfan blue (blue dye) through or alongside one of the localizing needles. The surgeon then excises the targeted breast lesion and localizes the sentinel node(s) using a handheld radiosensitive probe. The surgeon performs a transverse incision in an attempt to identify a blue lymphatic channel or a blue lymph node. The sentinel lymph node is then excised and submitted for meticulous histopathologic evaluation. Also, the excised breast lesion is carefully evaluated with specimen radiography and histopathologic techniques.

MAGNETIC RESONANCE IMAGING OF THE BREAST

Magnetic resonance imaging has 2 main roles in breast imaging: evaluation of prosthetic implants and evaluation of the extent and stage of known breast cancers. Recently, attention has also been focused on the use of MRI for breast cancer detection. The majority of breast MRI examinations at M. D. Anderson are performed to evaluate prosthetic implants.

Magnetic resonance imaging is more specific and more sensitive than sonography and mammography in detecting intracapsular and extracapsular implant rupture, and implant evaluation with MRI is well established. Intracapsular implant rupture is defined as rupture of the implant membrane with release of silicone gel within an intact fibrous capsule. Extracapsular rupture is defined as rupture of both the implant membrane and the fibrous capsule, resulting in extravasation of silicone gel into the adjacent breast parenchyma. Imaging of implants involves silicone-selective sequences, which take advantage of the differences between the resonance frequency of silicone and the resonance frequencies of fat and water. On MRI, the most reliable sign of intracapsular rupture is multiple curvilinear low-signal lines within the region of the silicone gel, the so-called "linguini sign." The curvilinear lines represent the collapsed implant membrane floating within the silicone gel. The "teardrop sign" is seen when silicone leaks out of a ruptured implant and enters into one of the radial folds at the exterior of the implant. This finding can be found in early implant rupture. Extracapsular rupture is characterized by the presence of free silicone in the breast parenchyma. On MRI, free silicone is seen as a focal area of high signal intensity outside the confines of the implant. In nearly all cases of extracapsular rupture, there is accompanying intracapsular rupture. Magnetic resonance imaging appears to be the most accurate imaging test for evaluating the integrity of silicone implants, with a sensitivity of 94% and a specificity of 97%.

Regarding the use of MRI for cancer staging and determination of the appropriate surgical treatment, we have chosen to focus first on techniques that will permit MRI-directed needle localization of lesions that are identified on MRI and not seen on mammography or sonography. Efforts are ongoing to develop techniques that will facilitate needle localization and core needle biopsy within the MRI unit. Eventually, after these localization techniques mature, MRI will be more readily available to be utilized in staging evaluations, especially in women with dense breasts. It is likely that MRI will be able to demonstrate multicentric and multifocal carcinoma that is not identifiable with mammography or sonography. In addition, it is thought that MRI will take on a greater role in surveillance of women who have undergone BCT.

The use of MRI for detection of breast cancer is in the developmental stage. Visualization of malignant breast tumors on MRI is based on rapid enhancement after the administration of gadolinium as well as morphologic characteristics. On dynamic scans, most breast cancers show rapid, intense enhancement. However, benign lesions occasionally enhance rapidly, and some malignant tumors, including DCIS, tubular carcinoma, and invasive lobular carcinoma, may have slower, less intense enhancement patterns than typical malignancies.

While enthusiasm for the development of breast MRI techniques is quite high, breast MRI does have some potential disadvantages. Magnetic resonance imaging remains costly, and a breast MRI examination takes more time than mammography or breast sonography. Also, women who are claustrophobic may not be well suited for MRI evaluation. Furthermore, from the imaging standpoint, MRI has limited utility in the detection of calcifications.

In summary, MRI is firmly established for breast implant evaluation, and in the future, MRI will play a greater role in screening for breast cancer (especially in women with dense breasts who are at high risk for developing cancer), detecting breast cancer, staging malignancy, and monitoring post-treatment changes. The expanded use of MRI will depend on quick, standardized pulse sequences as well as easy-to-use biopsy devices to facilitate MRI-guided needle localizations and MRI-guided core needle biopsies.

Sestamibi Breast Imaging

Technetium Tc 99m sestamibi breast imaging has recently been advocated for the evaluation of palpable and nonpalpable breast lesions. Currently, the precise niche for sestamibi breast imaging is uncertain. Although sestamibi imaging of palpable breast lesions has shown reasonable specificity and sensitivity, sestamibi breast imaging is thought to have only limited utility in the evaluation of nonpalpable breast lesions, especially small nonpalpable lesions.

While technetium Tc 99m sestamibi has properties similar to those of thallium, the exact mechanism of sestamibi uptake in cancer cells is unknown. It is believed that sestamibi tracer activity is concentrated in the mitochondria. When sestamibi studies are performed, 20 mCi of technetium Tc 99m sestamibi is injected intravenously in the arm (or sometimes the foot) contralateral to the breast with the palpable or the nonpalpable abnormality.

Sestamibi imaging has been shown to be reasonably accurate in the evaluation of palpable masses and large masses identified on mammography. A sensitivity of 93.7% and a specificity of 87.8% were reported in a series of 106 lesions (85 palpable and 21 nonpalpable) in which the average lesion size on mammography was 2.3 cm × 1.9 cm. In that study, sestamibi's negative predictive value was 97%, and the positive predictive value was 76.9%. It is thought that sestamibi breast imaging has little role in detecting nonpalpable tumors smaller than 1 cm, and sestamibi imaging may be unable to identify DCIS. Sestamibi breast imaging has limited utility for breast cancer screening because the sensitivity of sestamibi in the evaluation of nonpalpable breast lesions is low, ranging from 25% to 72%.

Sestamibi breast imaging does show some promise in helping to categorize nonpalpable mammographically detected lesions. Some investigators have used sestamibi breast imaging in evaluating mammographically detected lesions with an intermediate or a low probability of malignancy. With sestamibi breast imaging, false-negative results will occur, and a negative finding on sestamibi breast imaging should not serve as a reason to cancel a biopsy in the presence of suspicious mammographic findings.

Hillner (1997) used a decision analysis model and determined that compared with core needle biopsy, sestamibi would miss an additional 16 invasive cancers and an additional 12 in situ cancers per 1000 women. If sestamibi breast imaging could be developed to the point that it would aid in reducing the number of biopsies with benign findings without missing cancers, the use of sestamibi breast imaging would be advocated. However, in recent years, the relative ease and safety of performing percutaneous biopsies has strengthened breast imagers' interest in obtaining tissue diagnoses rather than performing additional imaging studies.

Sestamibi breast imaging may have a role in imaging the axillary lymph nodes and determining the presence of metastases in the axilla. Axillary lymph node involvement is an important prognostic indicator in breast cancer patients, and concomitant noninvasive evaluation of the axilla and the primary breast lesion is an appealing concept. Taillefer et al (1995) reported a sensitivity of 84% and a specificity of 91% for evaluation of axillary lymph nodes with sestamibi imaging.

Recent studies have reported that low sestamibi uptake may be associated with drug resistance in tumors. The low accumulation of sestamibi is thought to correlate with an overexpression of P-glycoprotein, a transmembrane protein that is believed to be involved in multidrug resistance. Further research is needed because P-glycoprotein expression may be heterogeneous. Studies have demonstrated that regions negative and positive for P-glycoprotein may coexist within the same tumor.

DIGITAL MAMMOGRAPHY

Film-screen x-ray mammography has been proven to be effective in the detection and diagnosis of breast cancers. However, current film-screen systems are limited by a relatively narrow dynamic range, low contrast resolution, film noise, and film processing artifacts. It is thought that digital mammography systems will allow for improved image quality and possibly reduced radiation dose.

In film-screen mammography systems, the film serves as an image acquisition detector and a storage and display device. With digital systems, the tasks of image acquisition, display, and storage are separated, and this arrangement allows for the potential optimization of each independent-function. Furthermore, digital mammography systems should allow for improved efficiency because delays due to film processing are eliminated. With digital systems, the technologist can verify positioning and check image quality on a monitor nearly immediately after an exposure is made. The digital image can then be routed to a workstation for "soft-copy" interpretation or to a printer for film printing and "hard-copy" interpretation. Soft-copy interpretation should result in fewer repeat studies because the window and level settings can be modified, the gray scale can be adjusted, and edge enhancement can be applied. With digital imaging, long-term image storage can be handled electronically and integrated into a picture archiving and communication system.

In the future, as digital technology evolves, we anticipate growth in telemammography, teleconsultations, and remote monitoring of diagnostic work-ups. In addition, direct digital data acquisition should result in improved (higher sensitivity and higher specificity) computer-aided diagnosis algorithms. These digital computer-aided diagnosis devices will serve as a "second reader," similar to the role of the computer-aided diagnosis systems that work with digitized film-screen mammograms.

Digital mammography offers new opportunities for acquiring, processing, and formatting anatomic and functional information. Three promising advanced digital applications are currently being developed: dual-energy subtraction mammography, tomosynthesis, and digital subtraction angiography. Dual-energy subtraction imaging involves the acquisition of 2 digital images with different x-ray spectra. The 2 images are combined, and a subtraction image is generated on a workstation, with the overlapping structures removed. Tomosynthesis involves acquiring volumetric digital information and then performing reconstructions in a prescribed plane. Tomosynthesis aims to remove superimposed structures, enhance contrast, and increase contour definitions. With rapid frame rates, digital subtraction angiography can be performed in digital mammographic units after injection of intravenous contrast material. Angiographic techniques are based on the premise that breast tumors demonstrate rapid enhancement due to angiogenesis. It is thought that digital angiographic techniques will be helpful in detecting cancers and in monitoring response to chemotherapy.

KEY PRACTICE POINTS

- Screening mammography can detect small, node-negative, nonpalpable cancers, resulting in decreased death rates from breast cancer.

- Detailed, focused diagnostic mammographic work-ups are helpful for characterizing findings identified on screening mammography and defining the extent of disease.

- In women who have undergone BCT, mammography is useful for monitoring the treated breast and screening the contralateral breast.

- Mammography can identify nonbreast primary cancers and metastases from other malignancies.

- Galactography is used to detect and localize intraductal lesions and to provide a presurgical map of the ductal system.

- Stereotactic core needle biopsy is a safe and accurate technique, and stereotactic techniques have allowed for a reduction in the number of surgical biopsies.

- Mammographically guided needle localizations are used to help guide surgical excision of targeted lesions along with a minimal amount of adjacent normal breast tissue.

- Peritumoral administration of technetium Tc 99m sulfur colloid with mammographic guidance can be performed to facilitate lymph node mapping.

- Magnetic resonance imaging is the most accurate technique for evaluating the integrity of breast implants, and MRI can be helpful in defining the extent of malignancy in women with known breast cancer.

- While technetium Tc 99m sestamibi imaging has demonstrated reasonable sensitivity and specificity in determining whether palpable breast lesions are malignant, the role of sestamibi imaging in the evaluation of nonpalpable breast lesions is thought to be limited.

- Digital mammographic systems should allow for improved image quality, a lower recall rate, and possibly reduced radiation dose. In addition, 3 advanced digital applications are being developed: dual-energy subtraction mammography, tomosynthesis, and digital subtraction angiography.

ACKNOWLEDGMENTS

We thank Mary Carr, Mary Ann Waggoner, Loretta F. Price, and Angela Lynch for secretarial assistance.

SUGGESTED READINGS

American College of Radiology. *Illustrated Breast Imaging Reporting and Data System (Illustrated BI-RADS)*. 3rd ed. Reston, VA: American College of Radiology; 1998.

Andersson I, Aspegren K, Janzon L, et al. Mammographic screening and mortality from breast cancer: the Malmo mammographic screening trial. *BMJ* 1988;297:943–948.

Baker KS, Davey DD, Stelling CB. Ductal abnormalities detected with galactography: frequency of adequate excisional biopsy. *AJR Am J Roentgenol* 1994;162:821–824.

Bassett LW, Gold RH, Mirra JM. Nonneoplastic breast calcifications in lipid cysts: development after excision and primary irradiation. *AJR Am J Roentgenol* 1982;138:335–338.

Bhatia S, Robison LL, Oberlin O, et al. Breast cancer and other second neoplasms after childhood Hodgkin's disease. *N Engl J Med* 1996;334:745–751.

Bjurstam N, Bjorneld L, Duffy SW, et al. The Gothenburg breast screening trial: first results on mortality, incidence, and mode of detection for women ages 39–49 years at randomization. *Cancer* 1997;80:2091–2099.

Canavese G, Gipponi M, Catturich A, et al. Sentinel lymph node mapping opens a new perspective in the surgical management of early-stage breast cancer: a combined approach with vital blue dye lymphatic mapping and radioguided surgery. *Semin Surg Oncol* 1998;15:272–277.

Cardenosa G, Eklund GW. Benign papillary neoplasms of the breast: mammographic findings. *Radiology* 1991;181:751–755.

Chu KC, Smart CR, Tarone RE. Analysis of breast cancer mortality and stage distribution by age for the Health Insurance Plan clinical trial. *J Natl Cancer Inst* 1988;80:1125–1132.

Daniel BL, Birdwell RL, Ikeda DM, et al. Breast lesion localization: a freehand, interactive MR imaging-guided technique. *Radiology* 1998;207:455–463.

Dao TH, Rahmouni A, Campana F, Laurent M, Asselain B, Fourquet A. Tumor recurrence versus fibrosis in the irradiated breast: differentiation with dynamic gadolinium-enhanced MR imaging. *Radiology* 1993;187:751–755.

Dershaw DD. Mammography in patients with breast cancer treated by breast conservation. *AJR Am J Roentgenol* 1995;164:309–316.

DiPiro PJ, Meyer J, Shaffer K, Denison CM, Frenna TH, Rolfs AT. Usefulness of the routine magnification view after breast conservation therapy for carcinoma. *Radiology* 1996;198:341–343.

Glass EC, Essner R, Giuliano AE. Sentinel node localization in breast cancer. *Semin Nucl Med* 1999;29:57–68.

Gorczyca DP, DeBruhl ND, Ahn CY, et al. Silicone breast implant ruptures in an animal model: comparison of mammography, MR imaging, US, and CT. *Radiology* 1994;190:227–232.

Gorczyca DP, Schneider E, DeBruhl ND, et al. Silicone breast implant rupture: comparison between three-point Dixon and fast spin-echo MR imaging. *AJR Am J Roentgenol* 1994;162:305–310.

Hillner BE. Decision analysis: MIBI imaging of nonpalpable breast abnormalities. *J Nucl Med* 1997;38:1772–1778.

Khalkhali I, Cutrone JA, Mena IG, et al. Scintimammography: the complementary role of Tc-99m sestamibi prone breast imaging for the diagnosis of breast carcinoma. *Radiology* 1995;196:421–426.

Khalkhali I, Cutrone J, Mena I, et al. Technetium-99m-sestamibi scintimammography of breast lesions: clinical and pathological follow-up. *J Nucl Med* 1995;36:1784–1789.

Kopans DB, Feig SA. The Canadian National Breast Screening Study: a critical review. *AJR Am J Roentgenol* 1993;161:755–760.

Landis SH, Murray T, Bolden S, Wingo PA. Cancer statistics, 1999. *CA Cancer J Clin* 1999;49:8–31.

Liberman L, Cohen MA, Dershaw DD, Abramson AF, Hann LE, Rosen PP. Atypical ductal hyperplasia diagnosed at stereotaxic core biopsy of breast lesions: an indication for surgical biopsy. *AJR Am J Roentgenol* 1995;164:1111–1113.

McCrea ES, Johnston C, Haney PJ. Metastases to the breast. *AJR Am J Roentgenol* 1983;141:685–690.

Mendelson EB. Evaluation of the postoperative breast. *Radiol Clin North Am* 1992;30:107–138.

Miller AB, Baines CJ, To T, Wall C. Canadian National Breast Screening Study. 2. Breast cancer detection and death rates among women aged 50 to 59 years. *CMAJ* 1992;147:1477–1488.

Miner TJ, Shriver CD, Jaques DP, Maniscalco-Theberge ME, Krag DN. Ultrasonographically guided injection improves localization of the radiolabeled sentinel lymph node in breast cancer. *Ann Surg Oncol* 1998;5:315–321.

Piwnica-Worms D, Chiu ML, Budding M, Kronauge JF, Kramer RA, Croop JM. Functional imaging of multidrug-resistant P-glycoprotein with an organotechnetium complex. *Cancer Res* 1993;53:977–984.

Reynolds HE. Core needle biopsy of challenging benign breast conditions: a comprehensive literature review. *AJR Am J Roentgenol* 2000;174:1245–1250.

Smart CR, Hendrick RE, Rutledge JH III, Smith RA. Benefit of mammography screening in women ages 40 to 49 years. Current evidence from randomized controlled trials. *Cancer* 1995;75:1619–1626.

Stomper PC, Recht A, Berenberg AL, Jochelson MS, Harris JR. Mammographic detection of recurrent cancer in the irradiated breast. *AJR Am J Roentgenol* 1987;148:39–43.

Tabar L, Fagerberg G, Duffy SW, Day NE, Gad A, Grontoft O. Update of the Swedish two-county program of mammographic screening for breast cancer. *Radiol Clin North Am* 1992;30:187–210.

Taillefer R, Robidoux A, Lambert R, Turpin S, Laperriere J. Technetium-99m-sestamibi prone scintimammography to detect primary breast cancer and axillary lymph node involvement. *J Nucl Med* 1995;36:1758–1765.

Waxman AD. A perspective on decision analysis modeling as it relates to sestamibi imaging of nonpalpable breast abnormalities. *J Nucl Med* 1997;38:1778–1780.

Woods ER, Helvie MA, Ikeda DM, Mandell SH, Chapel KL, Adler DD. Solitary breast papilloma: comparison of mammographic, galactographic, and pathologic findings. *AJR Am J Roentgenol* 1992;159:487–491.

5 BREAST SONOGRAPHY

Bruno D. Fornage and Beth S. Edeiken-Monro

Chapter Overview

Sonographic examination of the breast has recently come to maturity with the availability of high-frequency, handheld transducers. The technique is now routinely used in breast imaging centers as an essential complement to physical examination and mammography in the evaluation of breast masses. Sonography not only differentiates cystic from solid masses but also aids in discrimination between benign solid masses and malignant solid masses. In patients with known breast cancer, sonography of lymph node–bearing areas (with ultrasound-guided fine-needle aspiration of nodes) can reveal findings that help to more accurately define the pretherapeutic stage.

Although sonography can detect some nonpalpable carcinomas missed by mammography, sonography is not used for routine cancer screening because sonography cannot demonstrate microcalcifications and because the success of sonographic imaging is highly operator dependent. Because of its unique real-time capability, sonography is preferred to stereotaxy for guiding needle biopsy of nonpalpable breast masses, and sonography is being used more frequently for preoperative localization of such lesions. A new application of sonography is to guide and monitor percutaneous in situ destruction of small nonpalpable breast masses with techniques such as cryotherapy or radiofrequency ablation.

Introduction

Sonography is now routinely used as an adjunct to mammography in the evaluation and characterization of breast lesions. Sonography can differentiate cystic from solid breast masses; can reveal some breast lesions not visible on mammography; and can provide information about breast lesions that cannot be obtained with mammography. In addition, sonography can be used to guide interventional procedures in the breast, including percutaneous biopsy of nonpalpable breast lesions. This chapter will outline the technical details of sonographic examination of the breast and describe the many current applications of breast sonography at M. D. Anderson Cancer Center.

Instrumentation and Technique of Examination

When a breast mass is being evaluated, efforts should be made to have the physical examination, mammography, sonography, and—if needed—needle biopsy performed during a single visit to the breast center.

Except in very young patients, sonography of the breast should not be done without the benefit of a thorough review of recent mammograms. In addition, it is good practice to perform a targeted physical examination before starting the sonographic study.

Sonographic examination should be performed with state-of-the-art equipment, which includes a high-frequency linear-array transducer. The new extended-field-of-view technology is helpful. This technology allows the operator to "stretch" the standard sonogram to build a static picture with a field of view much wider than that available with standard real-time transducers (Fornage et al, 2000b). This feature allows the sonologist to obtain ultrasound scans of the entire breast and measure the distance between a lesion and the nipple (Figure 5–1).

Scans should be obtained longitudinally, transversely, and also radially around the nipple, along the orientation of the ducts. The scans must be carefully labeled. The labeling includes but is not restricted to the patient's demographic information, the location of the area examined, and the orientation of the scan.

Altering the amount of compression applied to the breast with the transducer is a key step in the real-time sonographic examination. This maneuver clears or confirms the presence of artifacts and demonstrates the compressibility of a lesion and its mobility in relation to the surrounding tissues, features that can be assessed only with real-time sonography.

In the case of palpable lesions, the use of a standoff pad during the sonographic examination is helpful. This practice allows the operator to

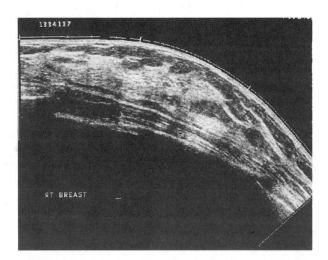

Figure 5–1. Extended-field-of-view (SieScape™ imaging, Siemens Ultrasound, Issaquah, WA) sonogram of normal breast displays a global cross section of the breast and underlying chest wall.

slide his or her fingers between the pad and the skin to palpate the abnormal area while the sonogram of this area is continuously displayed on the video monitor. This allows unequivocal correlation between findings on palpation and findings on sonography.

Whenever a mass is demonstrated on sonography, conventional color and power Doppler imaging should be used to assess its vascularity.

The concordance between sonographic and mammographic findings must be the primary preoccupation of the sonologist. The lesion's size, shape, and location (clock position, distance from the nipple, and depth) and the appearance of the surrounding tissues (fat vs glandular tissue) must correlate perfectly on sonograms and mammograms, although minimal differences in size—less than 10%—due to mammographic magnification and slight differences in clock location—about 1 hour—due to differences between the 2 modalities in breast positioning and compression are acceptable.

Although some have recommended that the sonographic examination be limited to the area of concern defined on the basis of palpation or mammographic findings ("targeted examination"), at M. D. Anderson we scan the entire breast. This approach does not take much longer and may demonstrate additional foci of cancer, especially in a dense breast, which may alter the treatment plan dramatically. In addition, at M. D. Anderson, the ipsilateral axilla and internal mammary chains are systematically included in the examination of the breast (Fornage, 1993).

Other recent technological developments in breast sonography include the use of tissue harmonic imaging, which improves the spatial and contrast resolution and has shown promising results when used in conjunction with an ultrasound contrast agent (Fornage et al, 2000a). Three-dimensional sonography is not yet widely available, but it is expected to change the way breast sonograms will be acquired, displayed, and interpreted in the not-too-distant future.

DIFFERENTIATION BETWEEN CYSTS AND SOLID MASSES

Differentiation between cysts and solid masses was the first successful application of sonography in general and remains the best and most widely used application of breast sonography (Figure 5–2). It must be borne in mind, however, that some cysts contain internal echoes and that inspissated cysts that are filled with echogenic material (Figure 5–3) may mimic a solid mass. In contrast to mammography, sonography can readily reveal the rare intracystic tumor.

In addition to demonstrating cysts, sonography can demonstrate other fluid collections, such as postoperative seromas or hematomas or lymphoceles, which may occasionally present as slowly enlarging firm masses, raising the possibility of residual or recurrent disease after seg-

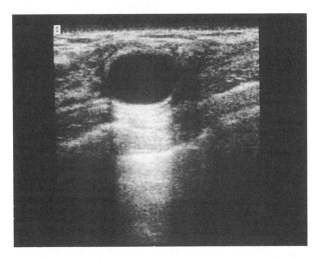

Figure 5–2. Typical cyst. Sonogram shows the smooth, rounded, anechoic cyst with characteristic distal sound enhancement.

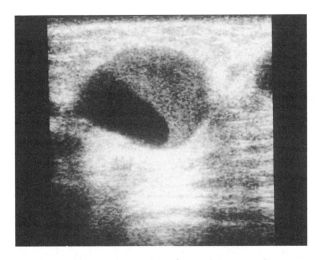

Figure 5–3. Inspissated cyst. Sonogram shows 2 intracystic components—one anechoic, the other homogeneously echogenic—separated by a flat interface. This 2-tone appearance is characteristic of an inspissated cyst.

mentectomy for breast cancer. The sonographic appearances of hematomas vary significantly, mostly with the age of the lesion. The presence of echogenic clots within a large hematoma is not uncommon. However, no flow signals should be detected inside a hematoma by color Doppler examination.

Sonography can also demonstrate abscesses, which appear as fluid-filled or complex masses that have an ill-defined, hypervascular wall and sometimes contain a small amount of gas (Figure 5–4).

EVALUATION OF THE QUESTIONABLE PALPABLE MASS OR THICKENING

A significant number of sonographic examinations are performed to rule out the possibility of an underlying palpable mass in women in whom self-examination or examination by a nurse or physician reveals some nodularity or "thickening." In this setting, sonography performed with state-of-the-art equipment by experienced operators has a very high negative predictive value and can rule out the presence of a mass. In most cases, the cause of the nodularity or thickening is a prominent fat lobule, a lipoma, or a prominent area of normal fibroglandular breast tissue, and the sonographic examination performed in combination with palpation (made possible with the use of a standoff pad) clearly identifies the culprit.

CHARACTERIZATION OF SOLID MASSES

Although the sonographic appearances of benign and malignant solid masses will always overlap, the improved resolution of modern, high-frequency transducers allows better discrimination between these lesions.

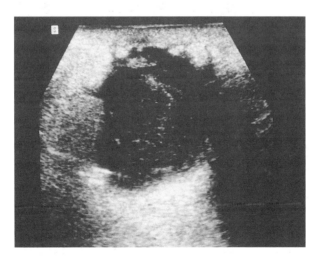

Figure 5–4. Abscess. Sonogram demonstrates a fluid collection with irregular margins and internal debris.

Fibroadenomas

Fibroadenomas typically appear as hypoechoic, homogeneous, smoothly marginated, oval-shaped solid masses (Figure 5–5). The coarse calcifications characteristic of fibroadenomas appear on sonograms as bright foci with acoustic shadowing. However, calcifications are always depicted better on mammograms than on sonograms. Fibroadenomas are typically elongated, with their greatest diameter oriented parallel to the skin and an average length-to-anteroposterior-diameter ratio of 1.8. On color Doppler examination, some increased vascularity can be seen, most often at the periphery of the mass, with vessels often retaining a smooth course and distribution.

About 25% of fibroadenomas show irregular or markedly lobulated margins. The finding of a solid mass with irregular margins indicates a potential malignancy and the need for further work-up. Small fibroadenomas in large fatty breasts may be difficult to differentiate from the surrounding fat on sonograms.

Small cystosarcoma phyllodes tumors cannot be differentiated from fibroadenomas on sonography. Large cystosarcoma phyllodes tumors often contain fluid-filled necrotic areas, which should suggest the correct diagnosis; however, a fast-growing carcinoma could have the same appearance.

Fat Necrosis

Fat necrosis usually displays a mild to moderate echogenicity, higher than that of cancer. The presence of a small oil cyst inside a mass is a useful

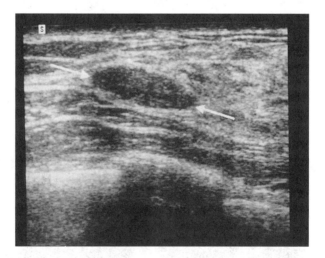

Figure 5–5. Typical fibroadenoma surrounded by dense breast tissue. Sonogram shows an elongated, well-defined, homogeneous, hypoechoic, solid mass (arrows). There is no sound attenuation or enhancement associated with the lesion.

clue suggesting fat necrosis. As a rule, the presence of cysts—even minute ones—in a mass suggests a benign etiology. Fat necrosis is the most common mass found in reconstructed breasts.

Other Benign Solid Lesions

Other benign solid lesions that may have a pathognomonic appearance on sonography include intramammary lymph nodes, which display a characteristic echogenic fatty hilum, and lipomas, which are typically hyperechoic (although lipomas can also be isoechoic or even hypoechoic). The fat component of hamartomas is usually better demonstrated on mammograms than on sonograms.

Some benign lesions may appear on sonograms as irregular masses with marked shadowing, 2 hallmarks of malignancy. These include sclerosing adenosis, granulomatous mastitis, granular cell tumor, and nipple adenoma.

Abnormalities of the Ducts

Although sonography clearly demonstrates dilated ducts and intraductal masses, ductography remains the gold standard in the evaluation of nipple discharge because ductography demonstrates a greater extent of the ductal network. When a dilated duct cannot be cannulated or is not associated with discharge, percutaneous ultrasound-guided ductography can be done.

Changes in Breasts with Implants

Sonography is superior to mammography in demonstrating changes associated with ruptured breast implants, but magnetic resonance imaging (MRI) provides a more global view of the implant and surrounding tissues and is currently considered the gold standard for the diagnosis of a ruptured implant. Sonography remains instrumental in the evaluation of the breast tissues surrounding an implant for masses or fluid collections and in the evaluation of complications of implant rupture—e.g., diagnosis of free silicone, which is anechoic, and silicone-induced granulomas, which are distinctively hyperechoic and associated with a characteristic "snowstorm" artifact (Figure 5–6). Sonography is the best technique with which to guide needle biopsy of lesions close to an implant.

Breast Cancer

Carcinomas, even those less than 1 cm in diameter, are routinely identified on sonograms with the use of state-of-the-art equipment. On sonograms, breast carcinoma typically appears as a focal hypoechoic mass that has irregular or spiculated margins and disrupts the architecture of the breast (Figures 5–7 and 5–8). In contrast to fibroadenomas and other benign

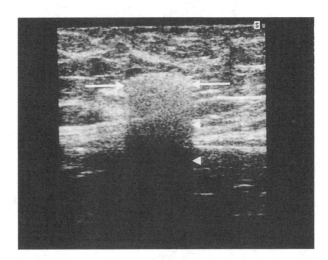

Figure 5–6. Silicone-induced granuloma in the tail of the breast in a patient with a history of a ruptured silicone-gel prosthesis. Sonogram shows the granuloma (arrows) associated with a typical "snowstorm" artifact (arrowheads).

masses, carcinomas may exhibit a "taller-than-wide" shape, with the tumor's longest diameter being perpendicular to the skin (length-to-anteroposterior-diameter ratio less than 1) (Figure 5–9). This shape is highly characteristic of carcinoma, although carcinomas may also be elongated like benign masses. If the mass is sufficiently large, some heterogeneity of the echotexture may be noted. Intratumoral clustered microcalcifications can be visualized as minute bright echoes within the hypoechoic tumor (Figure 5–9). Acoustic shadowing—once considered an essential diagnostic feature of cancer—is present in only about half of cases. Lack of compressibility and adherence of the tumor to the surrounding tissues during palpation are important clues suggesting malignancy.

Invasive lobular carcinomas are difficult to identify on sonography, as they are on mammography. The significant distortion and fibrosis seen on mammograms may appear on sonograms as areas of marked shadowing without a well-defined mass. If a mass is not clearly defined, percutaneous biopsy is better performed with stereotactic than with sonographic guidance.

Mucinous and medullary carcinomas are often relatively well circumscribed, sometimes with a frankly benign appearance. Medullary cancer may be markedly hypoechoic with significant sound through-transmission and may mimic a cyst; however, on closer inspection, the margins are irregular and microlobulated, and low-level internal echoes are present.

Carcinoma of the breast in men usually presents as a firm nodule, and the sonographic appearances are not different from those of breast cancer in women.

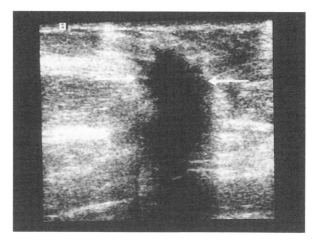

Figure 5–7. Typical invasive ductal carcinoma. Sonogram shows the 1-cm spiculated solid mass (arrows) disrupting the architecture of the breast. Note the taller-than-wide shape of the lesion and the marked associated shadow.

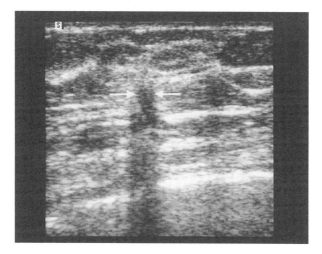

Figure 5–8. Minute (0.3-cm) carcinoma. Sonogram clearly shows a small hypoechoic round mass (arrows) with some shadowing.

Color and Power Doppler Imaging

Abnormal Doppler signals reflecting hypervascularity have been reported in the majority of malignant tumors but also in a significant number of benign masses. In malignant tumors, neovessels are typically tortuous and disorganized and penetrate the tumor at a 90° angle (Figure 5–10); in

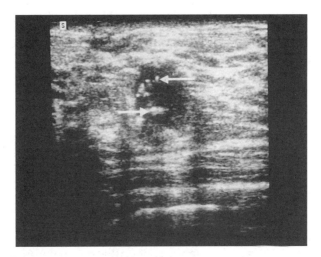

Figure 5–9. Typical invasive ductal carcinoma. Sonogram shows a smaller-than-1-cm, taller-than-wide, irregular, hypoechoic, solid mass containing microcalcifications (arrows).

contrast, the vessels associated with fibroadenomas are usually straight or curvilinear, often draping smoothly over the lesion. However, there is certainly an overlap between the flow mapping features of carcinomas and fibroadenomas, especially the fast-growing fibroadenomas. Other flow-positive benign masses include abscesses, other inflammatory conditions, and cystosarcoma phyllodes. Flow-negative benign masses include fibroadenomas, fibrocystic changes, areas of fibrosis, and scars.

Currently, there is no single Doppler spectral analysis parameter (e.g., resistance index, pulsatility index, or peak systolic velocity) that can discriminate between benign and malignant masses. With the advent of the highly sensitive power Doppler technique and the use of contrast agents, detailed analysis of the flow distribution inside and outside a tumor in conjunction with flow quantification techniques should provide information valuable for differentiating between benign and malignant lesions.

LOCAL-REGIONAL STAGING OF CANCER

The size of the primary breast tumor and the extent of lymphatic spread at presentation are the most important prognostic factors assessed during the local-regional staging of breast cancer. The size of the primary tumor can be accurately measured with sonography. When breast conservation therapy is planned, another crucial factor is the detection of unsuspected multicentric disease. Whole-breast—not targeted—sonographic exami-

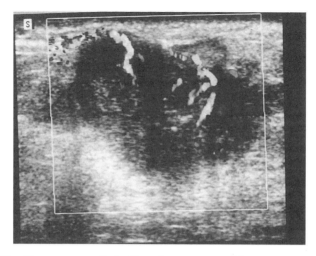

Figure 5–10.   Breast cancer. Color Doppler sonogram (shown in black and white) shows typical malignant internal hypervascularity with tortuous, branching neovessels penetrating the mass at a 90° angle.

nation can reveal additional foci of cancer not seen on mammography, especially in dense breasts.

The detection of clinically occult metastases in the regional nodal basins can have a significant impact on breast cancer staging. For example, if ipsilateral internal mammary lymphadenopathy is detected, the disease is classified as stage IIIB, and if a supraclavicular nodal metastasis is detected, the disease is classified as stage IV. Lymph nodes that are replaced by metastatic breast carcinoma appear as rounded or irregularly shaped, hypoechoic masses (Figure 5–11). Sonography is more sensitive than physical examination in the detection of axillary nodal metastases. Palpation and mammography cannot detect small or high (level III) axillary ("infraclavicular") lymph nodes, and neither technique can be used to assess the internal mammary lymphatic chains. Sonography overcomes these limitations and can detect nonpalpable lymph node metastases as small as 5 mm in diameter (Figure 5–12).

Documentation of lymph node metastasis is readily achieved with ultrasound-guided fine-needle aspiration (FNA); usually only a single needle pass is required because lymph nodes are highly cellular.

SONOGRAPHIC EVALUATION OF RESPONSE TO TREATMENT

For more than 10 years, sonography has been used routinely at M. D. Anderson to quantify the response of breast tumors and any regional

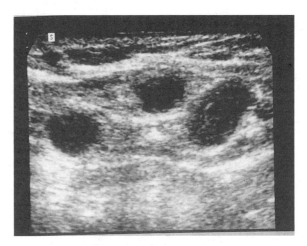

Figure 5–11. Axillary lymph node metastases. Sonogram shows 3 grossly rounded and completely hypoechoic nodes well demarcated from the surrounding echogenic fat.

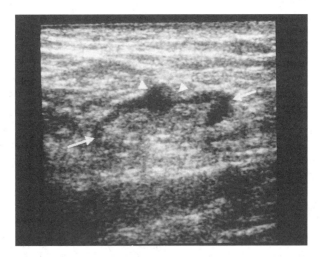

Figure 5–12. Minute axillary lymph node metastasis. Sonogram shows an elongated, mostly fat-replaced, echogenic node (arrows) with a focal, eccentric, markedly hypoechoic bulge (arrowheads) representing a metastatic deposit.

nodal metastases to chemotherapy (Fornage et al, 1990a). Sonography has the advantage of readily measuring the longest 3 diameters of any mass. The formula for calculating the volume of a prolate ellipsoid (0.52 times the product of the 3 longest diameters) can be used to calculate the volume of the mass, and the volume can be compared with the volume calculated on the previous study or studies. This allows the sonologist to provide the clinician with a percentage decrease in volume that accurately reflects the response of the tumor to chemotherapy.

COMPLEMENTARITY OF SONOGRAPHY AND MAMMOGRAPHY

The sensitivity of mammography is severely limited in patients with dense breasts (e.g., young, pregnant, or lactating women), patients with breast implants, and patients who have undergone surgery and radiation therapy for breast cancer. While mammography can detect microcalcifications in these women, it is widely accepted that it can miss relatively large masses.

Sonography is more sensitive than mammography in demonstrating small benign solid masses in dense breasts and can detect nonpalpable breast carcinomas not seen on mammograms. However, although this capability is increasingly being recognized, the cost-effectiveness of sonography remains to be evaluated, especially in the United States, where the cost of sonography is higher than in the rest of the world. Indeed, the increasing sonographic detection of nonpalpable, mammographically invisible, benign-appearing solid masses in dense breasts is posing the problem of rising costs due to additional tests required to confirm the benign nature of such masses. If sonography reveals a nonpalpable mass that is not seen on mammography, the radiologist has the option of recommending follow-up sonography, ultrasound-guided needle biopsy (with follow-up sonography), or ultrasound-guided surgical excision.

ULTRASOUND-GUIDED NEEDLE BIOPSY OF NONPALPABLE BREAST MASSES

Percutaneous needle biopsy has advantages over surgical biopsy, including significant cost savings and the absence of a residual scar that might impair the interpretation of subsequent diagnostic images. Percutaneous needle biopsy can be repeated as often as needed.

The goal of imaging-guided percutaneous needle biopsy is to obtain a 100% reliable tissue diagnosis of nonpalpable breast lesions and thereby reduce the number of unnecessary surgical biopsies. Virtually any nonpalpable breast lesion that is clearly demonstrated on sonograms can be sampled with a needle under sonographic guidance. Both FNA and core needle biopsy (CNB) are effectively guided by real-time sonography.

Ultrasound-guided needle biopsy is not without difficulty, and experience in every step is needed to yield optimal results. The success of ultrasound-guided biopsy of the breast depends on the skill of the operator in hitting the target lesion; successful tissue extraction, which depends on the operator's technique and the nature of the tumor; adequate preparation of the specimens; and interpretation by an expert pathologist or cytopathologist. Any factor compromising the success of any step will jeopardize the overall success of the procedure.

In the case of lesions that have been visualized with mammography, ultrasound-guided needle biopsy must be performed only after a meticulous review of recent mammograms to ensure that the targeted lesion is the same one that was demonstrated on mammograms. Performing an ultrasound-guided needle biopsy only after all imaging has been completed also avoids the risk of misinterpreting a postbiopsy hematoma on imaging performed after the biopsy.

Sonographic versus Stereotactic Guidance of Needle Biopsy

For masses that can be demonstrated with high-resolution sonography (the vast majority), the advantages of sonographic guidance over stereotactic guidance of needle biopsy include the ability to use the shortest route to the lesion, the unique real-time monitoring of both placement of the needle and sampling of the lesion, the ability to perform multidirectional sampling with FNA, the rapidity of the procedure, the comfort of the patient, the applicability to virtually any mass in the breast or in node-bearing regions, and the wide availability of sonographic equipment. For nonpalpable lesions visualized only with sonography, sonography is the only guidance technique to use.

In specialized breast centers, both sonography and stereotaxy must be available for guiding needle biopsy of nonpalpable lesions. In dedicated centers so equipped, the wave of popularity of stereotaxy has been reversed, and biopsy of the vast majority of nonpalpable masses is now guided by sonography rather than stereotaxy.

Although biopsy of microcalcifications without a mass is the domain of stereotactic guidance, microcalcifications are increasingly demonstrated with sonography when new state-of-the-art, high-frequency transducers are used. When stereotactically guided biopsies cannot be performed for technical reasons, careful attempts can be made to visualize the area of calcifications with sonography; if the operator judges that the calcifications are positively identified on the screen, then ultrasound-guided CNB of the area of calcifications can be performed, followed by radiographic confirmation of the presence of the calcifications in the cores.

Ultrasound-Guided Fine-Needle Aspiration

Although less popular than CNB in the United States, FNA, if performed by experienced practitioners and interpreted by well-trained cytopathologists, remains a powerful problem-solving tool in the evaluation of breast masses.

Equipment and Technique

Fine-needle aspiration is performed with standard 20- or 22-gauge (generally 20-gauge), 1.5-inch (3.8-cm) hypodermic needles. Rarely, a 2-inch needle is needed because of a deep lesion or large breast. If a needle guide is used, a longer needle (e.g., a spinal needle) must be used to compensate for the longer pathway. The ultrasound transducer is carefully cleansed and then soaked in rubbing alcohol (70% isopropyl alcohol) for several minutes before the procedure. After the procedure, the transducer is again carefully cleansed.

Informed consent is obtained, and the patient is asked about medications and possible impairment of coagulation. The skin is prepared with alcohol, which also serves as an acoustic coupling medium. Depending on the location of the tumor, the patient is placed in a dorsal decubitus or oblique lateral position to spread the breast on the chest wall and thus reduce the thickness of the breast parenchyma and consequently the length of the needle's pathway. In our experience, FNA of the breast and axilla can usually be performed without local anesthetization.

The standard technique of needle insertion for FNA is an oblique insertion, in which the needle is inserted from the end of the transducer along the scan plane, the obliquity of the needle depending on the depth of the target. With this technique, not only the tip but most of the distal portion of the needle is visualized from the moment it enters the scan plane (Figure 5–13). In experienced hands, the oblique insertion technique is 100% accurate and therefore safe. Although needle guides are available that attach to the transducer and maintain the needle within the scan plane, the freehand technique is often preferred for FNA because it allows reorientation of the needle at different angles and therefore permits a larger volume to be sampled during a single pass.

Solid masses are sampled with to-and-fro rotation (corkscrew movements) of the needle to dissociate the tumor tissue while a moderate but constant negative pressure is applied using a 20-mL syringe. The appearance of material in the needle's hub confirms that the lumen of the needle is loaded with aspirated material. Then the negative pressure is released, and the needle is withdrawn. Automatic aspiration devices are available that allow the negative pressure necessary for FNA to be applied with a single hand while the other hand is used to hold the transducer in place for continuous real-time monitoring of the entire procedure. It is recom-

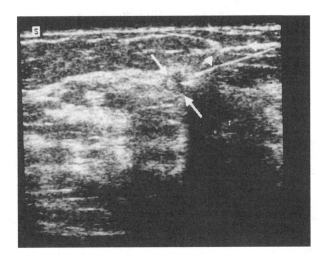

Figure 5–13. Sonogram obtained during ultrasound-guided FNA of a minute (0.3-cm) carcinoma shows the tip of the echogenic needle (arrowheads) reaching the small lesion (arrows).

mended that the entire biopsy procedure be videotaped to document un-equivocally that samples were obtained from within the lesion.

An insufficient smear represents a complete failure of the FNA procedure and should prompt another pass. Should a repeat FNA also fail, CNB should be performed. If for any reason the CNB is inconclusive, then a surgical excision after ultrasound-guided localization of the lesion must be considered.

Cysts and Fluid Collections

Cysts and other fluid collections can be readily aspirated with a fine needle. On occasion, an 18-gauge needle may be needed to drain an inspissated cyst, the contents of which typically appear as toothpaste-like material. In such a case, it may not be possible to drain the cyst completely.

When an intracystic tumor is suspected on the basis of sonograms, a pneumocystogram can be obtained after a volume of air equal to the volume of fluid aspirated is injected into the cyst. However, it may be argued that such a procedure is not necessary since intracystic tumors need to be excised anyway. Other collections that can be subjected to diagnostic FNA or percutaneous drainage in the proper clinical setting include postoperative hematomas, lymphoceles, and abscesses.

Solid Masses

Solid masses are sometimes difficult to sample with FNA. As a rule, an insufficient specimen must be regarded as a failure of the procedure and necessitates a second attempt at FNA. There is significant interindividual variation in the rate of inadequate FNA specimens. In a series of 254 surgically verified, nonpalpable, noncystic breast lesions that were subjected to ultrasound-guided FNA by various members of our ultrasound section, 11% of the specimens were inadequate (Sneige et al, 1994). In an early series of 36 carcinomas smaller than 1 cm^3 sampled by a single operator, only 3% of specimens were inadequate (Fornage et al, 1990b).

Fine-needle aspiration has high sensitivity and specificity in the diagnosis of breast cancer. In the series of 254 nonpalpable, noncystic breast lesions from M. D. Anderson, the sensitivity in the diagnosis of cancer was 91%, the specificity was 77%, the false-negative rate was 2%, and the false-positive rate was 1%. When only lesions diagnosed as definitely benign or malignant were considered, FNA had a sensitivity of 97% and a specificity of 98% (Sneige et al, 1994).

Fine-needle aspiration of ductal carcinomas usually yields highly cellular cytologic smears; in our experience, the diagnosis is established with examination of cytologic material from a single pass in the majority of cases. Other forms of breast malignancy, such as medullary or mucinous carcinomas, lymphomas, and metastases to the breast from extramammary primary cancers, can also be correctly diagnosed cytologically.

Although hormone receptor status and proliferation markers (e.g., Her-2/*neu*, DNA ploidy, Ki-67) are usually determined using a CNB specimen, these tests can also be performed on fine-needle aspirates if necessary.

The vast majority of radiologists across the nation have totally abandoned FNA in favor of CNB, but it is critical to keep in mind that with rigorous cytologic criteria, the diagnosis of fibroadenoma can be reliably established through examination of FNA specimens by experienced cytopathologists. The major limitation in the FNA diagnosis of fibroadenoma is the relatively high incidence of insufficient specimens, e.g., in the case of hyalinized lesions. When a fibroadenoma is suspected and FNA specimens are insufficient, the operator should switch to CNB. In experienced hands, cytologic examination can also readily establish the definitive diagnosis of a number of other benign conditions, such as fat necrosis, acute inflammation, and intramammary lymph nodes, thus obviating CNB (Fornage, 1999).

In experienced hands, errors in sampling the target lesion do not occur, and false-negative cytologic diagnoses are rare. They occur with paucicellular and markedly desmoplastic tumors such as infiltrating lobular carcinomas. Tubular carcinomas have also been reported as having the potential to mimic a fibroadenoma cytologically. False-positive cytologic results are even rarer; they have been reported mainly in cases of hypercellular benign lesions such as papillomas, some tubular adenomas, and atypical ductal hyperplasia. Radiation-induced changes can also mimic recurrent carcinoma cytologically.

Lymph Nodes

Whenever a definitive tissue diagnosis is needed, ultrasound-guided FNA readily confirms or rules out metastatic involvement of an abnormal lymph node in any of the nodal basins, including the internal mammary chains. Fine-needle aspiration of lymph nodes is easy because of the lymph nodes' rich cellularity. As a rule, a single pass is sufficient for obtaining an adequate specimen from a lymph node. The cytologic diagnosis of benign versus metastatic lymph node is easy to establish, and there is no need to perform CNB (Fornage, 1996).

In a patient with FNA-proven breast cancer that requires determination of invasiveness before therapy, confirmation by FNA of a metastatic lymph node in the axilla provides indirect proof of the cancer's invasiveness. This spares the patient a CNB of the primary breast tumor if determination of invasiveness was the only reason for the CNB to be done.

Advantages and Limitations

Advantages of ultrasound-guided FNA include its pinpoint accuracy, the excellent tolerance by patients, and the ability to aspirate or inject fluid or air. The outstanding accuracy is synonymous with total safety; lesions that lie close to the chest wall or to breast implants can be safely aspirated. Also, results can be obtained within minutes.

The disadvantages of FNA include the absolute requirement for an expert cytopathologist, the potential for inadequate sampling in cases of fibrous tumors, and the fact that it is not possible to differentiate between invasive and noninvasive breast carcinoma through examination of FNA specimens. This differentiation requires histopathologic examination of a CNB specimen.

Ultrasound-Guided Core Needle Biopsy

Interest in CNB has been revived with the advent of automated spring-loaded devices that activate a 14- to 18-gauge cutting needle in a fraction of a second. These devices are much easier to use than the original Tru-Cut biopsy needle.

Equipment and Technique

Numerous commercially available devices provide automatic propulsion of a cutting needle with a throw of about 2 cm. Successful use of these devices requires that the operator have a clear understanding of the mechanism of the device and know the location from which the core will be taken. Although the Biopty gun with a 14-gauge Tru-Cut-type needle has been considered a standard for CNB, other devices are available that cut full-cylinder cores and provide high-quality specimens with thinner (18-gauge) needles and therefore less trauma (Fornage, 1999).

The procedure is explained in detail to the patient, and informed consent is obtained. The site of entry and the path of the needle are carefully planned, keeping in mind that the needle must be inserted as horizontally as possible to avoid any injury to the chest wall and underlying lung, especially in women with small breasts. The skin is disinfected using povidone-iodine. A generous amount of local anesthetic is then administered from the skin to the mass under real-time sonographic guidance. Before the actual biopsy is started, the firing mechanism of the biopsy device is tested, and the device is cocked and locked in the safety position (if a safety lock is available). The small skin incision required when 14-gauge needles are used is not required with 18-gauge needles, which are easily advanced through the skin.

Because the needle is inserted nearly horizontally (i.e., perpendicular to the ultrasound beam), its visualization on the monitor is optimal. Because the needle is propelled automatically, the postfiring position of the needle tip must be anticipated before the biopsy "gun" is triggered. Thus CNB requires more experience in sonographic guidance of needles than does FNA, especially when very small lesions are targeted in small breasts. Under sonographic guidance and using the freehand technique, the tip of the needle is brought into contact with the mass. The perfect alignment of the needle with the scan plane is verified, and a hard copy of the prefiring position of the needle is printed. The biopsy gun is then fired, and a postfiring hard copy showing the needle traversing the target is also printed. In the case of a minute lesion, a transverse sonogram is obtained to ensure that the needle is actually traversing the lesion. The transducer is swiveled 90°, and a hard copy is printed showing the cross section of the needle inside the target (Figure 5–14). The needle is then withdrawn, and the tissue core is recovered. The procedure is repeated in different areas of the tumor until a sufficient number of satisfactory cores have been obtained. In our experience, when the transfixion of the target has been clearly documented with sonography and cores appear to be of satisfactory size, no more than 4 cores are needed for diagnosis when an 18-gauge cutting needle is used.

To avoid repeat passage through (and trauma to) the subcutaneous tissues when multiple cores are obtained, an introducer can be inserted through the skin down to the surface of the lesion before the cutting needle is inserted; this permits rapid reinsertion of the needle for repeat passes and may reduce the risk of seeding malignant cells along the needle track.

Processing of Cores

The cores are placed in a solution of formalin and left overnight to allow fixation. If the diagnosis of cancer needs to be ascertained more rapidly, an FNA pass with rapid staining can be done; this yields a diagnosis within minutes.

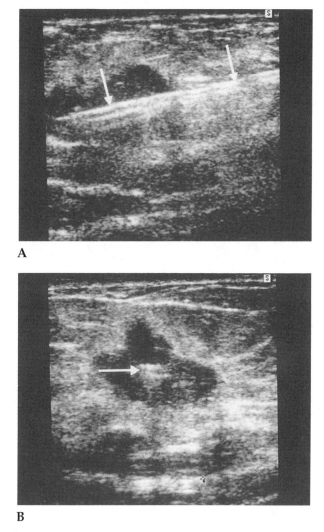

Figure 5–14. Ultrasound-guided CNB of a breast carcinoma. A, Postfiring sonogram shows that the echogenic cutting needle (arrows) has traversed the targeted mass. B, Confirmatory sonogram obtained after swiveling the transducer 90° shows the cross section of the needle (arrow) in the center of the tumor.

In rare cases, ultrasound-guided CNB is done to sample an extensive area of microcalcifications without a discrete mass. In this case, it is imperative to process the cores the same way they would be processed if the biopsy were done under stereotactic guidance—i.e., the cores must be radiographed using a mammographic unit and magnification technique (or dedicated equipment for specimen radiography) to document the presence of the calcifications.

Advantages and Drawbacks

Advantages of ultrasound-guided CNB include a near-100% tissue recovery rate even in fibrous masses, the ability to assess the invasiveness of the cancer, and the fact that tissue cores are readily interpreted by any pathologist. However, CNB is more invasive than FNA, with a higher rate of associated bleeding complications, and malignant seeding along the needle track has been reported with the use of 14-gauge needles.

Keys to Success of Ultrasound-Guided Biopsy

Ultrasound-guided needle biopsy of nonpalpable breast lesions requires teamwork. Progress can be made and experience can be accumulated only through ongoing communication between the radiologist, the pathologist, and the surgeon.

Ultrasound-guided interventional procedures require excellent eye-hand coordination and a significant amount of practice before the mandatory 100% accuracy level in hitting the target can be reached. Practicing with easy-to-make phantoms shortens the learning curve of beginners.

The golden rule in breast biopsy is the concordance between the biopsy results and the findings on imaging and clinical examination. Any discrepancy—e.g., a negative result of the needle biopsy in the face of a single suspicious finding on physical examination, mammography, or sonography—should be carefully reevaluated and should not delay surgical excision.

Other Ultrasound-Guided Interventional Procedures

Nonpalpable breast masses detected by mammography or sonography can be localized with sonography before surgery or in the operating room. The same localizing techniques used with mammographic guidance can be used with sonographic guidance.

Preoperative and Intraoperative Localization of Nonpalpable Masses

Nonpalpable masses can be localized preoperatively with a localizing needle or hookwire inserted under sonographic guidance. Sonography can be used whenever mammography cannot, e.g., when the breast is very small, when the mass is very close to the chest wall or to an implant, or when the lesion is not clearly seen on mammograms. Obviously, masses that have been detected by sonography alone must be localized with sonography.

At M. D. Anderson, for the past 10 years, we have been localizing nonpalpable breast masses in the operating room rather than in the radiology department. Because the procedure is done with the patient placed in the operating position, the risk of the localizing needle or hookwire being dislodged is eliminated. The localization is done while the patient is under anesthesia (general or local), which avoids stress and discomfort for the patient. Transportation-related delays between the radiology and the surgery departments are avoided, and the only timing issue is for the radiologist to arrive in the operating theater a few minutes before the surgeon.

Another significant advantage of intraoperative localization is that it allows the radiologist and the surgeon to communicate directly and discuss the actual real-time images of the tumor. As surgeons have become more familiar with this approach, the number of requests for placement of a localizing needle at the time of the intraoperative localization has decreased significantly; at present, most localizations in small to medium-sized breasts are done by simply marking the projection of the mass on the skin with an X and indicating the depth of the lesion to the surgeon (Fornage et al, 1994). In exceptional cases, further real-time guidance has been provided using a gowned transducer in the open wound.

Sonography of the Surgical Specimen

Sonographic confirmation of the successful excision of a lesion that was detected by sonography but not by mammography (and for which radiography of the specimen is therefore not relevant) can be obtained by scanning the freshly excised specimen placed in a container filled with saline. Failure to visualize the mass in the specimen should prompt the radiologist to scan the area of the wound to identify the residual mass and further guide the surgeon.

Localization of Tumors Responding to Neoadjuvant Chemotherapy

At M. D. Anderson, metallic markers are implanted under sonographic guidance in and/or adjacent to breast carcinomas that are responding dramatically to neoadjuvant (preoperative) chemotherapy (Edeiken et al, 1999). The goal of this practice is to allow the surgeon to locate and excise the tumor bed if the tumor disappears completely during chemotherapy. Markers are implanted as soon as the tumor is no longer palpable (usually after 2 courses of chemotherapy) but while it is still clearly seen on sonograms.

Using a 15-gauge needle, four 18-gauge, 5-mm-long stainless steel rods are inserted in or at the periphery of the shrinking tumor (Figure 5–15). After completion of the neoadjuvant chemotherapy, the breast is reassessed. If the clustered metallic markers can be identified on sonog-

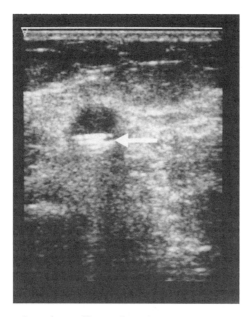

Figure 5–15. Insertion of metallic markers into a tumor responding to neoadjuvant chemotherapy. Sonogram shows the metallic markers (arrow) in the small residual tumor and the associated comet-tail artifact.

raphy through their distinctive comet-tail artifact, the tumor bed is localized in the operating room with sonography. If, however, the markers cannot be seen on sonography, then the markers are localized preoperatively with mammography.

Ultrasound-Guided Injections for Sentinel Node Mapping in Patients with Nonpalpable Breast Cancer

Examination of sentinel lymph nodes in the axilla has been proposed as a way to reduce the number of unnecessary axillary node dissections and eliminate the associated cost and morbidity. The principle underlying sentinel node mapping is that the histologic status of the sentinel node is expected to reflect that of the rest of the axilla. Two basic methods are used to identify sentinel nodes. One method involves lymphoscintigraphy after direct injection of approximately 2.5 mCi (in 4 mL) of technetium-labeled sulfur colloid around the primary tumor. Another method involves the injection of a vital dye (isosultan blue) around the tumor in the operating room just prior to surgery. Often the 2 methods are used in combination. In both techniques, the injection around nonpalpable lesions can be performed under real-time sonographic guidance, which allows

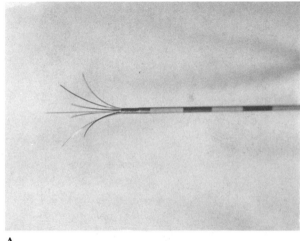

A

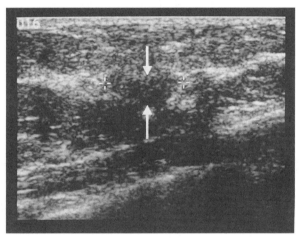

B

Figure 5–16. Ultrasound-guided radiofrequency ablation of a small breast carcinoma. A, View of the needle-electrode used for radiofrequency ablation with the
prongs deployed (RITA Medical Systems, Inc., Mountain View, CA). B, Prepro-
cedure sonogram shows a small carcinoma (arrows and calipers).

accurate distribution of the fluid at the periphery of the tumor (Fornage,
1998).

Ultrasound-Guided Percutaneous Ablation of Breast Masses

An exciting new field of investigation is the use of ultrasound to guide
and monitor percutaneous ablation of small nonpalpable breast masses.

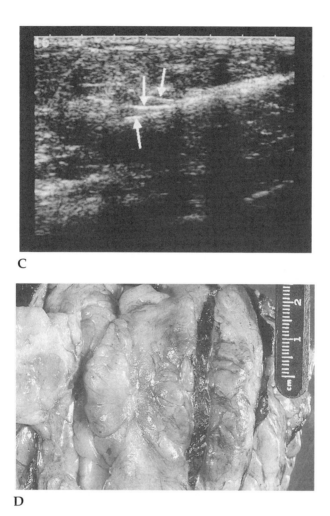

C

D

Figure 5–16. *(continued)*   C, Sonogram after placement of the electrode through the lesion shows the deployed prongs (antennas) (arrows). D, View of the resected specimen shows the ablated lesion (center) surrounded by a rim of hyperemia.

Pilot studies are currently under way that use cryotherapy, radiofrequency, or high-intensity focused ultrasound to ablate such masses and ultrasound to guide the accurate placement of the ablating device and to monitor the procedure. Our preliminary experience with ultrasound-guided radiofrequency ablation of small (< 2 cm in diameter) breast carcinomas indicates that 100% ablation is achievable with this technique (Figure 5–16).

KEY PRACTICE POINTS

- Sonography not only differentiates cysts from solid masses but also helps discriminate between benign and malignant solid masses.

- Sonography can reveal nonpalpable, mammographically occult carcinoma and reveal unsuspected multicentric disease.

- Sonography is helpful in evaluating breasts that contain implants.

- Sonography can confirm the absence of a mass in the case of indeterminate findings on physical examination.

- Sonography can reveal nonpalpable regional nodal metastases, which can alter the patient's staging. To ensure that any nodal disease is detected, the node-bearing areas must be scanned systematically.

- Sonography is routinely used at M. D. Anderson to quantify the response to chemotherapy of the primary tumor and nodal metastases.

- Sonography is the best guidance technique for percutaneous needle biopsy of masses that are seen on sonograms and, in rare selected cases, of clustered microcalcifications without an associated mass.

- Sonography is efficacious in localizing nonpalpable masses in the operating room and can be used to document successful excision of masses detected by sonography only.

- Sonography is used to guide percutaneous ablation of nonpalpable breast tumors.

SUGGESTED READINGS

Chopra S, Evans AJ, Pinder SE, et al. Pure mucinous breast cancer—mammographic and ultrasound findings. *Clin Radiol* 1996;51:421–424.

Cosgrove DO, Kedar RP, Bamber JC, et al. Breast diseases: color Doppler US in differential diagnosis. *Radiology* 1993;189:99–104.

Edeiken BS, Fornage BD, Bedi DG, et al. US-guided implantation of metallic markers for permanent localization of the tumor bed in patients with breast cancer who undergo preoperative chemotherapy. *Radiology* 1999;213:895–900.

Everson LI, Parantainen H, Detlie T, et al. Diagnosis of breast implant rupture: imaging findings and relative efficacies of imaging techniques. *AJR Am J Roentgenol* 1994;163:57–60.

Fornage BD. Intraoperative sonography of the breast. In: Kane RA, ed. *Intraoperative, Laparoscopic, and Endoluminal Ultrasound*. New York: Churchill Livingstone; 1998:142–147.

Fornage BD. Role of color Doppler imaging in differentiating between pseudocystic malignant tumors and fluid collections. *J Ultrasound Med* 1995;14:125–128.

Fornage BD. A simple phantom for training in ultrasound-guided needle biopsy using the freehand technique. *J Ultrasound Med* 1989;8:701–703.

Fornage BD. Sonographically guided needle biopsy of nonpalpable breast lesions. *J Clin Ultrasound* 1999;27:385–398.

Fornage BD. Ultrasound-guided percutaneous needle biopsy on nonpalpable breast masses. In: Harris JR, Lippman ME, Morrow M, Hellman S, eds. *Diseases of the Breast.* Philadelphia: Lippincott-Raven; 1996:152–158.

Fornage BD. Ultrasound of the breast. *Ultrasound Quarterly* 1993;11:1–39.

Fornage BD, Atkinson EN, Nock LF, Jones PH. US with extended field of view: phantom-tested accuracy of distance measurements. *Radiology* 2000b;214:579–584.

Fornage BD, Brown C, Edeiken BS, Bedi D. Contrast-enhanced breast sonography: preliminary results with gray-scale and contrast harmonic imaging of breast carcinoma. *J Ultrasound Med* 2000a;19(suppl):85A.

Fornage BD, Coan JD, David CL. Ultrasound-guided needle biopsy of the breast and other interventional procedures. *Radiol Clin North Am* 1992;30:167–185.

Fornage BD, Faroux MJ, Simatos A. Breast masses: US-guided fine-needle aspiration biopsy. *Radiology* 1987;162:409–414.

Fornage BD, Lorigan JG, Andry E. Fibroadenoma of the breast: sonographic appearance. *Radiology* 1989;172:671–675.

Fornage BD, Ross MI, Singletary SE, Paulus DD. Localization of impalpable breast masses: value of sonography in the operating room and scanning of excised specimens. *AJR Am J Roentgenol* 1994;163:569–573.

Fornage BD, Samuels BI, Paulus DD, Hortobagyi GN, Singletary SE. The use of sonography in the evaluation of the response of locally advanced breast carcinoma to preoperative chemotherapy. *J Ultrasound Med* 1990a;9:23A.

Fornage BD, Sneige N, Faroux MJ, Andry E. Sonographic appearance and ultrasound-guided fine-needle aspiration biopsy of breast carcinomas smaller than 1 cm³. *J Ultrasound Med* 1990b;9:559–568.

Fornage BD, Sneige N, Singletary SE. Masses in breasts with implants: diagnosis with US-guided fine-needle aspiration biopsy. *Radiology* 1994;191:339–342.

Fornage BD, Toubas O, Morel M. Clinical, mammographic, and sonographic determination of preoperative breast cancer size. *Cancer* 1987;60:765–771.

Gordon PB, Goldenberg SL. Malignant breast masses detected only by ultrasound. A retrospective review. *Cancer* 1995;76:626–630.

Gui GP, Allum WH, Perry NM, et al. One-stop diagnosis for symptomatic breast disease. *Ann R Coll Surg Engl* 1995;77:24–27.

Harris KM, Ganott MA, Shestak KC, Losken HW, Tobon H. Silicone implant rupture: detection with US. *Radiology* 1993;187:761–768.

Harter LP, Curtis JS, Ponto G, Craig PH. Malignant seeding of the needle track during stereotaxic core needle breast biopsy. *Radiology* 1992;185:713–714.

Kline TS, Joshi LP, Neal HS. Fine-needle aspiration of the breast: diagnoses and pitfalls. A review of 3545 cases. *Cancer* 1979;44:1458–1464.

Kolb TM, Lichy J, Newhouse JH. Occult cancer in women with dense breasts: detection with screening US—diagnostic yield and tumor characteristics. *Radiology* 1998;207:191–199.

McNicholas MM, Mercer PM, Miller JC, McDermott EW, O'Higgins NJ, MacErlean DP. Color Doppler sonography in the evaluation of palpable breast masses. *AJR Am J Roentgenol* 1993;161:765–771.

Mendelson EB. Imaging the post-surgical breast. *Semin Ultrasound CT MR* 1989;10:154–170.

Paramagul CP, Helvie MA, Adler DD. Invasive lobular carcinoma: sonographic appearance and role of sonography in improving diagnostic sensitivity. *Radiology* 1995;195:231–234.

Parker SH, Jobe WE, Dennis MA, et al. US-guided automated large-core breast biopsy. *Radiology* 1993;187:507–511.

Peters-Engl C, Medl M, Leodolter S. The use of colour-coded and spectral Doppler ultrasound in the differentiation of benign and malignant breast lesions. *Br J Cancer* 1995;71:137–139.

Peterse JL, Thunnissen FB, van Heerde P. Fine needle aspiration cytology of radiation-induced changes in nonneoplastic breast lesions. Possible pitfalls in cytodiagnosis. *Acta Cytol* 1989;33:176–180.

Reuter K, D'Orsi CJ, Reale F. Intracystic carcinoma of the breast: the role of ultrasonography. *Radiology* 1984;153:233–234.

Rissanen T, Typpö T, Tikkakoski T, Turunen J, Myllymäki T, Suramo I. Ultrasound-guided percutaneous galactography. *J Clin Ultrasound* 1993;21:497–502.

Scatarige JC, Hamper UM, Sheth S, Allen HA III. Parasternal sonography of the internal mammary vessels: technique, normal anatomy, and lymphadenopathy. *Radiology* 1989;172:453–457.

Sneige N, Fornage BD, Saleh G. Ultrasound-guided fine-needle aspiration of non-palpable breast lesions: cytologic and histologic findings. *Am J Clin Pathol* 1994;102:98–101.

Stavros AT, Thickman D, Rapp CL, Dennis MA, Parker SH, Sisney GA. Solid breast nodules: use of sonography to distinguish between benign and malignant lesions. *Radiology* 1995;196:123–134.

Venta LA, Dudiak CM, Salomon CG, Flisak ME. Sonographic evaluation of the breast. *Radiographics* 1994;14:29–50.

6 CORE NEEDLE BIOPSY AND NEEDLE LOCALIZATION BIOPSY OF NONPALPABLE BREAST LESIONS: TECHNICAL CONSIDERATIONS AND DIAGNOSTIC CHALLENGES

Nour Sneige

CHAPTER OVERVIEW

Ten percent to 30% of nonpalpable breast lesions that are submitted to open surgical biopsy are found to be malignant. Currently, these lesions are sampled using image-guided needle biopsy (fine-needle aspiration, core needle biopsy, or both) or needle localization excisional biopsy to obtain a tissue diagnosis. Accurate diagnosis is essential in determining the appropriate management of these early lesions. Diagnostic accuracy depends on several factors. Standardization of biopsy procedures and specimen handling and familiarity with diagnostic problems and solutions are necessary to optimize diagnostic results. It must be emphasized that accurate assessment of nonpalpable breast lesions requires correlating the histopathologic results with the imaging and clinical findings.

INTRODUCTION

The widespread use of screening mammography has resulted in an increase in the rate of detection of nonpalpable breast lesions and an increase in the number of biopsies done to evaluate such lesions. In many cases, these biopsies are performed using the needle localization excisional biopsy technique (see the section Mammographically Guided Needle Localization in chapter 4 for a description), but core needle biopsy (CNB) and fine-needle aspiration (FNA) are being used with increasing frequency to sample nonpalpable breast lesions.

With the increasing use of needle localization excisional biopsy and CNB, surgical pathologists are faced with new diagnostic challenges in their daily practice. For example, in CNB specimens, the histologic presentation of nonpalpable breast lesions, especially in the incomplete form and sometimes in the disrupted form, can complicate the diagnosis. Common diagnostic problems include differentiating infiltrating carcinoma from benign sclerosing lesions, differentiating carcinoma in situ from invasive carcinoma, and differentiating papilloma from papillary carcinoma. To ensure accurate pathologic assessment of nonpalpable breast lesions, it is necessary to use standardized biopsy techniques and methods of evaluating pathologic materials and to understand the diagnostic problems associated with needle biopsy specimens. In addition, in the case of needle localization excisional biopsy, accurate specimen assessment requires that the pathologist understand the histologic changes that can be induced by the needle localization excisional biopsy or by prior biopsies.

The first part of this chapter will describe needle localization excisional biopsy and CNB and how specimens obtained by these techniques are handled. The merits of CNB and FNA will be compared. Then the methods used to report results of CNB and needle localization excisional biopsy will be discussed. The second part of the chapter will present some of the problems commonly encountered in evaluating specimens obtained by CNB or needle localization excisional biopsy and will discuss the use of immuno-histochemical techniques as an adjunct to other methods of pathologic evaluation of such specimens.

TECHNICAL CONSIDERATIONS

Specimen handling and evaluation procedures differ for needle localization excisional biopsy and CNB. Several technical issues specific to each technique must be considered in order to ensure optimal diagnostic results.

Needle Localization Excisional Biopsy

Accurate evaluation and diagnosis of specimens of nonpalpable breast lesions that are excised using the needle localization excisional biopsy technique requires the coordinated efforts of the surgeon, pathologist, and radiologist. Before processing, the specimen must be oriented, and the presence of the lesion in the specimen must be confirmed. Our approach to handling and evaluating needle localization excisional biopsy specimens is illustrated in Figure 6–1.

When the needle localization biopsy specimen is received from the operating room, it is oriented by the surgeon as to location and margins of excision. A radiograph of the intact specimen is obtained and immediately compared with the preoperative mammogram or sonogram. A sonogram of the specimen may be necessary if specimen mammography does not show the lesion in question. The purpose of this initial step is to confirm the presence of the suspicious microcalcifications or atypical soft-tissue density within the excised specimen. The surface of the oriented specimen is then marked with multiple colors of ink to identify the 6 margins: lateral, medial, inferior, superior, anterior, and posterior. Because there is no palpable lesion, if the radiograph of the intact specimen shows the area containing suspicious microcalcifications or the atypical soft-tissue density, the radiograph can be used to select the optimal opposing orientation sites (poles) farthest from the area of concern. The specimen is sectioned sequentially from 1 of these poles to the opposite pole in 3- to 5-mm intervals along a plane parallel to the chosen opposing orientation sites.

The individual tissue sections are then placed in order on a radiographic plate (orientation is maintained between sections), and a second radiograph is obtained. Lesions identified by specimen radiography and on gross examination should be compared with preoperative mammographic findings. If suspicious microcalcifications or an atypical soft-tissue density appears close to or at a tissue margin on the radiograph, additional tissue from this area can then be obtained by the surgeon to ensure an adequate margin.

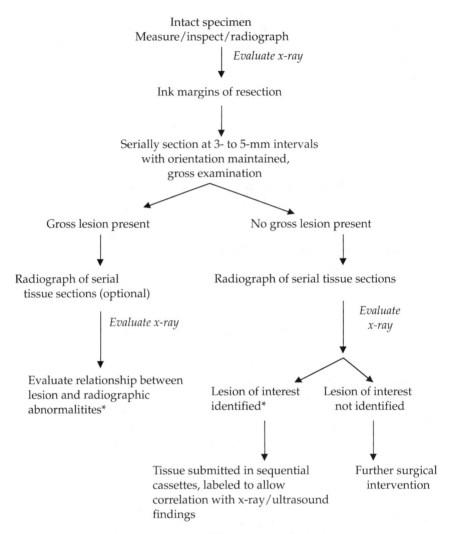

*Lesion at margin: Additional tissue should be removed and submitted as a new margin

Figure 6–1. M. D. Anderson approach to pathologic evaluation of breast specimens obtained by needle localization excisional biopsy.

If the radiograph of the sequential tissue sections fails to show the mammographic abnormality, the surgeon and radiologist must proceed to relocate the suspicious abnormality within the breast tissue.

Sections of the specimen are submitted for permanent section evaluation. The locations of all sections submitted are mapped on the radiograph of the serial sections. Frozen section evaluation is not recommended for diagnosis of tissue containing microcalcifications or a nonpalpable, grossly unapparent radiographic soft-tissue density or for lesions less than 1 cm in diameter. If the specimen is small (< 5 cm), it can be submitted in its entirety for permanent section evaluation. For specimens 5 cm in diameter or larger, all areas containing microcalcifications or atypical soft-tissue densities should be submitted in their entirety. Margins closest to the microcalcifications and areas of fibrosis should also be submitted. If permanent sections of a larger specimen show only carcinoma in situ or atypical hyperplasia, additional sampling of any residual tissue in the specimen is recommended.

Core Needle Biopsy

The goals of CNB in the evaluation of breast lesions are to identify benign lesions with a high degree of accuracy, thus eliminating unnecessary surgery in the majority of cases; to distinguish carcinoma in situ from invasive carcinoma; and to identify high-risk lesions and determine appropriate therapy. To attain these goals, however, many standards must be met with regard to the size of the needle, number of cores, type of biopsy device, specimen handling procedures, and correlation of pathologic and radiologic findings.

Needle Size

The gauge and length of the biopsy needle are important factors in CNB. Early in the practice of CNB, it became apparent that small-gauge needles (i.e., 20- or 18-gauge) produced insufficient tissue samples, and as a result, Parker et al (1994) advocated the use of 14-gauge needles for breast biopsies. In a study of 57 surgically removed mass breast lesions that were sampled using a short-throw, automated biopsy gun with 18-, 16-, and 14-gauge needles, Nath et al (1995) found that the most accurate diagnoses were made with the samples obtained with the 14-gauge needle.

In addition to the needle gauge, the length of the needle excursion into the mass is also important. A short-throw needle results in shorter tissue cores than a long-throw needle (1.3 cm vs 2.3 cm). In a study by Liberman et al (1997), the likelihood of not diagnosing carcinoma because of insufficient tissue sampling was shown to be significantly higher in biopsies performed with the short-throw needle compared with the long-throw needle (60% vs 18%). At M. D. Anderson Cancer Center, we use 11- or 14-gauge needles for sampling calcifications under stereotactic guidance. Our experience with 18-gauge, long-throw needles for ultrasound-guided biopsies of solid masses has been satisfactory, resulting in near 100% adequacy.

Number of Cores

Multiple tissue cores are needed to assess nonpalpable breast lesions. The number of cores may vary from case to case, but on average, accurate diagnosis of solid masses can be accomplished with 4 cores, whereas accurate diagnosis of microcalcifications requires 10 cores. In a study of 145 mammographically detected lesions (53 calcifications and 92 masses) that were sampled using 14-gauge needles, the authors found that diagnostic material was present in the first core in 70% of the lesions and that obtaining more cores increased the diagnostic yield (Liberman et al, 1994). In that study, obtaining 5 cores enabled a diagnosis in 87% of the calcifications and 99% of the masses. When the number of cores obtained increased to 6, the diagnostic yield increased for calcifications but did not increase for masses. On the basis of these findings, the authors recommended that a minimum of 5 cores be obtained in cases of masses and more than 6 cores be obtained in cases of microcalcifications. Several other studies have resulted in similar findings (Brenner et al, 1996).

Type of Biopsy Device

The revival of the use of CNB can be credited to the advent of automated spring-loaded devices that activate a 14- to 18-gauge needle in a fraction of a second. These devices are much easier to use than the traditional Tru-Cut biopsy needle. Ultrasound-guided biopsies are performed using these devices.

The directional vacuum-assisted biopsy device (Mammotome, Ethicon Endo-Surgery, Cincinnati, OH) uses 11- or 14-gauge needles connected to a vacuum chamber that sucks tissue into a cutting notch. This device has several advantages compared with the automated cutting core biopsy device, especially when differentiation between ductal carcinoma in situ (DCIS) and atypical ductal hyperplasia (ADH) is the issue. The directional vacuum-assisted biopsy device is also most suitable for sampling of calcifications under stereotactic guidance.

Burbank (1997) compared the results of 2 stereotactic-guidance breast-biopsy protocols. One study used an automated needle device to obtain an average of 17 and 19 specimens per ADH or DCIS lesion, respectively. The other study used a directional vacuum-assisted device to obtain an average of 27 and 26 specimens per ADH or DCIS lesion, respectively. Fourteen-gauge needles were used in both protocols. Burbank found that underestimation of ADH or DCIS could be essentially eliminated with no clinical complications with use of the directional vacuum-assisted biopsy device. Eight of 18 lesions diagnosed as ADH using an automated needle device were determined at surgery to be breast cancer (DCIS or invasive ductal carcinoma [IDC]), whereas none of the 8 lesions diagnosed as ADH using the directional vacuum-assisted device was determined at surgery to be breast cancer. Nine of 55 lesions diagnosed as DCIS using the automated needle device were diagnosed as IDC at surgery, whereas none of the 32 lesions diagnosed as DCIS using the directional vacuum-assisted device were determined to be IDC at surgery. A few other studies have shown similar results using the directional vacuum-assisted device; however, in those studies, underestimation of DCIS and ADH could not be totally eliminated.

The improved performance of directional vacuum-assisted devices has been attributed to ease of obtaining a large number of specimens, higher average specimen weights, a higher percentage of breast tissue versus clotted blood per specimen, and contiguous breast tissue samples.

Specimen Handling Procedures

When calcifications are sampled by CNB, it is essential to confirm that calcifications are indeed present in the CNB specimen. For this purpose, CNB specimens are placed in a petri dish and kept moist with a drop of sterile water on a small Telfa pad (Kendall Co., Milford, OH). After they are magnified and radiographed, the tissue cores with calcifications are either marked with India ink before fixation in 10% normal buffered formalin (Figure 6–2) or placed in a separate container to localize the calcifications for pathologic correlation. Multiple tissue levels of the tissue block are often required for histologic examination. We routinely obtain 6 levels and use the first and last levels for histologic evaluation; the unstained slides are reserved for any marker studies that may be needed. If calcifications are not found on specimen radiography as expected, a repeat biopsy should be done. If more than 1 mammographically detected lesion is biopsied, tissue cores from each lesion should be submitted and evaluated separately.

Comparison of Core Needle Biopsy and Fine-Needle Aspiration

Comparisons of CNB and FNA should be made in the same breast lesions, although this practice has only been documented in a few studies. Dowlatshahi et al (1991) reported 250 cases of nonpalpable breast lesions that were sampled under stereotactic guidance using 20-gauge biopsy needles (a Franzen-type device for FNA; a Biopty device [C. R. Bard, Inc., Covington, GA] or Monopty device [Radiplast, Uppsala, Sweden] for CNB).

About 54% of the cancers were diagnosed using both FNA and CNB, 41% with CNB alone, and 32% with FNA alone. Of 125 lesions characterized as slightly suspicious, 85 (68%) were definitively diagnosed using 1 or both of these techniques. Fine-needle aspiration was more accurate than CNB in diagnosing mammographic calcifications: the false-negative rates were 45% for CNB and 10% for FNA. The authors concluded that FNA and CNB are complementary. Both FNA and CNB are highly specific for low-risk lesions, and high-risk lesions should be sampled by open biopsy even when FNA and CNB results are negative.

In a multi-institutional study conducted by the Radiologic Diagnostic Oncology Group (RDOG-5), 377 breast lesions were sampled using 22- to 25-gauge needles for FNA and 14-gauge needles for CNB. In this RDOG-5 study, sampling was performed under stereotactic or ultrasound guidance. The only results reported so far relate to the insufficient sample rate for FNA (Pisano et al, 1998). Among 18 participating institutions, the

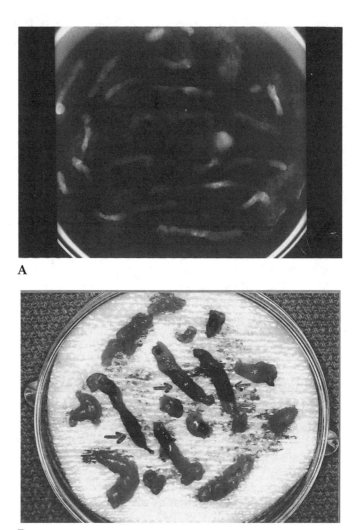

A

B

Figure 6–2. A, Specimen radiograph demonstrating the presence of calcifications in some of the tissue cores. B, CNB specimen with India ink indicating the tissue cores with calcifications.

insufficient sample rate averaged 33% (range, 3% to 82%). The rate varied significantly by lesion type (significantly higher for calcified lesions than for masses), image-guidance method (higher for stereotactic guidance than for ultrasound guidance), and histologic diagnosis (higher for benign lesions than for malignant lesions). Because FNA could not be consistently applied in multiple practices around the United States using the same

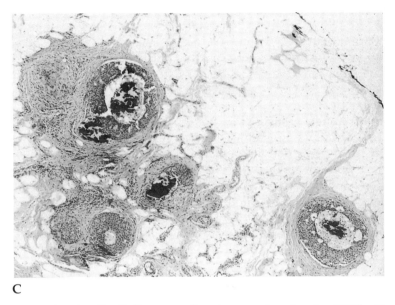

C

Figure 6–2. *(continued)*   C, Corresponding tissue section showing DCIS with calcifications. The black ink at the edge of the tissue core corresponds to the core
with calcifications identified in panel B.

protocol, the National Cancer Institute's RDOG-5 Data Safety and Monitoring Board convened to oversee the progress of the study and decided
to stop enrolling patients in the FNA arm of this trial. It is unfortunate
that this decision meant that FNA was also discontinued in institutions
with insufficient sample rates of less than 10%. The findings from this
study indicate that FNA should be limited to sampling of solid lesions
amenable to ultrasound-guided biopsy.

In our study (Ballo and Sneige, 1996), 124 palpable breast carcinomas
were sampled with FNA and CNB performed in succession by the same
operator. For FNA, an average of 3 needle passes were made with a 23-
or 25-gauge needle. For CNB, 3 biopsies were performed on each lesion
using an 18-gauge needle (Bard Monopty device). Three additional cores
were obtained if the first 3 were deemed inadequate after examination of
frozen sections. Both FNA and CNB showed a specificity of 100% when
consideration was given to the accepted limitations of each method; that
is, FNA cannot establish the presence of invasive disease, and CNB cannot
determine relative amounts of invasive or in situ carcinoma. A specific
diagnosis of carcinoma was made in 114 specimens by FNA and in 112
specimens by CNB. The sensitivity of CNB was 90% (lesions viewed as
"suspicious" after FNA was performed were considered positive for the
calculation of sensitivity). Twelve lesions had a false-negative diagnosis

by 1 or both methods. The 3 specimens for which FNA results were false-negative also had negative CNB results. Of the remaining 9 lesions, which had false-negative CNB results, 6 had positive FNA results and 3 had suspicious FNA results. On the basis of our findings, we concluded that FNA is more sensitive than CNB for detecting malignancy in palpable breast lesions. Several reasons were given for the higher false-negative rate for CNB than for FNA. These included lesions close to the chest wall, which necessitate a longer pathway (i.e., parallel to the chest wall) for the needle than would normally be used with FNA, and small lesion size, in which case a coring device (compared with a 23- or 25-gauge needle) may, in effect, push the lesion out of the path of the needle.

Other studies have also shown that FNA is equal or superior to CNB in detecting carcinoma. Reports from the late 1970s and early 1980s showed that CNB was more reliable than FNA in evaluating palpable breast lesions; however, these reports are likely to have been influenced by the fact that FNA was a new procedure at that time.

Core Needle Biopsy versus Fine-Needle Aspiration: Points and Counterpoints

Core needle biopsy and FNA provide different but complementary information. Depending on the patient scenario and the diagnostic situation, FNA may be adequate. In some cases, however, CNB is needed for definitive surgical treatment planning.

Proponents of CNB believe that it is more advantageous than FNA because CNB provides a more specific diagnosis for most benign abnormalities, eliminates problems with atypical cytologic diagnoses, and distinguishes carcinoma in situ from invasive carcinoma. However, there are several drawbacks to CNB. As to the benign diagnoses, results reported from the multi-institutional study by Parker et al (1994) using CNB (41% of the lesions diagnosed as fibrocystic change, 20.6% diagnosed as fibroadenoma, and 19% diagnosed as other disease) are not more accurate than those reported by experienced cytopathologists using FNA. Furthermore, in the study by Parker and colleagues, no histologic or adequate clinical follow-up was available to determine the specificity of the benign diagnoses rendered.

Similarly, atypical histologic diagnoses rendered by CNB are no less problematic than those rendered by FNA. In the CNB series by Jackman et al (1994) and Liberman et al (1995a), ADH was diagnosed in 3.6% and 9% of the cases, respectively. On excision, 56% and 52% of the cases thought to be ADH in the Jackman and Liberman studies, respectively, were found to be malignant. Recent advances in CNB and the development of directional vacuum-assisted needle devices have markedly reduced but have not eliminated the rate of underdiagnosis of DCIS and invasive carcinoma. Because a diagnosis of ADH on CNB is associated with a significant false-negative rate, it is recommended that such cases be followed by surgical biopsy. In the FNA series reported by Mitnick et al (1996) and Boerner et al (1999), a cytologic diagnosis of atypia was reported in 9.5% and 8% of cases, respectively. Similar to findings in the CNB series, 60% of the cases diagnosed as atypia were found to be malignant on subsequent surgical biopsy, indicating that a cytologic diagnosis of atypia is significant and should be followed by excisional biopsy.

Finally, CNB cannot reliably indicate the absence of invasive disease when only DCIS is found. Liberman et al (1995b) reported 92% accuracy of CNB in predicting invasive disease. In that series, among the diagnostic results of the CNB as to the absence or presence of invasive carcinoma, 1 result was false-positive; 3 were false-negative; and in 1 case, there was no residual tumor on excisional biopsy (total mastectomy was required). In other studies, up to 30% of the DCIS cases were found to be invasive on subsequent excisional biopsy. Fine-needle aspiration cannot distinguish in situ from invasive carcinoma, but it is not always necessary to make this distinction in FNA specimens if axillary lymph nodes show metastatic carcinoma on FNA.

Another advantage of CNB cited by its proponents is the fact that CNB eliminates the added cost of having a cytopathologist on site. However, when the costs of the CNB needle and histologic tissue preparation are compared with those of FNA needles and smear preparation, the savings realized with FNA are enough to cover the cost of having a cytopathologist on site for immediate interpretation. At M. D. Anderson, the cost of CNB is similar to the cost of having a cytopathologist on site for immediate assessment of FNA material.

From a technical point of view, FNA is favored by clinicians skilled in both FNA and CNB because FNA is better tolerated by patients, is less invasive (it uses finer needles: 20- to 25-gauge vs 14- to 18-gauge), and is safer in cases in which lesions are close to the chest wall. In addition, FNA allows the clinician to maintain tactile sensitivity, which enhances accurate localization of the lesion.

At M. D. Anderson, FNA is used as a first-line test for evaluating nonpalpable and palpable breast lesions. Nonpalpable breast masses are aspirated under ultrasound guidance; microcalcifications and mammographic abnormalities that cannot be visualized on sonography are sampled under stereotactic guidance using CNB. Fine-needle aspiration of palpable breast lesions is performed by the cytopathologists in the FNA clinic, whereas ultrasound-guided FNA of nonpalpable lesions is performed by radiologists. The FNA material is immediately smeared, stained, and evaluated as to specimen adequacy while the patient is still in the clinic. In the case of a nondiagnostic aspirate, CNB is performed for definitive diagnosis. Core needle biopsy is also performed for carcinomas requiring determination of tumor invasiveness prior to chemotherapy or sentinel lymph node biopsy.

Generally, the decision whether to use CNB or FNA takes into account the clinical presentation of the lesion and whether it is palpable. For palpable lesions and lesions for which imaging guidance is not justified, FNA is the most efficient, cost-effective, and reliable procedure. For non-palpable lesions, ultrasound-guided FNA is used as the first-line test. Ultrasound-guided CNB is reserved for cases that require determination of tumor invasiveness and cases with insufficient or nondiagnostic aspirates. Stereotactic guidance is used for calcifications, which cannot be visualized on sonography, and for lesions that are not clearly seen on sonography. When mammographic and clinical findings do not correlate with FNA or CNB results, a surgical biopsy should be performed. Finally, the benefits of a team approach to the success of FNA and CNB cannot be overemphasized. Breast lesions are best managed when the radiologist, pathologist, and surgeon are all involved in the decision-making process.

Reporting of Pathology Results

Pathology reports for CNB and needle localization excisional biopsy specimens should describe several specific features in addition to stating the main pathologic diagnosis. This information may be helpful for future treatment decisions.

Core Needle Biopsy Specimens

In cases of malignancy, the histologic evaluation of CNB specimens should include determination of the histologic type and nuclear/histologic grade of the tumor for both invasive and in situ carcinomas. Because of limited tissue sampling, the extent of tumor invasion cannot be reliably determined from CNB specimens. At M. D. Anderson, prognostic-marker studies (e.g., determination of estrogen and progesterone receptor status, proliferation rate [MIB-1], and HER-2/*neu* status) are performed on samples from patients who are considered candidates for preoperative chemotherapy. Reports comparing standard prognostic factors and marker-study results of CNB specimens to those of the excised tissue showed that histologic tumor type could be accurately determined with CNB in most cases, whereas histologic grade was discordant in a substantial minority (~30%). Discrepant results were usually due to tumor heterogeneity. On the other hand, marker studies showed excellent correlation.

On microscopic examination of tissue sections from blocks containing microcalcifications, the microcalcification density on radiographs and that observed in the tissue section should always be correlated to ensure that the densities are similar. A marked disparity in the number or density of microcalcifications often indicates the need for deeper sections within the block to reach and evaluate the area of greatest concern. In some cases, the initial histologic sections of the breast specimens may fail to reveal microcalcifications. There are several possible explanations for this. First, the microcalcifications may be composed of calcium oxalate rather than the usual calcium phosphate. Both types of calcium deposits appear as microcalcifications on mammograms, but they appear differently when examined histologically. When these specimens are examined under polarized light, however, this type of calcification is readily demonstrated. If, after examination under polarized light, there is still no microscopic evidence of calcifications, other possibilities must be considered. For example, the blocks may not have been cut deeply enough to provide histologic sections that can demonstrate the calcifications. To investigate this possibility, the blocks can be radiographed, and any blocks containing calcifications can be cut deeper until the calcifications are microscopically identifiable. Finally, in some cases, calcifications may shatter out of the block during sectioning and therefore will not be demonstrable on histologic sections.

The location of calcifications within the breast tissue (e.g., benign acini, blood vessels, stroma, and ducts) should be specified. In cases sampled with CNB, the correlation between the presence of calcifications on a specimen radiograph and at pathologic analysis is not always 100%. Calcifications were seen on histologic examination in 86% of the cases evaluated by Mainiero et al (1996). As stated earlier, there are a number of possible explanations for the absence of calcifications on histologic evaluation. In addition, it has been shown that calcifications may dissolve within 3 days when the specimens are preserved in aqueous solutions such as 10% formaldehyde, whereas a mixture of 74% ethanol plus 10% propanol can maintain calcifications for up to 2 weeks.

Histologic findings should always be correlated with imaging findings. A copy of the specimen radiographs together with a requisition form indicating radiologic findings should be provided to the pathologist with each specimen (Figure 6–3).

Needle Localization Excisional Biopsy Specimens

In needle localization excisional biopsy specimens showing DCIS or IDC, the margin status and the closest distance from the DCIS or invasive carcinoma to the margin is indicated. In the case of nonpalpable lesions, tumor volume or extent of disease is described by indicating the number of tumor blocks involved by tumor as well as the largest dimension of tumor on the glass slide. In specimens with prior CNB, in which no residual tumor or only small areas of tumor are found, the extent of DCIS or invasive cancer is best determined by providing the maximum dimension of the lesion on the CNB or excisional biopsy specimen and the number of cores and tissue blocks involved and by correlating these findings with the mammographic description.

Invasive carcinomas are categorized according to histologic type and nuclear grade (Table 6–1). The size or extent of the invasive component and presence of vascular involvement are also indicated. Hormone receptor status (estrogen and progesterone receptors) and tumor proliferation

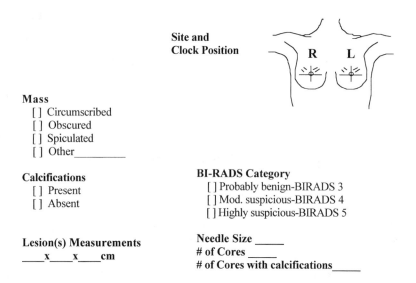

Figure 6–3. A prototype of the radiology evaluation form accompanying CNB specimens submitted to pathology laboratory.

rate are evaluated by immunohistochemical techniques, and the results are reported as the percentage of positive tumor nuclei. Tumors are considered hormone receptor positive when more than 10% of the tumor nuclei are stained. The proliferation rate is categorized as low (< 17%), intermediate (18% to 34%), or high (> 34%) on the basis of the percentage of positive tumor nuclei. HER-2/*neu* status is evaluated by immunohistochemistry as a first-line test. Cases that are positive for membranous staining are confirmed for gene amplification by fluorescence in situ hybridization (Hoang et al, 2000).

Ductal carcinoma in situ lesions are evaluated according to 6 features: nuclear grade (Table 6–1); presence or absence of necrosis (defined by the presence of ghost cells and necrotic debris and categorized as central or punctuate); architectural pattern (i.e., comedo, cribriform, papillary, micropapillary, or solid); size or extent of DCIS (number of sections containing DCIS as well as the largest dimension of the DCIS lesion on the glass slide); margins of resection (closest margin is recorded; if reexcision is performed to obtain new margin, then this will be stated in the report as being positive or negative for DCIS); and presence of calcifications.

For a discussion of the evaluation criteria for calcifications, see the preceding section on CNB specimens.

When lymph node tissue is provided as part of the specimen, axillary lymph node status is also evaluated. All excised lymph nodes are serially sectioned along the long axis of the node at 2- to 3-mm intervals and submitted for histologic evaluation. Immunohistochemical studies for cy-

Table 6–1. Modified Black's Nuclear Grading System for Invasive Carcinoma

Grade	Nuclear Size in Relation to Normal Duct (Red Blood Cells)	Nuclear Shape	Chromatin	Nucleoli	No. of Mitoses per 10 High-Power Fields
I	Similar, minimal enlargement (1.5–2.0)	Monomorphic round	Uniform, fine	–	<1
II	Twofold variation; uniformity is the rule with only slight variation	Round, smooth	Uniform, fine	Micronucleoli ±	2–5
III	Threefold variation in nuclear size (>2.5)	Markedly pleomorphic, irregular	Hyperchromatic, coarse	Macronucleoli ±	>5–10

tokeratin are performed on sections with atypical cytologic findings to confirm or dispute the presence of malignant cells within the node.

Diagnostic Challenges Encountered with Core Needle Biopsy

Because the results of a CNB often determine the next step in patient management, it is essential that the CNB specimen be properly assessed so an accurate diagnosis can be made. Generally, when a pathologist evaluates CNB specimens, the following questions must be addressed: Is the lesion malignant or benign? If malignant, is it invasive or in situ? If the lesion is in situ, is it ductal or lobular? Is the specimen adequate for the questions being asked?

Tubular Carcinoma versus Adenosis

Tubular carcinomas are encountered with increasing frequency as a result of the growing use of mammography. In the Breast Cancer Detection Demonstration Project, 8% of invasive carcinomas 1.0 cm or smaller in diameter were of the tubular variety. On mammographic examination, most tubular carcinomas are spiculated. Rounded lesions (i.e., densities with indistinct borders or calcifications in the absence of a mass) rarely prove to be tubular carcinoma. Patient age at diagnosis of tubular carcinoma ranges from 24 to 83 years, with a mean age of 46 years, which is slightly younger than that of women with breast cancer in general. Most tubular carcinomas are 2 cm or smaller in diameter.

Microscopically, tubular carcinoma is composed of small glands or tubules distributed largely in a haphazard manner within a reactive-appearing, fibroblastic stroma. The tubules may have virtually any shape, but angulated and rounded forms with distinctly open lumina are common. Typically, these structures are formed from a single layer of neoplastic epithelial cells; myoepithelial cells are absent. The cells are cuboidal or columnar, with round or oval hyperchromatic nuclei. Mitoses are rare to nonexistent. Apical snouts are often evident at the luminal cell border. The cytoplasm is usually amphophilic. Intracytoplasmic mucin droplets are rare but may be found. Almost all tubular carcinomas are positive for estrogen receptors.

Stroma between the glands is characterized by the presence of dense collagenous tissue, abundant elastic tissue, or both. Although notable elastosis has been regarded as a hallmark of tubular carcinoma, it may also be a prominent feature of some benign lesions, particularly those with the radial scar pattern. Other stromal features may include fibroblastic, reactive-appearing, or loosening stroma due to accumulation of metachromatic ground substances.

The primary consideration in the differential diagnosis of tubular carcinoma is sclerosing adenosis, a lesion composed of varying proportions of compressed glands with interlacing spindly myoepithelial cells. In contrast to tubular carcinoma, sclerosing adenosis has a lobulocentric proliferation pattern (best appreciated on low-power magnification) and is not infiltrative. In sclerosing adenosis, the glands are compact, whorled, elongated, and largely compressed, with interlacing spindly myoepithelial cells that can be easily highlighted by immunohistochemical stains for smooth-muscle actin (Figure 6–4; Table 6–2). Some tubular carcinomas may be entirely composed of round or oval glands of mostly uniform caliber. These cases may be mistaken for microglandular adenosis. The latter is extremely rare and can be distinguished from tubular carcinoma on the basis of the absence of stromal reaction and characteristic clear-cell changes and luminal secretion. As in tubular carcinoma, however, myoepithelial cells are absent (Table 6–2).

Calcifications are found microscopically in at least 50% of tubular carcinomas either within the lumens of the neoplastic tubules or within the stroma. Intraductal carcinoma has been described in 62% to 84% of cases. This tumor typically has a papillary or cribriform pattern or a mixture of the 2 patterns. Lobular neoplasia is present in the immediate vicinity of the tubular lesion in a median of 15% (range, 0.7% to 40%) of cases. Associated pretubular or columnar-cell hyperplasia, a recently described finding, is commonly found in association with tubular carcinoma.

Papillary Carcinoma versus Papilloma

Papillary lesions may be categorized as those that can be seen grossly and those that are only evident microscopically. The line of distinction with respect to size is usually in the range of 3 to 5 mm. The grossly evident lesions are papillomas and intracystic papillary carcinomas. The microscopic lesions are papillomatosis and intraductal carcinoma of a papillary or micropapillary type. In women, about 1% to 2% of breast carcinomas can be classified as papillary; in men, a slightly greater percentage of breast carcinomas are papillary. Although the majority of papillary carcinomas are noninvasive, a distinction should be made between invasive and noninvasive papillary carcinoma.

The median age at diagnosis for intracystic papillary carcinoma of the breast is older than the median age at diagnosis for other types of breast cancer; a majority of intracystic papillary carcinomas are diagnosed in women in the fifth and sixth decades of life. Nearly 50% of papillary carcinomas arise in the central part of the breast; as a consequence, nipple discharge has been described in 22% to 34% of patients. Bleeding from the nipple occurs in a higher percentage of patients with papillary carcinoma than in those with papilloma. The average size of an intracystic papillary carcinoma as assessed clinically is 2 to 3 cm in diameter.

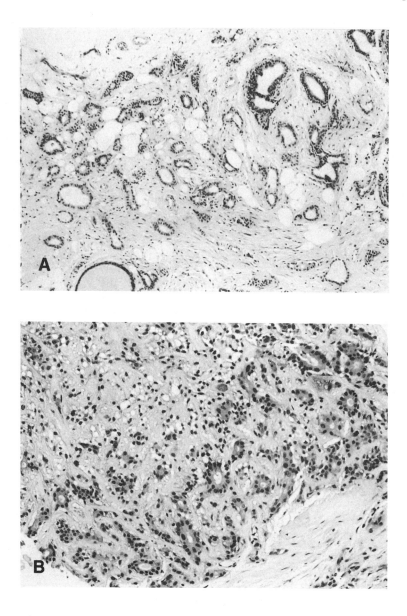

Figure 6–4. A, Tubular carcinoma. B, Microglandular adenosis.

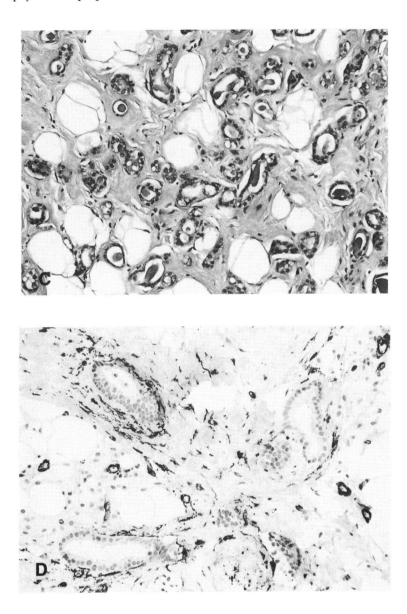

Figure 6–4. *(continued)*   C, Sclerosing adenosis. These 3 lesions are distinguished on the basis of a combination of histologic features and immunohistochemical characteristics (see Table 6–2). D, Immunostains for smooth-muscle actin showing the absence of the myoepithelial cell layer in the case of tubular carcinoma.

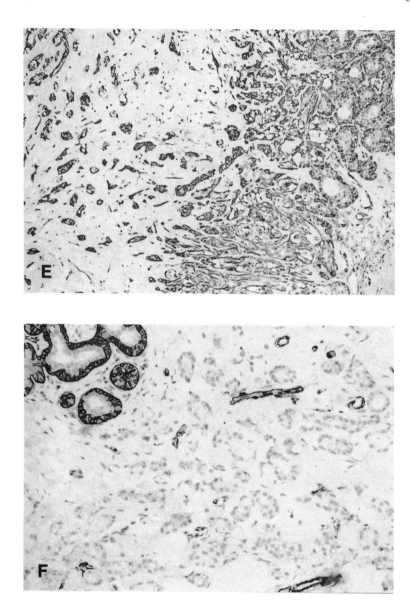

Figure 6–4. *(continued)* E, The absence of myoepithelial cells is also evident in microglandular adenosis. F, Contrast the example of tubular carcinoma in panel D with this case of sclerosing adenosis, in which prominent myoepithelial cells surrounding the epithelial structures are identified.

Table 6–2. Comparison of Features of Tubular Carcinoma, Microglandular Adenosis, and Sclerosing Adenosis

Tubular Carcinoma	Microglandular Adenosis	Sclerosing Adenosis
Stellate lesion with defined margins	Random nonlobular	Expanded lobular architecture
Distended oval to round or angular ductules (majority)	Rounded open ducts	Elongated compressed ducts
No myoepithelial layer	No myoepithelial layer	Prominent myoepithelial layer
Apocrine snouts	Clear epithelial cells	Crowding of ducts and stroma
Marked elastosis	Colloid-like secretion	Thickened basement membrane
	No stromal reaction	

Papillary carcinoma often appears as a rounded, circumscribed lesion on mammograms; on sonograms, its appearance is characterized by the presence of a solid, irregular area in a hypoechoic cystic lesion. Calcifications are not abundant, and when present, they tend to be punctate. Coarse, irregular calcifications may develop in areas of sclerosis or resolved hemorrhage.

The neoplastic growth pattern is predominantly frond-forming, but other minor arrangements may include micropapillary, cribriform, reticular, and solid appearances. Solid papillary carcinoma is a variant of papillary carcinoma in which the papillary character is determined on the basis of the presence of a supporting network of fibrovascular stroma; separate epithelial fronds are minimal or absent.

Microscopically, the distinction between a papilloma and a papillary carcinoma is based primarily on the criteria of Kraus and Neubecker (1962). However, of these criteria, the presence of a myoepithelial cell layer documented by immunoreactivity for smooth-muscle actin is the only reliable distinguishing feature.

In papillomas, myoepithelial cells are regularly distributed along the branches and at the base of the epithelium. In contrast, in papillary carcinomas, myoepithelial cells are absent except in areas where multiple papillomas are present and associated with ductal or papillary cancer. Apocrine metaplasia is commonly encountered in papillomas; however, when it is present in a papillary carcinoma, there are usually cytologic atypia consistent with the rest of the tumor and therefore different from the bland foci of apocrine metaplasia. In addition to the eosinophilic columnar cells, some papillary carcinomas may exhibit cuboidal cells with abundant clear or faintly eosinophilic cytoplasm that mimic myoepithelial cells. These clear cells are of epithelial origin with no reactivity for S-100 protein or smooth-muscle actin. Other features include the presence of conspicuous intracytoplasmic mucin vacuoles or apical snouts. Mucin may accumulate between the papillary fronds (Figure 6–5).

Because of the difficulty in distinguishing papillary carcinoma from papilloma lesions on CNB specimens, most pathologists believe that diagnosis of a papillary lesion on CNB should always be followed by an excisional biopsy to obtain a more definitive diagnosis. Recent reports have suggested that papillary lesions can be distinguished with confidence by CNB, with surgical excision being limited to those lesions with atypical and carcinomatous features (Liberman et al, 1999a).

The diagnosis of true stromal invasion in papillary carcinoma may be difficult, especially in CNB specimens. Many papillary carcinomas are bounded by zones of fibrosis, recent or resolved hemorrhage, and chronic inflammation with entrapped glandular or epithelial cells. Similar alterations may also occur within the lesion. Stromal invasion is, therefore, best evaluated in completely excised specimens and not on samples obtained by CNB. The growth patterns of the invasive component may appear papillary or similar to that of the garden variety of IDC.

Mucocele-Like Tumors versus Mucinous Carcinoma

Most mucocele-like lesions of the breast are palpable tumors that appear well circumscribed and lobulated on mammography. Small, nonpalpable, mucocele-like tumors have been detected by mammography alone because of the presence of calcifications. Histologically, the lesion is made up of multiple aggregated cysts containing viscous, often transparent mucinous material. The cyst may rupture, and the secretion may discharge into the adjacent stroma. The epithelium that lines the cysts in the typical mucocele-like tumor is largely flat or cuboidal, but low columnar and minor papillary elements may be present. Detached epithelial cells are almost never found in secretion that has been discharged into the stroma. Histiocytes and inflammatory cells may be present in the extruded mucin.

Mucinous carcinoma presents as a palpable (in most cases), moderately firm to soft lesion and appears on mammography as a lobulated mass lesion. In its pure form, mucinous carcinoma accounts for 2% of mammary carcinomas. Focal mucinous differentiation may be found in up to 2% of other carcinomas. Mucinous carcinoma is characterized by the accumulation of abundant extracellular mucin around invasive tumor cells. The proportions of secretion and neoplastic epithelium vary from case to case. In a recent study, the proportion of extracellular mucin in tumors classified as pure mucinous carcinoma varied from slightly less than 40% to 99.8%, with a mean percentage of 83.5%. Delicate bands of fibrovascular connective tissue are evident within the mucus lakes. Tumor cells are arranged in a variety of patterns in the mucinous secretion, including strands, alveolar nests, and papillary structures, as well as large sheets of cells that may have cribriform areas or focal comedo necrosis.

Intraductal carcinoma has been found to be associated with about 75% of mucinous carcinoma, generally at the periphery of the lesion. The amount of intracellular mucin in mucinous carcinoma varies. Some lesions have prominent signet-ring cells. Argyrophilic cells with the ultrastructural features of endocrine secretory granules have been detected in 25% to 50% of mucinous carcinomas.

In CNB specimens, mucin should be distinguished from interstitial fluid, necrotic debris, or myxoid stroma. The presence of individual or detached strands of bland-appearing cells reflects the epithelial lining of disrupted ducts and is characteristic of mucocele-like lesions. The epithelium may have been hyperplastic and therefore may present as nests of cells. Invariably, however, in some of these nests, the myoepithelial cells are readily apparent or may be detected by immunostaining for actin. The presence of adjacent ducts in various stages of disruption is a helpful clue in identifying the lesion as a mucocele. A diagnosis of mucinous carcinoma should be based on the finding of several clusters of cells or cell balls surrounded by pools of mucin with the characteristic branching capillary vessels within the mucinous stroma. Because mucocele-like lesions may contain areas of ADH, DCIS, or invasive mucinous carcinoma, complete excision of these lesions is essential for accurate assessment.

Fibroadenoma versus Phyllodes Tumor

Cellular fibroadenoma may mimic phyllodes tumor on CNB specimens. Conversely, stromal heterogeneity in phyllodes tumor may create diagnostic difficulty in accurately categorizing CNB specimen of these lesions. Dershaw et al (1996) reported 7 cases in which the CNB specimen was interpreted as fibroadenoma rather than phyllodes tumor. At surgery, 4 specimens proved to be fibroadenomas, and 3 were phyllodes tumors. In our series of 20 CNB specimens diagnosed as fibroadenomas, 2 were found to be low-grade phyllodes tumors when excised. When CNB specimens have features that raise concern about a possible phyllodes tumor, excisional biopsy is recommended. Abnormalities that suggest an indeterminate diagnosis in CNB samples include noteworthy stromal cellularity and mitosis and atypia of stromal cells. It must be noted that fewer than 1% of fibroadenomas detected by CNB may actually represent benign or low-grade phyllodes tumors.

Spindle Cell Carcinoma

Spindle cell carcinoma of the breast is a rare neoplasm in which the spindle cell component predominates. This tumor resembles a low-grade sarcoma or a reaction process such as fasciitis or tissue granulation. In a report by Wargotz et al (1989) in which 100 samples of spindle cell carci-

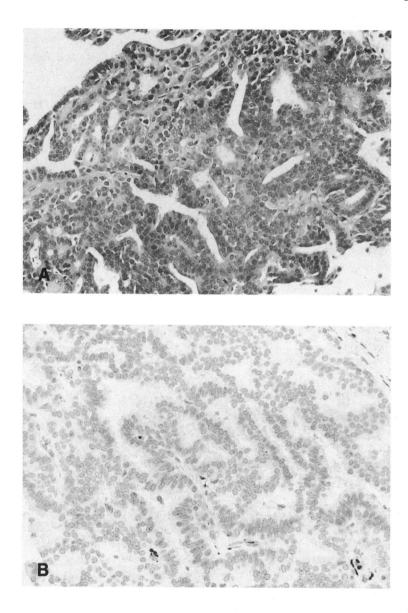

Figure 6–5. Papillary carcinoma versus papilloma. A, Core needle biopsy specimen showing papillary fragments with atypical cell proliferation. The limited biopsy material precludes further categorization. B, Papillary carcinoma showing absence of myoepithelial cells demonstrated by negative immunostaining for smooth-muscle actin.

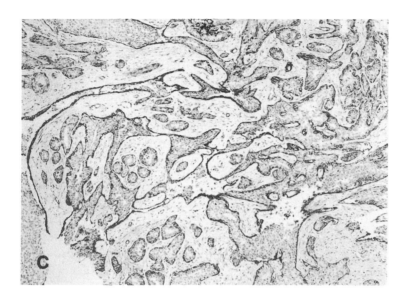

Figure 6–5. *(continued)* C, In this example, the benign nature of the papillary lesion is confirmed by the presence of a myoepithelial cell layer along the branches and at the base of the epithelium. Compare this panel with panel B.

noma were evaluated, 83 contained an overt carcinoma component (65 IDC, 7 pure DCIS, and 11 pure squamous carcinomas), and 17 consisted of bland spindle cell proliferation and were keratin positive but with no overt carcinoma component. The spindle cell components were predominantly fibrocollagenous, with the spindle cells arranged in wavy, interlacing, and overlapping fascicles that resembled the feathered pattern of fasciitis in some areas and the storiform pattern of dermatofibrosarcoma protuberans and malignant fibrous histiocytoma in others. Some neoplasms resembled cellular examples of fibromatosis or low-grade fibrosarcoma with finger-like extensions into adjacent fat. Areas appearing to be angioid, fibromyxoid, or both are frequently-occurring minor components and are the predominant component in a few neoplasms.

Cellular pleomorphism is usually minimal. Focal inflammatory cells consisting of lymphocytes and plasma cells are often found along the periphery of the lesion. Mitotic figures of the spindle cell component range from 0 to 11 per 10 high-power fields; abnormal forms are rarely found.

Our cases of spindle-cell carcinoma (total 30 cases) are similar to those reported by Wargotz et al and Gobbi et al (1999). Unlike in the Gobbi study, however, 2 patients in our study had lung metastasis within 3 years of the initial breast lesions; therefore, we believe spindle cell carcinomas should be treated as carcinoma with the potential for distant metastasis.

Spindle cell carcinoma might easily be confused with fasciitis, fibro-matosis, or a low-grade sarcoma of the breast. One third of our cases referred for consultation had benign diagnoses. Immunoreactivity studies for cytokeratin should establish the correct diagnosis. Keratin-positive cells are seen as cords or sheets of polygonal cells with a few isolated cells. Immunoreactivity with smooth-muscle actin is often confined to the spindle cells, with the epithelioid cells being negative. Strong co-expression of keratin and smooth-muscle actin may be noted in a mi-nority of cases. Fasciitis, fibromatosis, and low-grade sarcoma of the breast are very rare and should only be diagnosed after the possibility of spindle cell carcinoma is excluded.

Lobular Carcinoma In Situ versus Ductal Carcinoma In Situ

In situ carcinoma of the breast is categorized histologically as either ductal (DCIS) or lobular (LCIS) depending on the cytologic features and growth pattern. With the advent of screening mammography, the reported inci-dence of noninvasive lesions, especially DCIS, has increased markedly. In the Breast Cancer Detection Demonstration Project, for example, 31% of the cancers detected only by screening mammography were noninvasive. It is now well recognized that the natural histories of DCIS and LCIS are different. Whereas DCIS is associated with the development of invasive cancer at or near the biopsy site in the ipsilateral breast, LCIS appears to be a marker for increased risk of developing invasive cancer at any site in either breast at nearly equal rates.

Although distinguishing between DCIS and LCIS is usually not diffi-cult, there is overlap between these 2 types of lesions. Ductal carcinoma in situ may extend into recognizable lobules; LCIS may involve extralob-ular ducts. Some lesions may have cytologic features intermediate be-tween these 2 disorders. However, this problem is more challenging in CNB specimens and more so with the introduction of the pleomorphic variants of LCIS. Recent studies have shown that immunostaining for E-cadherin is useful in distinguishing between LCIS and DCIS; however, long-term studies are needed to determine the clinical significance of this finding. We recommend that an excisional biopsy be done when lesions cannot be categorized with confidence as LCIS or DCIS after examination of CNB specimens.

Carcinoma In situ versus Invasive Carcinoma

One of the most important goals in the histologic examination of carci-noma is the identification of stromal invasion because, in general, the therapeutic algorithm for patients with pure carcinoma in situ differs from that of patients with stromal invasion.

Most of the mistaken diagnoses are overdiagnoses of in situ lesions as invasive or microinvasive carcinoma. Lesions and conditions that are com-monly mistaken for invasion or microinvasion include DCIS involving

---

KEY PRACTICE POINTS

- Image-guided biopsies represent important advances in the diagnosis and management of breast lesions.

- Standardization in the processing and pathologic evaluation of specimens from image-guided biopsies is essential for optimizing diagnostic results.

- A correlation between radiologic, pathologic, and clinical findings is necessary in every case.

- Breast lesions are best managed when the clinician, radiologist, pathologist, and surgeon are all involved in diagnosis and treatment.

---

lobules (cancerization of lobules); branching of ducts; distortion or entrapment of involved ducts or acini by fibrosis; inflammation obscuring involved ducts or acini; crush or cautery artifacts; artifactual displacement of DCIS cells into the surrounding stroma or adipose tissue due to tissue manipulation or a prior needling procedure; and DCIS or LCIS involving benign sclerosis, such as radial scars, complex sclerosing lesions, and sclerosing adenosis.

There are a number of ways to resolve these diagnostic issues to distinguish the lesions or conditions that mimic stromal invasion from true stromal invasion. Obtaining further levels through the block is often useful in defining the nature of the process. Immunohistochemical staining to identify myoepithelial cells is the most reliable method for determining the absence or presence of invasion. In our experience, as well as that of others, the use of smooth-muscle actin antibodies can reliably identify myoepithelial cells. The presence of myoepithelial cells around nests of tumor cells confirms an in situ lesion. However, caution must be exercised in the interpretation of actin stains because myofibroblasts will also stain positive. Some researchers have recommended the use of more specific markers, such as calponin and the smooth-muscle actin heavy chain, for identifying myoepithelial cells.

When CNB specimens are used, a conservative approach to the diagnosis of stromal invasion, especially microinvasion, should be exercised. If there is doubt, the final determination is best made after an excisional biopsy is performed.

SUGGESTED READINGS

Acs G, Lawton TJ, LiVolsi VA, Zhang PJ. Differential expression of E-cadherin in ductal and lobular carcinoma of the breast. *Mod Pathol* 2000;13:17A. Abstract 77.
Baker LH. Breast Cancer Detection Demonstration Project: five-year summary report. *CA Cancer J Clin* 1982;32:194–225.

Ballo MS, Sneige N. Can core needle biopsy replace fine-needle aspiration cytology in the diagnosis of palpable breast carcinoma. A comparative study of 124 women. *Cancer* 1996;78:773–777.

Boerner S, Fornage B, Singletary E, Sneige N. Ultrasound-guided fine needle aspiration of non-palpable breast lesions: a review of 1,885 FNA cases using the NCI-supported recommendations on the uniform approach to breast FNA. *Cancer Cytopathology* 1999;87:19–24.

Brenner RJ, Fajardo L, Fisher PR, et al. Percutaneous core biopsy of the breast: effect of operator experience and number of samples on diagnostic accuracy. *AJR Am J Roentgenol* 1996;166:341–346.

Burbank F. Stereotactic breast biopsy of atypical ductal hyperplasia and ductal carcinoma in situ lesions: improved accuracy with directional, vacuum-assisted biopsy. *Radiology* 1997;202:843–847.

Chinyama CN, Davies JD. Mammary mucinous lesions: congeners, prevalence and important pathological associations. *Histopathology* 1996;29:533–539.

Coady AT, Shousha S, Dawson PM, Moss M, James KR, Bull TB. Mucinous carcinoma of the breast: further characterization of its three subtypes. *Histopathology* 1989;15:617–626.

Dershaw DD, Morris EA, Liberman L, Abramson AF. Nondiagnostic stereotaxic core breast biopsy: results of rebiopsy. *Radiology* 1996;198:323–325.

Dowlatshahi K, Yaremko ML, Kluskens LK, Jokich PM. Nonpalpable breast lesions: findings of stereotaxic needle-core biopsy and fine-needle aspiration cytology. *Radiology* 1991;181:745–750.

Ely K, Carter B, Page D, Jensen RA, Simpson J. Core biopsy of the breast with atypical ductal hyperplasia: probabilistic approach to reporting. *Mod Pathol* 2000;13:21. Abstract 101.

Flotte TJ, Bell DA, Greco MA. Tubular carcinoma and sclerosing adenosis: the use of basal lamina as a differential feature. *Am J Surg Pathol* 1980;4:75–77.

Fornage BD, Coan JD, David CL. Ultrasound-guided needle biopsy of the breast and other interventional procedures. *Radiol Clin North Am* 1992;30:167–185.

Fraser JL, Raza S, Chorny K, Connolly JL, Schnitt SJ. Columnar alteration with prominent apical snouts and secretions: a spectrum of changes frequently present in breast biopsies performed for microcalcifications. *Am J Surg Pathol* 1998;22:1521–1527.

Gala I, Fisher P, Hermann GA. Usefulness of Telfa pads in the histologic assessment of stereotactic-guided breast biopsy specimens. *Mod Pathol* 1999;12:553–557.

Gobbi H, Simpson JF, Borowsky A, Jensen RA, Page DL. Metaplastic breast tumors with a dominant fibromatosis-like phenotype have a high risk of local recurrence. *Cancer* 1999;85:2170–2182.

Hamele-Bena D, Cranor ML, Rosen PP. Mammary mucocele-like lesions. Benign and malignant. *Am J Surg Pathol* 1996;20:1081–1085.

Hoang MP, Sahin AA, Ordonez NG, Sneige N. HER-2/neu gene amplification compared with HER-2/neu protein overexpression and interobserver reproducibility in invasive breast carcinoma. *Am J Clin Pathol* 2000;113:852–859.

Hull MT, Warfel KA. Mucinous breast carcinomas with abundant intracytoplasmic mucin and neuroendocrine features: light microscopic, immunohistochemical, and ultrastructural study. *Ultrastruct Pathol* 1987;11:29–38.

Ioffe OB, Berg WA, Silverberg SG, Kumar D. Mammographic-histopathologic correlation of large-core needle biopsies of the breast. *Mod Pathol* 1998;11:721–727.

Ioffe OB, Silverberg SG, Simsir A. Lobular lesions of the breast: immunohistochemical profile and comparison with ductal proliferations. *Mod Pathol* 2000;13:23. Abstract 115.

Jackman RJ, Nowels KW, Shepard MJ, Finkelstein SI, Marzoni FA Jr. Stereotaxic large-core needle biopsy of 450 nonpalpable breast lesions with surgical correlation in lesions with cancer or atypical hyperplasia. *Radiology* 1994;193: 91–95.

Jacobs TW, Siziopikou KP, Prioleau JE, et al. Do prognostic marker studies on core needle biopsy specimens of breast carcinoma accurately reflect the marker status of the tumor? *Mod Pathol* 1998;11:259–264.

Komaki K, Sakamoto G, Sugano H, et al. The morphologic feature of mucus leakage appearing in low papillary carcinoma of the breast. *Hum Pathol* 1991;22:231–236.

Kraus FT, Neubecker RD. The differential diagnosis of papillary tumors of the breast. *Cancer* 1962;15:444–455.

Landercasper J, Gundersen Jr SB, Gundersen AL, Cogbill TH, Travelli R, Strutt P. Needle localization and biopsy of nonpalpable lesions of the breast. *Surg Gynecol Obstet* 1987;164:399–403.

Liberman L, Bracero N, Vuolo MA, et al. Percutaneous large-core biopsy of papillary breast lesions. *AJR Am J Roentgenol* 1999a;172:331–337.

Liberman L, Cohen MA, Dershaw DD, Abramson AF, Hann LE, Rosen PP. Atypical ductal hyperplasia diagnosed at stereotaxic core biopsy of breast lesions: an indication for surgical biopsy. *AJR Am J Roentgenol* 1995a;164:1111–1113.

Liberman L, Dershaw D, Glassman JR, et al. Analysis of cancers not diagnosed at stereotactic core breast biopsy. *Radiology* 1997;203:151–157.

Liberman L, Dershaw DD, Rosen PP, et al. Stereotaxic core biopsy of breast carcinoma: accuracy at predicting invasion. *Radiology* 1995b;194:379–381.

Liberman L, Evans WP III, Dershaw DD, et al. Radiography of microcalcifications in stereotaxic mammary core biopsy specimens. *Radiology* 1994;190:223–225.

Liberman L, Sama M, Susnik B, et al. Lobular carcinoma in situ at percutaneous breast biopsy: surgical biopsy findings. *AJR Am J Roentgenol* 1999b;173:291–299.

Mainiero MB, Philpotts LE, Lee CH, et al. Stereotactic core needle biopsy of breast microcalcifications: correlation of target accuracy and diagnosis with lesion size. *Radiology* 1996;198:665–669.

McDivitt RW, Boyce W, Gersell D. Tubular carcinoma of the breast. Clinical and pathological observations concerning 135 cases. *Am J Surg Pathol* 1982;6:401–411.

Mitnick JS, Vazquez MF, Pressman PI, Harris MN, Roses DF. Stereotactic fine-needle aspiration biopsy for the evaluation of nonpalpable breast lesions: report of an experience based on 2,988 cases. *Ann Surg Oncol* 1996;3:185–191.

Nath ME, Robinson TM, Tobon H, Chough DM, Sumkin JH. Automated large-core needle biopsy of surgically removed breast lesions: comparison of samples obtained with 14-, 16-, and 18-gauge needles. *Radiology* 1995;197:739–742.

Oberman HA, Fidler WJ Jr. Tubular carcinoma of the breast. *Am J Surg Pathol* 1979;3:387–395.

Page DL, Salhany KE, Jensen RA, Dupont WD. Subsequent breast carcinoma risk after biopsy with atypia in a breast papilloma. *Cancer* 1996;78:258–266.

Papotti M, Eusebi V, Gugliotta P, Bussolati G. Immunohistochemical analysis of benign and malignant papillary lesions of the breast. *Am J Surg Pathol* 1983;7:451–461.

Parker SH. Percutaneous large core breast biopsy. *Cancer* 1994;74(suppl 1):256–262.

Parker SH, Burbank F, Jackman RJ, et al. Percutaneous large-core breast biopsy: a multi-institutional study. *Radiology* 1994;193:359–364.

Peters GN, Wolff M, Haagensen CD. Tubular carcinoma of the breast. Clinical pathologic correlations based on 100 cases. *Ann Surg* 1981;193:138–149.

Pisano ED, Fajardo LL, Tsimikas J, et al. Rate of insufficient samples for fine-needle aspiration for nonpalpable breast lesions in a multicenter clinical trial: the Radiologic Diagnostic Oncology Group 5 Study. *Cancer* 1998;82:679–688.

Raju UB, Lee MW, Zarbo RJ, Crissman JD. Papillary neoplasia of the breast: immunohistochemically defined myoepithelial cells in the diagnosis of benign and malignant papillary breast neoplasms. *Mod Pathol* 1989;2:569–576.

Reynolds HE, Jackson VP, Gin FM, et al. Large-gauge core needle biopsy of the breast. *Breast J* 1996;1:370–373.

Ro JY, Sneige N, Sahin AA, Silva EG, del Junco GW, Ayala AG. Mucocelelike tumor of the breast associated with atypical ductal hyperplasia or mucinous carcinoma. A clinicopathologic study of seven cases. *Arch Pathol Lab Med* 1991;115:137–140.

Rosen PP. Mucocele-like tumors of the breast. *Am J Surg Pathol* 1986;10:464–469.

Rosen PP, Obermann HA. *Atlas of Tumor Pathology, Tumors of the Mammary Gland. Third Series, Fascicle 7.* Armed Forces Institute of Pathology, Washington, DC, 1993.

Schwartz GF, Feig SA, Patchefsky AS. Significance and staging of nonpalpable carcinomas of the breast. *Surg Gynecol Obstet* 1988;166:6–10.

Scopsi L, Andreola S, Pilotti S, et al. Mucinous carcinoma of the breast. A clinicopathologic, histochemical, and immunocytochemical study with special references to neuroendocrine differentiation. *Am J Surg Pathol* 1994;18:702–711.

Sharifi S, Peterson MK, Baum J, et al. Assessment of standard prognostic factors in breast core needle biopsies (CNB). *Mod Pathol* 1999;12:941–945.

Skinner MA, Swain M, Simmons R, McCarty Jr KS, Sullivan DC, Iglehart JD. Nonpalpable breast lesions at biopsy. A detailed analysis of radiographic features. *Ann Surg* 1988;208:203–208.

Sneige N, Tulbah A. Accuracy of cytologic diagnoses made from touch imprints of image-guided needle biopsy specimens of nonpalpable breast abnormalities. *Diagn Cytopathol* 2000;23:29–34.

Wargotz, ES, Deos, PH, Norris, HJ. Metaplastic carcinomas of the breast. II. Spindle cell carcinoma. *Hum Pathol* 1989;20:732–740.

Wong AY, Salisbury E, Bilous M. Recent developments in stereotactic breast biopsy methodologies: an update for the surgical pathologist. *Adv Anat Pathol* 2000;7:26–35.

World Health Organization. *Histological Typing of Breast Tumors.* 2nd ed. Geneva: World Health Organization, 19, 1981.

Wright CJ. Breast cancer screening: a different look at the evidence. *Surgery* 1986;100:594–598.

Yaziji H, Sneige N, Mandavilli S, et al. Spindle cell carcinoma (SpCC) of the breast: a clinicopathologic study of 30 cases. *Mod Pathol* 1999; Abstract 178.

7 SURGICAL OPTIONS FOR BREAST CANCER

Funda Meric and Kelly K. Hunt

Chapter Overview

Over the past decade, the surgical management of breast disease has evolved significantly, and the trend has been towards less invasive approaches. The introduction of stereotactic core needle biopsy has allowed less invasive diagnosis of nonpalpable breast lesions. Breast conservation therapy has become accepted as an alternative to mastectomy for most patients with ductal carcinoma in situ and early-stage invasive breast cancer. The use of preoperative chemotherapy has made breast conservation therapy feasible for selected locally advanced tumors. The use of sentinel lymph node biopsy has allowed surgeons to avoid axillary lymph node dissection and its associated morbidity in many patients with early-stage breast cancer. Postoperative hospital stays have shortened such that most patients now recuperate at home after a short observation period in the hospital.

Introduction

Breast cancer remains a major cause of mortality in women. It is crucial for surgeons and oncologists to keep up with the rapidly changing diagnostic approaches and treatment strategies for breast cancer. This chapter will summarize the basic algorithm and the rationale for the surgical approach used at M. D. Anderson Cancer Center. We believe a similar treatment approach would also be beneficial to patients receiving treatment outside a comprehensive cancer center.

Surgical Approach to Diagnostic Biopsies

The widespread use of screening mammography has led to increased detection of nonpalpable mammographic abnormalities. The traditional approach to diagnosis of these lesions is needle-localization excisional biopsy. Recently, stereotactic core needle biopsy (SCNB), a less invasive technique, has been introduced as an alternative to excisional biopsy.

Stereotactic Core Needle Biopsy

The introduction of SCNB has altered the diagnostic approach to both nonpalpable and palpable abnormalities of the breast. The use of SCNB has been shown to shorten the time from detection of a mammographic abnormality to pathologic diagnosis, reduce the incidence of positive margins and the reexcision rate, and reduce cost per patient compared with the routine use of needle-localization excisional biopsy (Lind et al, 1998). At M. D. Anderson, SCNB is the preferred method of diagnosis for nonpalpable mammographic abnormalities that are not visualized on breast sonography.

Core needle biopsy is the preferred diagnostic approach for palpable breast lesions as well because it can establish the diagnosis of invasive cancer and thus facilitate surgical planning (Figure 7–1). Among patients with palpable breast lesions, fine-needle aspiration biopsy is mainly used to establish the diagnosis of metastases in patients with palpable lymph nodes.

Stereotactic core needle biopsy is not possible in patients who weigh more than the weight limit of the stereotactic system. Patients who cannot remain prone or cannot cooperate for the duration of the procedure are also not candidates for SCNB. Bleeding disorders and concomitant use of anticoagulants are relative contraindications for SCNB. Patients who have very small breasts or mammographic abnormalities immediately under the skin surface are difficult to biopsy with the stereotactic system and are usually referred for surgical biopsy. When small mammographically detected lesions are biopsied with a stereotactic approach, a metallic marker is placed at the same time if biopsy will lead to excision of all microcalcifications or complete removal of a mass lesion.

The pathologic diagnosis obtained by SCNB dictates whether further intervention is needed (Figure 7–2). Fifty percent of patients with an SCNB diagnosis of atypical ductal hyperplasia and 20% of patients with an SCNB diagnosis of radical scar are found to have a coexistent carcinoma near the site of the SCNB. Therefore, these diagnoses on SCNB should be followed by surgical excisional biopsy. During operative planning, it should also be kept in mind that 20% of patients who have an SCNB diagnosis of ductal carcinoma in situ (DCIS) are found to have invasive carcinoma on excisional biopsy.

Excisional Biopsy

When SCNB cannot be performed, when further evaluation is required because of a diagnosis of atypical ductal hyperplasia or radial scar, or when the SCNB results are discordant with findings on imaging studies,

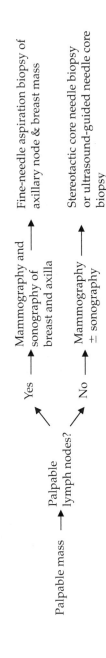

Figure 7–1. Approach to diagnostic biopsies for palpable breast masses.

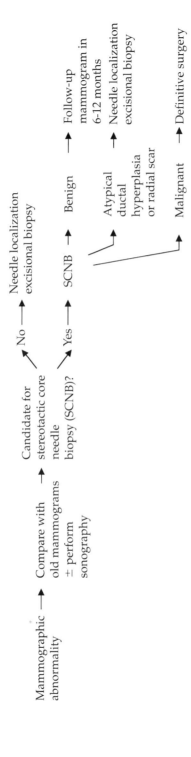

Figure 7–2. Approach to diagnostic biopsies for mammographically detected breast lesions.

an excisional biopsy is performed for diagnosis and, potentially, for treatment as well. At the time of excisional biopsy, the goal is to resect the lesion with margins of at least 1 cm so that the biopsy can also serve as definitive local therapy.

For nonpalpable lesions that can be visualized on sonography, intraoperative sonographic localization can be used to guide the excisional biopsy. For nonpalpable lesions that cannot be visualized by sonography, preoperative needle localization with a self-retaining hookwire is performed under mammographic guidance. The guidewire will usually enter the breast at an angle several centimeters from the lesion. Good communication between the radiologist and surgeon helps the surgeon determine the location of the lesion in the breast with respect to the wire.

After the excisional biopsy, the surgeon orients the specimen and hand-delivers it to the pathology department. The pathologist inks the lateral, medial, superior, inferior, superficial, and deep margins of the specimen in a color-coded fashion. A radiograph of the specimen is obtained to confirm the adequacy of the excision. Rarely, the targeted mass or microcalcifications are not demonstrated on the specimen radiograph. This may occur when the breast parenchyma in the excised specimen is very dense. In this scenario, the mammographic abnormality can usually be demonstrated if the specimen is sectioned serially and repeat specimen radiographs are obtained. If the mass or microcalcifications are not noted on repeat radiographs, further excision is performed. It is our standard at M. D. Anderson to obtain radiographs of both the whole specimen and the serial sections.

Great care is taken to ensure the best possible cosmetic outcome after excisional biopsy. The biopsy incision is oriented along the lines of skin tension (Langer's lines) to optimize the cosmetic outcome. The incision should be placed directly over the lesion being excised since this will result in less removal of uninvolved breast tissue. The biopsy incision may be placed so that it can be encompassed in a future mastectomy incision if mastectomy is ultimately necessary. The breast tissues—especially the skin edges—are handled gently to avoid formation of excessive scar tissue. Meticulous hemostasis of the biopsy cavity is crucial because a postoperative hematoma not only will affect the cosmetic result but also may make follow-up by physical examination more difficult. After hemostasis is achieved, the incision is closed with dermal and subcuticular sutures. Deep parenchymal sutures, which might cause distortion of the breast, are not placed. Some breast surgeons at M. D. Anderson fill the biopsy cavity with saline solution before finishing the skin closure. Although filling the cavity with saline solution results in a normal breast contour immediately after the procedure, no studies have been done to determine if this procedure leads to a better long-term aesthetic outcome.

SURGICAL MANAGEMENT OF DUCTAL CARCINOMA IN SITU

The management of DCIS is controversial. The traditional treatment for DCIS is total mastectomy, and cure rates with this approach are near 100%. However, because lumpectomy followed by radiation therapy (breast conservation therapy) has been shown to be equivalent to mastectomy for treatment of early-stage invasive breast cancer, the need for mastectomy for DCIS has been questioned. The recent National Surgical Adjuvant Breast and Bowel Project (NSABP) B-17 trial update demonstrated that patients with localized DCIS can be successfully treated with lumpectomy and postoperative radiation therapy (Fisher et al, 1998). In the B-17 trial, at a median follow-up of 90 months, the rate of ipsilateral breast tumors detected after treatment of DCIS was 1.9 per 100 patients per year. Thirty of the 47 ipsilateral breast tumors were noninvasive; the other 17 were invasive breast cancer.

The results of a recent study called into question the role of postoperative radiation therapy after resection of DCIS with negative margins (Silverstein et al, 1999). This retrospective study evaluated the outcome of 469 patients with DCIS who had been treated with lumpectomy with or without radiation therapy according to the choice of the patient and her physician. Among patients with margins of excision of at least 10 mm, postoperative radiation therapy was not found to lower the local recurrence rate. Among patients with margins of 1 to 10 mm, the relative risk of local recurrence in patients who did not receive radiation therapy compared with patients who did was 1.49 ($P = 0.24$); when the margin width was less than 1 mm, the relative risk was 2.54 ($P = 0.01$). In contrast, in the NSABP B-17 trial, even on reanalysis, all patient cohorts benefited from radiation therapy regardless of clinical or mammographic tumor characteristics.

Selection of Therapy

At M. D. Anderson, the surgical treatment plan for patients with DCIS is based on several factors, including tumor size, tumor grade, margin width, mammographic appearance, and patient preference. Lumpectomy alone is considered in selected patients with small (<1 cm) lesions of low nuclear grade that have been excised with margins of at least 5 mm.

Most patients with DCIS are candidates for lumpectomy and radiation therapy. Patients for whom postoperative radiation therapy is planned are evaluated by the radiation oncologist before surgery to confirm that there are no contraindications to radiation. For patients with collagen vascular disease or previous radiation therapy and patients who are pregnant, postoperative radiation therapy is contraindicated, and total mastectomy is a more appropriate surgical treatment option.

Mastectomy is indicated in patients with diffuse, malignant-appearing calcifications in the breast and in patients with persistent positive margins after repeated attempts at surgical excision. Although certain histologic subtypes of DCIS are associated with an increased likelihood of multicentric disease, histologic subtype alone is not used to determine surgical treatment. Large tumor size is not an absolute indication for mastectomy; however, mastectomy is often preferred for patients with high-grade DCIS larger than 3 to 4 cm. Few studies have addressed the efficacy of breast conservation therapy for DCIS larger than 4 cm.

Patient preference is a crucial determinant in the choice of surgical treatment. The benefits and risks of mastectomy and breast conservation therapy are discussed in detail with each patient. Compared with mastectomy, breast conservation therapy is associated with a higher risk of local recurrence, including a higher risk of invasive breast cancer. However, the literature to date indicates that the choice of treatment—mastectomy versus breast conservation therapy—does not influence overall survival. The choice of treatment, then, is based on the patient's anxiety about recurrent disease and the projected impact of mastectomy on the patient's self-esteem, sexuality, and quality of life. Immediate breast reconstruction is considered for all patients who require or elect mastectomy.

Operative Strategy

Most patients with DCIS present with microcalcifications on mammography. Stereotactic core needle biopsy is the preferred diagnostic approach. Definitive surgical treatment consists of either mastectomy or lumpectomy following preoperative needle localization of the microcalcifications.

In patients treated with lumpectomy, a specimen radiograph is obtained while the patient is still under anesthesia. If the radiograph shows that microcalcifications extend to the cut edge of the specimen, further excision is performed immediately. To facilitate postoperative radiation therapy planning and mammographic follow-up, the extent of the lumpectomy cavity is marked with radio-opaque clips. A postoperative mammogram is obtained as soon as the patient can tolerate the required compression of the breast. If the mammogram reveals residual calcifications in the breast, a reexcision is performed. Reexcision is also indicated if the margins are deemed inadequate on pathologic analysis; postoperative radiation therapy should not be used as a substitute for good surgical treatment.

Patients who have mastectomy for treatment of DCIS are considered for skin-sparing mastectomy and immediate breast reconstruction. Extensive DCIS is not considered a contraindication for the skin-sparing approach. In patients with extensive DCIS or DCIS close to the skin surface, a radiograph of the sliced mastectomy specimen is obtained to confirm the adequacy of the margins of excision. If the radiograph demonstrates microcalcifications on the superficial (anterior) aspect, further skin can be excised.

The role for axillary dissection in DCIS is limited. In theory, because DCIS is noninvasive, lymph node involvement would not be expected. However, in patients with larger tumors or extensive microcalcifications, the possibility of missing a focus of invasion because of pathologic sampling error exists. In patients treated with mastectomy for large, high-grade DCIS, a low-level axillary dissection is often performed for staging purposes. Because DCIS diagnosed by SCNB is associated with concomitant invasive cancer in 20% of cases, sentinel lymph node biopsy is considered for patients with large, high-grade DCIS who are undergoing lumpectomy. (For more information, see the section Sentinel Lymph Node Biopsy later in this chapter.)

Postoperative Surveillance

In patients who are treated with lumpectomy and postoperative radiation therapy, another mammogram of the treated breast is obtained 6 months after the completion of radiation therapy. This mammogram serves as the new baseline mammogram. After all treatment is complete, patients have twice-yearly physical examinations and annual mammograms for 5 years and annual physical examinations and mammograms thereafter. Patients treated with mastectomy are followed with twice-yearly physical examinations and annual mammography of the contralateral breast for 5 years and with annual physical examination and mammography thereafter. The use of tamoxifen to reduce the risk of ipsilateral breast cancer recurrence and for chemoprevention of contralateral breast cancer should be discussed with the patient.

SURGICAL MANAGEMENT OF EARLY-STAGE INVASIVE BREAST CANCER

Early-stage invasive breast cancer (stage I or II disease) can be successfully managed with either mastectomy or breast conservation therapy (lumpectomy followed by radiation therapy). Over the past 20 years, the efficacy of breast conservation therapy has been studied in several prospective trials. One of the most widely cited studies is the NSABP B-06 trial (Fisher et al, 1989). In this trial, women with tumors up to 4 cm in size with N0 or N1 nodal status were randomly assigned to one of 3 treatment strategies: modified radical mastectomy, lumpectomy and axillary lymph node dissection followed by radiation therapy, or lumpectomy and axillary lymph node dissection alone. Patients who had lumpectomy specimens with positive margins were excluded. There were no differences in overall survival between the 3 treatment groups. However, patients who had radiation therapy in addition to lumpectomy had significantly lower local recurrence rates than did patients treated with lumpectomy and axillary dissection alone.

Selection of Therapy

Because mastectomy and breast conservation therapy appear to be equivalent in terms of patient survival, the choice of surgical treatment for stage I and stage II disease is individualized. Patients who desire breast conservation must be willing and able to attend postoperative radiation treatment sessions and to undergo close postoperative surveillance of the breast. These patients must also be willing to accept a 10% to 12% long-term risk of local recurrence.

Patients interested in breast conservation therapy see the radiation oncologist before the planned surgery. A mastectomy is recommended for patients who have contraindications to radiation therapy. Patients are advised about the risks of radiation therapy.

Factors related to the tumor also must be considered in the selection of surgical treatment. A key factor in determining whether breast conservation therapy is feasible is the relationship between tumor size and breast size: the tumor must be small enough in relation to the breast to permit the tumor to be resected with adequate margins and acceptable cosmesis. Breast conservation therapy is generally reserved for tumors smaller than 4 cm; however, it can be performed for larger tumors in patients with larger breasts. The use of preoperative chemotherapy may decrease the tumor size sufficiently to permit breast-conserving surgery in patients who would not otherwise appear to be good candidates. This strategy is used commonly at M. D. Anderson. Another strategy for patients with tumors that are large in relation to the size of the breast is the use of a latissimus dorsi flap to fill the defect resulting from lumpectomy. Thus a multidisciplinary approach optimizes the chance of breast conservation in patients with larger tumors. Patients with multicentric tumors are usually served best by mastectomy because recurrence rates may be higher and it is difficult to perform more than one lumpectomy in the same breast with acceptable cosmesis. Although high nuclear grade, lymphovascular invasion, and negative hormone receptor status have all been linked to increased local recurrence rates, none of these factors are considered contraindications to breast conservation.

Mastectomy and Breast Reconstruction

Many patients with early-stage breast cancer who undergo mastectomy at M. D. Anderson elect to undergo breast reconstruction. Most of these patients are candidates for immediate reconstruction, which allows for a better cosmetic result and provides substantial psychological benefit to the patient. Either an autologous tissue flap or implants may be used for reconstruction, although flap reconstruction usually gives a better cosmetic outcome. A skin-sparing mastectomy is often performed because preservation of the breast envelope allows for a more natural contour for the reconstructed breast. No increase in the risk of local recurrence has been found with the use of the skin-sparing technique in patients with early-stage disease (Kroll et al, 1999).

SURGICAL MANAGEMENT OF LOCALLY ADVANCED BREAST CANCER

Patients who present with locally advanced breast cancer—a tumor 5 cm or larger (T3), a tumor that involves the skin or chest wall (T4), or fixed or matted axillary lymph nodes (N2)—have traditionally been treated with mastectomy in addition to chemotherapy and radiation therapy. However, we have found that with preoperative chemotherapy, a significant number of patients with locally advanced breast cancer at presentation can become candidates for breast conservation therapy.

Breast Conservation Therapy after Tumor Downstaging

In M. D. Anderson's initial feasibility study of breast-conserving surgery in patients with locally advanced breast cancer, the mastectomy specimens of 143 patients with locally advanced disease who received preoperative chemotherapy were analyzed (Singletary et al, 1992). Of these 143 patients, 33 (23%) had complete resolution of skin edema, had a residual tumor smaller than 5 cm, had lesions that were not multicentric, and had no extensive lymphatic invasion or extensive suspicious microcalcifications. These 33 patients would have been appropriate candidates for segmental mastectomy and axillary lymph node dissection rather than a modified radical mastectomy.

In our current practice, patients with locally advanced breast cancer are examined by a multidisciplinary team at presentation and then begin preoperative chemotherapy. Clinical response to preoperative chemotherapy is monitored after each cycle of chemotherapy. Patients are usually converted from inoperable to operable status after 3 or 4 cycles of chemotherapy; patients who do not respond after 3 to 4 cycles are considered for alternate chemotherapeutic regimens.

Patients with significant clinical tumor shrinkage after the first or second chemotherapy cycle undergo sonography and placement of metallic markers to facilitate subsequent localization of the tumor under ultrasound or mammographic guidance and to facilitate specimen radiography. At the conclusion of preoperative chemotherapy, these patients undergo repeat breast imaging and are then reevaluated by the multidisciplinary team to determine the options for local treatment. Patients who desire breast conservation therapy and who have had an adequate response to preoperative chemotherapy are considered for segmental mastectomy followed by radiation therapy. It is preferable that the residual tumor size after preoperative chemotherapy be 4 cm or less, but the size of the tumor in relation to the size of the breast is also taken into consideration. Patients who have extensive microcalcifications on mammography, multicentric disease on physical examination or mammography, or persistent skin edema on physical examination are not considered to be candidates for breast conservation therapy.

Recently, a review was done of 93 patients who underwent breast conservation therapy after preoperative chemotherapy at M. D. Anderson (Peoples et al, in press). Approximately 50% of the patients had stage IIA or IIB disease at presentation, and approximately 50% had stage IIIA or IIIB disease; 4 patients had disease classified as stage IV because of supraclavicular adenopathy. At a median follow-up of 73 months, 9 patients had had local recurrence, for an overall local recurrence rate of 9.7%. In 6 of these patients, local recurrence was the first type of recurrence; in the other 3 patients, disease recurred locally after distant metastases were detected. These results confirm that selected patients with locally advanced breast cancer at presentation can undergo breast conservation therapy after tumor downstaging with acceptable risk of local recurrence.

Modified Radical Mastectomy and Integration of Plastic Surgery for Chest Wall Coverage

Patients with locally advanced breast cancer whose tumors have enlarged after 3 courses of preoperative therapy undergo chemotherapy with a different drug regimen and are then considered for surgical resection (Figure 7–3) or radiation therapy followed by surgical resection. The goal of surgery in patients with locally advanced breast cancer is to achieve the best possible local control in order to avoid chest wall recurrence. In most patients, local control can be achieved with a standard modified radical mastectomy. For some stage IIIB tumors, however, invasion of the skin or chest wall may necessitate a more extensive skin excision or an en bloc chest wall resection. These more radical surgical resections are possible because M. D. Anderson has a highly skilled reconstructive surgery team.

Most soft tissue and skin defects are repaired with the use of autologous myocutaneous flaps. When the defect is limited to the skin, simple skin grafts can theoretically provide adequate coverage, but this approach has 2 disadvantages: a poorer cosmetic outcome and an extended healing period for both the donor and recipient areas, which delays initiation of postoperative adjuvant therapy. Thus, myocutaneous flaps are preferred for most patients.

The 2 most commonly used flaps are the latissimus dorsi flap and the rectus abdominis flap. The latissimus dorsi flap has less donor site morbidity relative to rectus flaps and has a reliable blood supply; however, this flap is limited in size. The transverse rectus abdominis myocutaneous (TRAM) flap can be much larger owing to the laxity of abdominal wall skin. The pedicled TRAM flap relies for its viability on perforators from the superior epigastric vessel. Alternatively, a free TRAM flap can be used; with this option, blood supply is based on the deep inferior epigastric vessels, and a microvascular anastomosis is performed to establish blood flow to the flap. The flap loss rate for free TRAM flaps is less than 1% at M. D. Anderson.

When a chest wall resection is performed, pedicled flaps are preferred in order to avoid complications that could occur in the rare scenario of loss of a free flap. A latissimus dorsi flap is the best choice for small defects, and a pedicled or bipedicled TRAM flap is used for larger defects or defects low on the chest wall. Reconstruction of the rib cage is usually not necessary if only 1 or 2 ribs are removed. For larger defects, Marlex or Prolene mesh is used to reconstruct the chest wall, and the participation of a thoracic surgery team may also be required. This multispecialty surgical approach optimizes the chance for margin-negative resection of chest wall tumors and thus optimizes the chance for local control.

AXILLARY STAGING

Axillary staging has 2 major goals. One goal is to obtain prognostic information. Axillary lymph node status—whether lymph node metastases are present and, if they are present, the number of lymph nodes involved and the extent of the involvement—is a powerful prognostic factor. The prognostic value of axillary lymph node status is not diminished in patients who have received preoperative chemotherapy. With our increasing understanding of cancer biology, several molecular markers that are prognostic have been identified, but no single marker or combination of markers to date reliably predicts patient prognosis as well as axillary lymph node status does.

The other goal of axillary staging is to obtain information that can affect decisions about treatment. Patients with tumors smaller than 1 cm would not be offered chemotherapy on the basis of the primary tumor characteristics alone. However, if the axillary nodes were determined to contain occult disease, these patients would be offered chemotherapy. In any patient with invasive breast cancer, if macroscopic extracapsular extension and involvement of several lymph nodes were detected, the patient would be treated with radiation therapy in addition to surgery because these findings are known to increase the risk of local-regional recurrence.

Axillary staging is usually performed in patients with invasive breast cancer, and axillary staging is considered for patients with DCIS who have large, high-grade lesions. In patients with microinvasion, the decision whether axillary staging is necessary is based on prognostic factors such as the patient's age and the size, histologic features, and hormone receptor

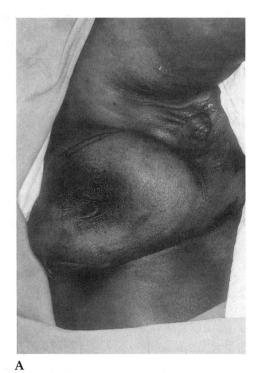

A

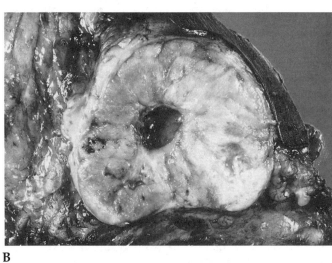

B

Figure 7–3. Mastectomy for locally advanced breast cancer. A, Locally advanced breast cancer that showed minimal response to preoperative chemotherapy. B, Resected specimen demonstrating an 11-cm invasive ductal carcinoma.

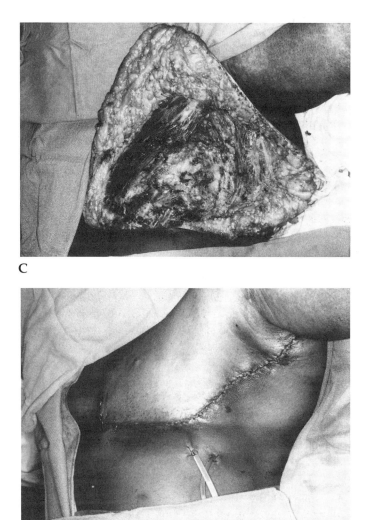

C

D

Figure 7–3. *(continued)* C, Defect after modified radical mastectomy with en bloc pectoral muscle resection. D, Closure of the mastectomy defect with a rotational flap.

status of the tumor. In patients with small (<1 cm) tubular carcinomas, axillary involvement is rare; thus axillary staging is not usually performed in this setting.

Axillary staging has traditionally been accomplished with axillary lymph node dissection. However, because of the recent introduction of the technique of sentinel lymph node biopsy, axillary staging can now be accomplished with only selective nodal dissection in many patients.

Traditional Axillary Lymph Node Dissection

Traditional axillary lymph node dissection involves the removal of level I and II axillary lymph nodes. The level III axillary nodes are no longer included in the dissection because removal of these nodes may increase the risk of lymphedema without providing significant additional information. Level III lymph node involvement occurs in fewer than 1% of patients when no metastasis is detected in level I or II lymph nodes.

The need to perform a level I and II axillary lymph node dissection in all patients with invasive breast cancer has recently been questioned for several reasons. Axillary dissection is associated with more potential morbidity than any other part of breast surgery. The most common complications are lymphedema, decreased range of motion in the shoulder, and sensory deficits in the upper arm due to disruption of the intercostobrachial nerves. Another drawback is the formation of seromas within the axilla, which can delay postoperative therapy. Another important reason to consider the more selective use of axillary dissection is the increasing rate of detection of DCIS and small invasive cancers, which have a very low rate of axillary lymph node metastases. Finally, decisions regarding the use of adjuvant chemotherapy and hormonal therapy are increasingly being made on the basis of the size of the primary tumor. Many patients are now treated with chemotherapy in the preoperative setting regardless of the axillary lymph node status. The introduction of lymphatic mapping with sentinel lymph node biopsy allows for a more selective approach to the axilla without the need for complete lymph node dissection in all patients.

Sentinel Lymph Node Biopsy

The first node to receive lymphatic drainage from a specific area of the breast is termed the sentinel node. This node is the node most likely to contain metastases if the tumor has indeed metastasized. Thus, when properly identified, the sentinel lymph node should indicate whether metastases are present in a lymph node basin. Feasibility studies have confirmed the proof of concept, and numerous subsequent studies have shown that the technique is accurate.

Sentinel lymph node biopsy allows the selective use of axillary lymph node dissection: patients with positive sentinel lymph nodes undergo completion axillary lymph node dissection, but patients with negative sentinel lymph nodes can be spared complete axillary dissection and the associated morbidity. Furthermore, the sentinel lymph node technique may increase the chance that metastases, if present, will be detected. With an axillary lymph node dissection, detailed analysis of all the lymph nodes removed is usually not possible. In contrast, the sentinel lymph node technique directs attention to a smaller number of nodes, allowing more careful analysis of the lymph node most likely to have a positive yield. Careful analysis requires step-sectioning of the lymph node. Immunohistochemical techniques can further enhance sensitivity by allowing detection of micrometastases. However, the clinical relevance of micrometastases detected by immunohistochemical techniques alone or reverse transcriptase–polymerase chain reaction is not yet understood.

Technique

The current approach to lymphatic mapping at M. D. Anderson involves the use of both technetium-labeled sulfur colloid and a vital blue dye (lymphazurin) for localization of the sentinel lymph node. The radiolabeled colloid and blue dye are injected around the tumor into the breast parenchyma (Figure 7–4). In patients with nonpalpable tumors, the radiolabeled colloid and blue dye are delivered under ultrasonographic or mammographic guidance.

A preoperative lymphoscintigram is obtained in almost all patients treated with sentinel node biopsy regardless of tumor location (Figure 7–5). The lymphoscintigram can provide information on the specific nodal basins draining the primary tumor, the number of sentinel nodes in each nodal basin, and the necessary time required before a node can be detected within the basin. Approximately 1 to 4 hours before surgery, filtered sulfur colloid labeled with 0.5 to 1.0 mCi of technetium is injected around the tumor. The time between injection of the radiolabeled colloid and identification of a lymph node in the nodal basin on preoperative lymphoscintigraphy can be used to help plan the timing of the sentinel lymph node biopsy after injection of radiolabeled colloid on the day of surgery. If preoperative lymphoscintigraphy demonstrates drainage to internal mammary lymph nodes, an internal mammary node biopsy can be considered. The inability to demonstrate a sentinel lymph node on preoperative lymphoscintigraphy does not preclude the success of intraoperative lymph node mapping. To avoid the inconvenience for the patient of having technetium-labeled sulfur colloid injections performed on 2 separate days, we recently started injecting a higher dose (2.5 mCi) of technetium the day before the operation, thus eliminating the need for a repeat injection the day of the operation.

The patient is brought to the operating suite between 1 and 4 hours after the preoperative technetium injection. The delay allows time for the colloid to travel to the nodal basin. In the operating room, 5 mL of blue dye is injected peritumorally, and then the injection site is massaged to facilitate passage of dye through the lymphatics. Next, transcutaneous localization of an area of increased radioactivity is attempted with a gamma probe. Localization may be difficult due to the radioactivity from the injection site, especially if the injection site is located in the lateral aspect of the breast. After an incision is made, localization of an area of increased radioactivity is again attempted with the gamma probe. If no such area can be found with the gamma probe, the surgeon relies on the

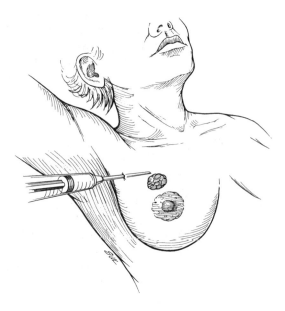

A

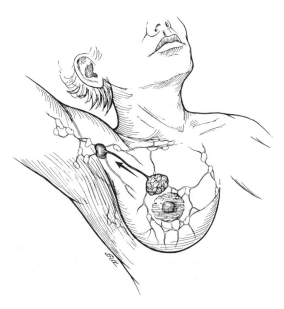

B

Figure 7–4. Sentinel lymph node biopsy for breast cancer. A, Peritumoral injection of blue dye. B, Blue dye draining into the sentinel lymph node.

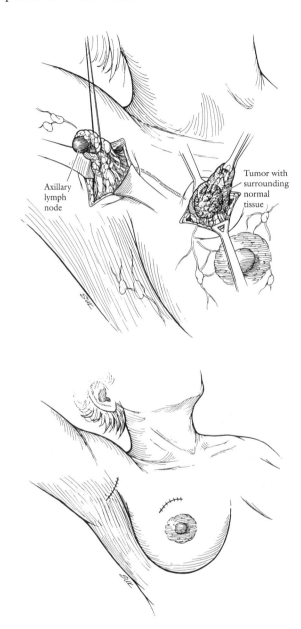

Axillary
lymph
node

Tumor with
surrounding
normal
tissue

C

D

Figure 7–4. *(continued)* C, Sentinel lymph node biopsy and wide local excision of the primary tumor. D, Skin closure at the conclusion of sentinel lymph node biopsy and breast-conserving surgery.

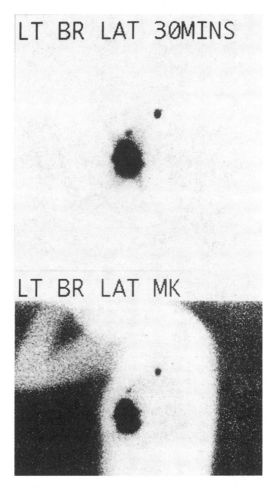

Figure 7–5. Lymphoscintigram demonstrating drainage into 2 axillary lymph nodes.

visualization of blue dye alone to identify the sentinel node. The surgeon traces the path of the blue-stained lymphatics leading away from the tumor. Dissection is done carefully to avoid prematurely disrupting the afferent lymphatic channel and staining of the surgical field with blue dye or blood. If a blue-stained lymphatic channel cannot be identified, a segmental mastectomy is performed to remove the site of injection of the radiolabeled colloid and thus decrease the background "shine through" radioactivity, thus facilitating localization of the sentinel node with the gamma probe. In most cases the blue node that is identified is also highly radioactive, as demonstrated by the probe. Once the sentinel node is excised, the axilla is checked again to confirm that the level of radioactivity has decreased. If the level of radioactivity remains high, this may indicate that additional sentinel nodes are present. Most studies have demonstrated an average of 2 sentinel nodes per patient.

Patient Selection

Our current practice at M. D. Anderson is to perform sentinel lymph node biopsy in all patients with clinically negative axillary nodes. Surgeons experienced in the technique of sentinel node biopsy can identify a sentinel lymph node in 95% of patients. The false-negative rate for sentinel lymph node biopsy ranges from 0.2% to 5%. The appropriateness of sentinel lymph node biopsy alone without completion axillary dissection must be determined for each individual patient, with this false-negative rate taken into consideration. Patients who present with clinically palpable axillary nodes are treated with complete axillary node dissection or considered for preoperative chemotherapy.

In patients who have undergone previous excisional biopsy of the primary tumor, accurate identification of the sentinel lymph node may be difficult. The lymphatics may have been disrupted by the biopsy, and the drainage pattern of the area surrounding the excisional biopsy site might be different from the drainage pattern of the original tumor. If an excisional biopsy has already been performed for a tumor at high risk for lymph node involvement, an axillary dissection is considered in addition to a sentinel lymph node biopsy. Ideally, this scenario should be avoided from the start by planning the sentinel lymph node biopsy at the time of excisional biopsy for highly suspicious lesions. The use of core needle biopsy prior to an open surgical biopsy would allow for planning of a sentinel lymph node biopsy at the time of tumor excision.

PROPHYLACTIC MASTECTOMY

Prophylactic mastectomy can reduce the risk of breast cancer in women who are at high risk for the disease, and it can reduce the risk of contralateral breast cancer in women who have already been diagnosed with unilateral breast cancer. However, the degree of benefit depends on patient and tumor factors. Careful evaluation of the potential risks and benefits and careful patient counseling are essential in the case of any woman considering prophylactic mastectomy.

Bilateral Prophylactic Mastectomy in Women at High Risk for Breast Cancer

The efficacy of bilateral prophylactic mastectomy was demonstrated by Hartmann et al in a study published in 1999. In this retrospective study,

639 women with a family history of breast cancer who had undergone bilateral prophylactic mastectomy were followed for a median of 14 years. The women were divided into 2 groups, high-risk and moderate-risk, on the basis of family history. According to the Gail model, 37.4 breast cancers were expected in the moderate-risk patients; 4 breast cancers actually occurred in this group (a risk reduction of 89.5%). Women in the high-risk group were compared with their sisters who had not undergone prophylactic surgery, and a risk reduction of at least 90% was found.

Survival Benefit

Using a decision analysis model, Schrag and colleagues calculated that on average, a 30-year-old woman who carries *BRCA1* or *BRCA2* mutations gains between 2.9 and 5.3 years of life expectancy from prophylactic mastectomy (Schrag et al, 1997). In this analysis, gains in life expectancy were expected to decline with age and were minimal for 60-year-old women. In another decision analysis, quality-of-life adjustment was performed, taking into account the perceived negative features of prophylactic surgery (Grann et al, 1998). For a 30-year-old high-risk woman, the improvement in survival with bilateral prophylactic mastectomy was calculated to be 2.8 to 3.4 years, with 1.9 quality-adjusted life-years saved compared with surveillance alone.

Although breast cancers have been reported after bilateral prophylactic mastectomy, it is clear that this surgery is indeed effective in decreasing the risk of breast cancer in young women at high risk. In young women with *BRCA1* and *BRCA2* mutations, no data are currently available regarding the efficacy of chemopreventive agents, and surveillance is difficult because the breasts tend to be denser and theoretical concerns exist about the safety of mammograms. In this population, then, bilateral prophylactic mastectomy may be a valid preventive option. Patients, however, should be advised that alternatives may be available in the near future.

In patients with a moderate risk of breast cancer, the utility of bilateral prophylactic mastectomy decreases with decreases in predicted cancer risk. In the study by Hartmann et al (1999), 33.4 cancers were prevented among the 425 women at moderate risk for breast cancer who underwent prophylactic surgery. The lower the expected breast cancer risk, the more bilateral prophylactic mastectomies must be performed to prevent 1 case of breast cancer. Thus in any clinical scenario, a woman's decision as to whether she is willing to undergo bilateral prophylactic mastectomy depends on how much risk she is willing to assume.

Patient Counseling

At M. D. Anderson, women with a family history of breast cancer who are interested in genetic testing undergo extensive counseling before and after such testing. If a genetic predisposition is confirmed by genetic testing or is highly suspected on the basis of analysis of the patient's pedigree, the possibility of prophylactic bilateral mastectomy is raised, and its potential benefits and risks are explained. The individual preferences of such women for bilateral prophylactic mastectomy versus close observation can be affected by several factors, including the patient's age, education, occupation, self-image, cultural and religious beliefs, and prior experience with surgery and disease.

Patients who are identified as being at increased risk for breast cancer because of a diagnosis of lobular carcinoma in situ or atypical ductal hyperplasia are told of their increased risk and given advice on close surveillance and chemoprevention. Prophylactic surgery is presented as an option but is usually not encouraged. This approach is supported by a survey of 370 women in the National Prophylactic Mastectomy Registry. In this study, regrets about prophylactic surgery were found to be most common in women with whom discussion about prophylactic mastectomy was initiated by a physician (Borgen et al, 1998).

Surgical Approach

Most patients who undergo bilateral prophylactic mastectomy choose to undergo immediate reconstruction. In such cases, a skin-sparing mastectomy is performed to achieve a better cosmetic outcome. The breast tissue left behind after a skin-sparing approach has not been found to be different from the amount of breast tissue left behind after traditional total mastectomy in terms of the associated breast cancer risk. The role of preservation of the nipple-areola complex, which might further enhance cosmetic outcome, remains to be determined.

Elective Contralateral Mastectomy

Elective contralateral mastectomy can be performed in women already diagnosed with unilateral breast cancer to reduce the risk of cancer development in the contralateral breast. As is the case with bilateral prophylactic mastectomy, the benefit of elective contralateral mastectomy depends on patient and tumor factors.

Survival Benefit

The utility of elective contralateral mastectomy depends on the risk of cancer development in the contralateral breast and on the prognosis associated with second breast tumors. The risk of developing carcinoma in the second breast is estimated to be 0.5% to 1% per year from the time of the initial diagnosis of breast cancer. In a review of 1036 patients with operable breast cancer treated at M. D. Anderson, the prognosis of patients with bilateral disease (44 synchronous and 17 metachronous) was similar to the prognosis of patients with unilateral carcinoma (Berte et al, 1988).

Invasive lobular carcinoma has been associated with an increased risk of contralateral breast disease. In a series of 133 patients with invasive lobular carcinoma treated at M. D. Anderson, 18 patients had undergone elective contralateral mastectomy (Babiera et al, 1997). None of the 18 patients had occult carcinoma in their mastectomy specimens. Three of these patients developed distant metastases from their original breast tumor. At a median follow-up of 68 months, 3 (3%) of the 115 patients who were managed with close observation had developed contralateral disease. No survival difference was noted between the 2 groups.

Patients diagnosed with unilateral breast cancer will most likely be followed closely after treatment is complete, and this close follow-up should facilitate the timely detection of any contralateral breast cancer. Given the possibility of recurrence and death from the original carcinoma, while elective contralateral mastectomy will most likely reduce the risk of contralateral breast cancer, it is not likely to significantly affect survival in most patients.

The only group identified to date in which elective contralateral mastectomy may confer a significant survival benefit is young patients who are diagnosed with early-stage ipsilateral disease and who are at high risk for contralateral disease because of genetic predisposition. It has been predicted that a 30-year-old woman with lymph node–negative breast cancer associated with *BRCA1* or *BRCA2* mutations would gain 0.6 to 2.1 years of life expectancy with elective contralateral mastectomy (Schrag et al, 2000). Older age and higher-risk primary breast cancer would attenuate the gains.

Patient Counseling

In patients diagnosed with unilateral breast cancer, it is crucial to discuss the risk of contralateral breast cancer and its potential impact on survival. Careful surveillance with physical examination and yearly mammograms is a reasonable plan for most patients with the exception of young women with a genetic predisposition. In patients who receive hormonal treatment for their initial tumor, this treatment may reduce the risk of cancer development in the contralateral breast. However, elective contralateral mastectomy may be used selectively on the basis of the emotional needs of the patient.

At M. D. Anderson, 155 patients with unilateral breast cancer and negative findings in the contralateral breast on physical examination and mammography chose to undergo elective contralateral mastectomy and immediate reconstruction between 1987 and 1995. On careful review of patient records, factors that appeared to influence the use of prophylactic surgery were family history of breast cancer in first-degree relatives (30%), any family history of breast cancer (56%), anticipated difficulty in contralateral breast surveillance (48%), associated lobular carcinoma in situ (23%), multicentric primary tumor (28%), reconstructive issues (14%), and failure of mammographic detection of the primary tumor (16%) (Gershenwald et al, 1998).

Surgical Approach

Women treated for breast cancer at M. D. Anderson often choose to undergo reconstruction with a TRAM flap, which can produce excellent cosmetic results. When TRAM flap reconstruction is performed, patients with large breasts may also need a reduction mammoplasty of the contralateral breast to achieve symmetry with the reconstructed breast, while patients with small breasts may need a breast augmentation of the contralateral breast. Women who require a surgical procedure on their contralateral breast may opt for an elective contralateral mastectomy to decrease their risk of contralateral breast cancer.

Bilateral TRAM flap reconstructions are possible, but only if both breasts are reconstructed at the same time. To reduce the possibility of subsequently developing contralateral breast cancer and having to undergo breast reconstruction with a different technique, which will most likely result in asymmetrical reconstructed breasts, some patients choose to undergo elective contralateral mastectomy with bilateral TRAM flap reconstruction.

In patients who choose elective contralateral mastectomy, the procedure is performed at the same time as the mastectomy performed for treatment of breast cancer. In patients who require postoperative radiation therapy, reconstruction is usually deferred until radiation therapy is complete. These patients may elect to undergo elective contralateral mastectomy at the time of delayed breast reconstruction.

OUTPATIENT SURGERY FOR BREAST CANCER

Over the past decade, hospital stays after most operative procedures have decreased. Prior to that, patients often remained in the hospital until their drains were removed, which generally occurred 2 to 3 weeks after surgery. Edwards et al examined the M. D. Anderson experience in 1988 and found that institution of a policy by which patients were admitted to the hospital on the day of surgery and discharged earlier (fourth postoperative day) resulted in a 34% reduction in hospital charges. This resulted in a change in the preoperative and postoperative stays for patients undergoing breast cancer surgery. In 1993, M. D. Anderson established a 23-hour "short stay" program for patients undergoing breast surgery. Currently, patients who undergo axillary dissections are observed for a short time (generally under 24 hours) before being discharged for recovery at home. Patients who undergo segmental mastectomy without an axillary procedure are treated on an outpatient basis. Patients who undergo immediate breast reconstruction usually require longer hospital stays to allow for the monitoring of the tissue flaps used in the reconstruction. Preoperative admissions are reserved for patients with underlying major medical problems requiring preoperative management and stabilization.

The success of the short-stay program depends in large part on the preoperative teaching and counseling process. Patients and their caregivers attend preoperative classes during which they receive instructions about the preoperative and postoperative care plan, including demonstrations on mannequins of postoperative incision and drain care. Patients also receive general instructions about postoperative diet and ambulation and specific instructions regarding arm exercises and lymphedema precautions. Patients and caregivers who are unable to manage the postoperative care are identified, and in such cases, arrangements are made for the assistance of a home-health nurse. Patients are also seen by a Reach to Recovery representative before surgery. These volunteers have all had breast cancer surgery and provide instruction on postoperative rehabilitation needs.

After the surgery, patients are admitted to short-stay observation units. After the observation period, patients are discharged home provided they have stable vital signs, intact wounds, an acceptable volume of output from their drains, and adequate pain control and that they are able to ambulate, void on their own, and tolerate food. Hospital discharge may be delayed in patients with underlying medical problems or special social circumstances. In a review of 187 patients treated in the ambulatory setting at M. D. Anderson, 17 patients (9.1%) were hospitalized longer than the planned 23-hour observation period. The major reasons for extended hospitalization were management of postoperative nausea and vomiting, pain control, and social factors.

A theoretical concern whenever duration of hospitalization is decreased is the impact of early discharge on quality of care and patient safety. After axillary procedures, the most worrisome postoperative complication is that of postoperative bleeding. In the review of the M. D. Anderson experience, the incidence of postoperative bleeding was found to be 2.7%. Most instances of postoperative bleeding occurred within 4 hours of the operation, and all occurred within 8 hours of the operation. These results confirm that patients can indeed be discharged home after a period of observation without compromise of patient safety.

Evaluation of our short-stay program at M. D. Anderson has shown that most patients are highly satisfied with their overall experience. In a survey, 52 patients were interviewed 24 to 72 hours after discharge and again 7 to 10 days after discharge (Burke et al, 1997). Most patients reported no difficulty with drain and incision care (84%), reported adequate pain control with the prescribed analgesic regimen (>95%), and felt prepared to leave the hospital on the first postoperative day (85%). Thus the practice of ambulatory surgery for breast cancer is well accepted by patients.

Special Situations

The following special situations are encountered less frequently but represent interesting management problems.

Patients with Prior Breast Augmentation

Patients who have undergone prior breast augmentation represent a special group with regard to both diagnostic and therapeutic planning. Mammographic screening is more difficult in patients who have had previous breast augmentation, especially if the implant was placed in a retroglandular rather than a submuscular position. Magnetic resonance imaging can be especially helpful in detecting implant-related problems such as prosthesis rupture or silicone leakage but is inferior to mammography in detecting DCIS and small carcinomas. Once an abnormality is detected in a woman with breast implants, the diagnostic approach needs to be carefully selected to avoid injury to the implant. In patients with an adequate amount of breast tissue between the breast lesion and the implant, image-guided needle biopsy can be used for diagnosis. Real-time sonography allows for continuous visualization of the needle during insertion and sampling, with pinpoint accuracy and safety (Fornage et al, 1994). Otherwise, surgical excisional biopsy would be the diagnostic approach of choice.

After breast cancer is diagnosed in a woman with implants, a choice needs to be made between mastectomy and breast conservation therapy. Breast conservation therapy may be problematic because of the increased risk of capsular contracture with postoperative radiation therapy. The risk of capsular contracture in the irradiated breast is reported to be as high as 65% (Handel et al, 1996). Patients with implants who desire breast conservation need to either accept the higher risk of cosmetic failure and the possible need for subsequent revisions or consider implant removal before radiation therapy.

Breast augmentation also affects axillary staging. Anecdotal evidence suggests that lymphatic mapping is often unsuccessful in patients with implants. This probably reflects a disruption of lymphatics during implant placement. Patients with implants should be considered for axillary dissection rather than, or in addition to, sentinel lymph node biopsy if axillary staging is deemed necessary.

Patients with Bilateral Breast Cancer

Women with breast cancer have an increased risk of developing a second primary breast cancer in the contralateral breast. The incidence of metachronous contralateral cancer is estimated to be 0.5% to 1% per year. Careful physical examination and mammography of the contralateral breast are crucial parts of the preoperative assessment of all patients with primary breast cancer.

Patients with synchronous bilateral breast cancer may choose the option of bilateral mastectomy with or without reconstruction. This option decreases both the risk of local recurrence and the risk of a subsequent new primary cancer. In patients who strongly desire breast conservation therapy, this approach can be pursued if both tumors can be treated with breast-conserving surgery.

Patients with metachronous bilateral breast cancer also may be treated with either mastectomy or breast conservation therapy. Of 1328 patients treated with breast conservation therapy at M. D. Anderson between 1958 and 1994, 63 developed contralateral breast cancer (Heaton et al, 1999). Eight patients had bilateral breast cancers, and the others developed contralateral breast cancer at a median of 63 months after the first tumor was diagnosed. The contralateral tumor tended to be smaller than the initial tumor at the time of diagnosis. Breast conservation therapy remained the preferred method of treatment for the contralateral tumor. Of the 45 patients in whom breast conservation therapy was judged appropriate, 39 (87%) elected this method of treatment for their contralateral tumor. Five of the 18 patients who had mastectomy chose to have a simultaneous prophylactic mastectomy. Recurrence rates for patients who underwent breast conservation therapy for a second tumor were not different from recurrence rates for patients who had breast conservation therapy for an initial tumor. Therefore both breast conservation and mastectomy are acceptable treatment options for bilateral breast cancer, and the treatment choice should be individualized.

Patients with Other Malignancies

Diagnosis of a breast mass in a patient with another known malignancy raises 2 issues. First, the origin of the breast mass must be determined to exclude the possibility of metastasis to the breast. Second, the extent of treatment to be rendered to the breast must be determined, taking into consideration the patient's other malignancy.

In a series of 1034 breast fine-needle aspiration biopsies performed at M. D. Anderson, 389 revealed malignancy, and in 20 cases (5.1%), the breast lesion represented metastasis to the breast from another site (Sneige et al, 1989). In patients with metastasis to the breast, the most common primary cancer is contralateral breast cancer, followed by melanoma, lymphoma, ovarian cancer, and lung cancer.

On physical examination, metastases in the breast are often superficial and mobile. On mammography, they may be well circumscribed and thus may resemble a benign process. Metastases in the breast may also be infiltrative, suggesting a primary breast carcinoma. Multiple or bilateral nodules of uniform size and density are especially suggestive of metastatic disease. Accurate diagnosis relies on pathologic evaluation and requires communication of the patient's history to the pathologist. Review of the patient's previous pathologic samples is invaluable.

   Metastasis to the breast usually indicates diffuse metastatic disease and poor prognosis. Accurate diagnosis of metastatic disease is important to avoid unnecessary radical surgery. The outcome of patients with metastases to the breast is dependent on the aggressiveness of the underlying disease. Similarly, the treatment of a primary breast cancer in a patient with another active malignancy should be tailored to the expected outcome of both diseases.

Patients with Nipple Discharge

Nipple discharge in women, although a frequent cause of concern, is rarely due to breast cancer. In contrast, nipple discharge in men is very suggestive of malignancy. The evaluation of nipple discharge starts with a careful history, including the duration of the discharge; whether it is unilateral or bilateral, cyclic, or spontaneous; any other symptoms; and medication use. Nipple discharge that is persistent, spontaneous, unilateral, and from a single duct is of special concern. In addition to palpating the breast and nodal basins, the physician should try to induce the discharge and localize the breast quadrant and duct associated with the discharge. Testing of the discharge for hemoglobin is especially helpful. Nipple aspirate cytology is often of low yield; however, ductal lavage, which yields a much higher number of cells, will be possible in the near future. Mammography and sonography should be performed, along with ductography of the suspicious duct. Ductography may reveal an intraductal lesion. Even if a lesion is not identified on ductography, however, an excisional biopsy is indicated in patients with bloody or persistent discharge. The excisional biopsy is facilitated by injecting methylene blue into the duct before surgery. The operation is started with a periareolar incision and elevation of the areola to allow identification of the blue duct. The identified ductal system with surrounding breast tissue is removed. The extent of the excision can be tailored to encompass the findings on the preoperative ductogram. If a single ductal system cannot be identified before surgery, the ducts emanating from the quadrant of the breast identified can be excised, or, in patients who do not plan to nurse children in the future, a subareolar central biopsy can be performed.

Inflammatory Breast Cancer

Inflammatory breast cancer is a rare but especially aggressive form of locally advanced breast cancer. Patients with inflammatory breast cancer present with an erythematous, warm, edematous breast. The clinical picture is often confused with cellulitis or mastitis, leading to a delay in diagnosis. The presentation is due to involvement of the subdermal lymphatics with tumor emboli, and the diagnosis can be made with biopsy of the involved skin. Treatment of inflammatory breast cancer begins with chemotherapy. Patients who have significant resolution of the erythema and edema with chemotherapy proceed to surgery, followed by additional chemotherapy and radiation therapy. Patients who do not experience significant improvement in the skin and breast with preoperative chemotherapy receive an alternate chemotherapy regimen and are considered for preoperative radiation therapy.

Breast Cancer in Men

Men with breast cancer usually present with a palpable mass. Breast cancer needs to be differentiated from gynecomastia, the most frequent abnormality in the male breast. A thorough history, including medication and drug use and family history of breast cancer, is crucial. Diagnosis can often be made with a fine-needle aspiration biopsy. The surgical treatment is usually a modified radical mastectomy. If there is chest wall invasion, en bloc chest wall resection may be necessary to achieve negative margins. Adjuvant radiation therapy is considered for tumors that invade the skin or chest wall. In the absence of clinical trials addressing breast cancer in men, the criteria used for making decisions about adjuvant chemotherapy and hormonal therapy in men are the same as the criteria used in women.

Paget's Disease of the Nipple

Paget's disease of the nipple most often presents with erythema and scaly eczematous change in the nipple and areola. This may be accompanied by a change in sensation of the nipple and nipple discharge. The diagnosis of Paget's disease is obtained with full-thickness biopsy of the nipple or nipple-areola complex. Mammography and a thorough physical examination of the underlying breast are required because of the high rate of ipsilateral carcinoma in cases of Paget's disease. The surgical treatment needs to be tailored according to whether ipsilateral carcinoma is present and, if so, its location. Paget's disease of the nipple is treated with a central segmentectomy for local control. Associated ipsilateral breast carcinoma can be treated with a central segmentectomy rather than a mastectomy if there are no contraindications to breast conservation therapy. Postoperative radiation therapy is recommended in patients who elect to undergo breast-conserving surgery.

Cystosarcoma Phyllodes

Phyllodes tumors usually present as a palpable breast mass in women in their 40s. Mammography and sonography often demonstrate features suggestive of a fibroadenoma. The surgical treatment of choice is a wide local excision with negative margins. Larger tumors may necessitate a total mastectomy. An axillary lymph node dissection is not necessary for phyllodes tumors. About 20% to 25% of phyllodes tumors are malignant. Adjuvant radiation therapy should be considered in patients with malignant tumors if margins are inadequate. Adjuvant chemotherapy is usually reserved for recurrences.

INTEGRATION OF SURGERY WITH OTHER TREATMENT STRATEGIES

Over the past 2 decades, the role of adjuvant therapy in the treatment of breast cancer has been expanding. Systemic therapy is now recommended not only for patients with positive lymph nodes but also for patients with node-negative disease if their tumors are larger than 1 cm.

Another area of change has been in the sequencing of adjuvant chemotherapy and surgery. Preoperative chemotherapy has become the standard of care for inoperable locally advanced breast cancer. The trend at M. D. Anderson has been to also deliver preoperative chemotherapy to patients with operable breast cancer. Preoperative chemotherapy has 3 advantages. The first is that preoperative regression of tumor can allow breast-conserving surgery in patients who otherwise would have required a mastectomy. The second is the treatment of micrometastases without the delay necessary for recovery after surgery. The third advantage is the ability to assess a patient's response to treatment clinically, after several courses of chemotherapy, as well as pathologically, after surgical resection.

Preoperative chemotherapy at M. D. Anderson has resulted in excellent response rates (Figure 7–6). A 1988 study at M. D. Anderson found that 3 preoperative cycles of 5-fluorouracil, doxorubicin, and cyclophosphamide produced a complete pathologic response in 16.7% of patients and a partial response in 70.7% of patients (Hortobagyi et al, 1988). Disease progression during preoperative chemotherapy is rare; thus, the opportunity for definitive surgical treatment is not lost by giving preoperative chemotherapy to patients with operable tumors.

Surgery performed after preoperative chemotherapy is as safe as primary surgery. Rates of postoperative wound infection, flap necrosis, and delays in postoperative adjuvant therapy do not differ between patients who are treated with mastectomy after preoperative chemotherapy and patients who are treated with surgery first (Broadwater et al, 1991). Surgery is usually performed 3 weeks after the completion of preoperative chemotherapy to allow for recovery of chemotherapy-induced bone marrow suppression. White blood cell and platelet counts are routinely measured preoperatively. If the absolute neutrophil count is less than 1500 at 3 weeks after completion of preoperative chemotherapy, the operation is delayed, and consideration is given to the use of filgrastim (granulocyte colony-stimulating factor) to facilitate bone marrow recovery.

Chemotherapy is resumed 3 weeks after the operation. In patients who had preoperative chemotherapy, crossover to alternate chemotherapy

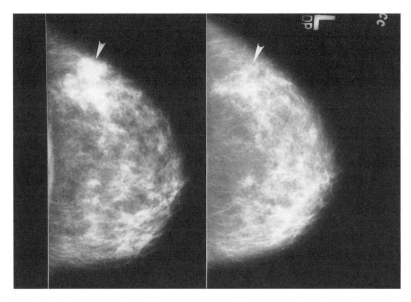

Figure 7–6. Downstaging of breast cancer with preoperative chemotherapy. The arrows point to the tumor on mammograms obtained before (left) and after chemotherapy (right).

regimens is considered if adequate pathologic response was not observed in the surgical specimen. Hormonal therapy, if appropriate, is also initiated after surgery.

Most patients who undergo breast-conserving surgery for DCIS or invasive disease at M. D. Anderson receive postoperative radiation therapy. Adjuvant postoperative chest wall irradiation is considered in patients treated with a mastectomy if the patient had a T4 primary tumor, 4 or more positive lymph nodes, positive ipsilateral supraclavicular lymph nodes, fixed or matted (N2) axillary lymph nodes, or macroscopic extranodal extension. Preoperative radiation therapy is usually reserved for patients with inoperable locally advanced breast cancer with progression of disease during preoperative chemotherapy.

The sequencing of postoperative radiation therapy and postoperative chemotherapy has received significant attention. Delaying postoperative chemotherapy raises concern about increased risk of systemic relapse, while delaying postoperative radiation therapy raises concern about local failure. In 2 studies, the outcome in patients who received postoperative chemotherapy followed by radiation therapy was compared with the outcome of patients who received postoperative radiation therapy followed by chemotherapy (Buzdar et al, 1993; Buchholz et al, 1999). In both studies, delay of irradiation in an effort to reduce the risk of sys-

---

KEY PRACTICE POINTS

- Preoperative diagnosis with SCNB can assist in operative planning and decrease reexcision rates.

- For DCIS, mastectomy is reserved for large, high-grade tumors and multicentric tumors; most other tumors are treated with lumpectomy and radiation therapy.

- Preoperative chemotherapy may achieve enough tumor downstaging to make breast conservation therapy feasible in selected locally advanced tumors.

- Skin-sparing mastectomy results in improved cosmetic outcome with no increase in local recurrence rates.

- Increased understanding of breast cancer biology and advances in genetic testing may allow us to determine which patients benefit from a prophylactic mastectomy.

- Sentinel lymph node biopsy provides accurate staging of the lymph node basin in patients with early-stage disease.

---

temic relapse was not associated with an increased risk of local failure. Currently at M. D. Anderson, for patients who are scheduled to receive postoperative chemotherapy, radiation therapy is deferred until the completion of chemotherapy.

IN SITU TUMOR ABLATION

A new treatment approach—in situ tumor ablation—is being actively investigated at M. D. Anderson as well as other institutions. Options being investigated for in situ tumor ablation include radiofrequency ablation, cryotherapy, and in situ laser ablation. These techniques are aimed at in situ destruction of a tumor detectable by an imaging modality (sonography, magnetic resonance imaging, or computed tomography), along with a surrounding rim of normal tissue. In situ ablation has the appeal of potential improvement in cosmetic outcome; its disadvantage is the lack of pathologic confirmation of cell death and negative margins. Surgical treatment is the gold standard with which in situ tumor ablation will be compared. The exact role for such in situ ablation techniques remains to be determined.

ACKNOWLEDGMENTS

The authors are grateful to Abigail Corona and Jacquilyn Valentine for assistance in preparation of the manuscript.

Suggested Readings

Babiera GV, Lowy AM, Davidson BS, Singletary SE. The role of contralateral prophylactic mastectomy in invasive lobular carcinoma. *The Breast Journal* 1997;3:2–6.

Bassett L, Winchester DP, Caplan RB, et al. Stereotactic core-needle biopsy of the breast: a report of the Joint Task Force of the American College of Radiology, American College of Surgeons, and College of American Pathologists. *CA Cancer J Clin* 1997;47:171–190.

Berte E, Buzdar AU, Smith TL, Hortobagyi GN. Bilateral primary breast cancer in patients treated with adjuvant therapy. *Am J Clin Oncol* 1988;11:114–118.

Borgen PI, Hill AD, Tran KN, et al. Patient regrets after bilateral prophylactic mastectomy. *Ann Surg Oncol* 1998;5:603–606.

Broadwater JR, Edwards MJ, Kuglen C, Hortobagyi GN, Ames FC, Balch CM. Mastectomy following preoperative chemotherapy: strict operative criteria control operative morbidity. *Ann Surg* 1991;213:126–129.

Buchholz TA, Hunt KK, Amosson CM, et al. Sequencing of chemotherapy and radiation in lymph node-negative breast cancer. *Cancer J Sci Am* 1999;5:159–164.

Burke CC, Zabka CL, McCarver KJ, Singletary SE. Patient satisfaction with 23-hour "short-stay" observation following breast cancer surgery. *Oncol Nurs Forum* 1997;24:645–651.

Buzdar AU, Kau SW, Smith TL, et al. The order of administration of chemotherapy and radiation and its effect on the local control of operable breast cancer. *Cancer* 1993;71:3680–3684.

Cox CE, Haddad F, Bass S, et al. Lymphatic mapping in the treatment of breast cancer. *Oncology* 1998;12:1283–1292.

Edwards MJ, Broadwater JR, Bell JL, Ames FC, Balch CM. Economic impact of reducing hospitalization for mastectomy patients. *Ann Surg* 1988;208:330–336.

Feig BW, Singletary SE, Ross MI, Kluger M, Ames FC. 23-hour observation is safe following breast surgery. *Proceedings of the Society of Surgical Oncology 48th Annual Cancer Symposium*, 1995;27 (abstract).

Fleming J, Breslin T, Delpassand A, et al. The utility of preoperative lymphoscintigraphy in the management of early stage breast cancer patients receiving sentinel node biopsy. *Proc Am Soc Clin Oncol* 1999;18:76 (abstract).

Fisher B, Dignam J, Wolmark N, et al. Lumpectomy and radiation therapy for the treatment of intraductal breast cancer: findings from National Surgical Adjuvant Breast and Bowel Project B-17. *J Clin Oncol* 1998;16:441–452.

Fisher B, Redmond C, Poisson R, et al. Eight-year results of a randomized clinical trial comparing total mastectomy and lumpectomy with or without irradiation in the treatment of breast cancer. *N Engl J Med* 1989;320:822–828.

Fornage BD, Sneige N, Singletary SE. Masses in breasts with implants: diagnosis with US-guided fine-needle aspiration biopsy. *Radiology* 1994;191:339–342.

Gershenwald JE, Hunt KK, Kroll SS, et al. Synchronous elective contralateral mastectomy and immediate bilateral breast reconstruction in women with early-stage breast cancer. *Ann Surg Oncol* 1998;5:529–538.

Grann VR, Panageas KS, Whang W, Antman KH, Neugut AI. Decision analysis of prophylactic mastectomy and oophorectomy in BRCA1-positive or BRCA2-positive patients. *J Clin Oncol* 1998;16:979–985.

Handel N, Lewinsky B, Jensen JA, Silverstein MJ. Breast conservation therapy after augmentation mammaplasty: is it appropriate? *Plast Reconstr Surg* 1996;98:1216–1224.

Hartmann LC, Schaid DJ, Woods JE, et al. Efficacy of bilateral prophylactic mastectomy in women with a family history of breast cancer. *N Engl J Med* 1999;340:77–84.

Heaton KM, Peoples GE, Singletary SE, et al. Feasibility of breast conservation therapy in metachronous or synchronous bilateral breast cancer. *Ann Surg Oncol* 1999;6:102–108.

Hortobagyi GN, Ames FC, Buzdar AU, et al. Management of stage III primary breast cancer with primary chemotherapy, surgery, and radiation therapy. *Cancer* 1988;62:2507–2516.

Hunt KK, Ames FC, Singletary SE, Buzdar AU, Hortobagyi GN. Locally advanced noninflammatory breast cancer. *Surg Clin North Am* 1996;76:393–410.

Hunt KK, Feig BW, Ames FC. Ambulatory surgery for breast cancer. *Cancer Bulletin* 1995;47:292–297.

Hunt KK, Kroll SS, Pollock RE. Surgical procedures for advanced local and regional malignancies of the breast. In: Bland KI, Copeland EM (eds). *The Breast: Comprehensive Management of Benign and Malignant Diseases.* Vol 2. Philadelphia: WB Saunders Co, 1998:1234–1243.

Hunt KK, Ross MI. Discussion of Cox CE, Haddad F, Bass S, et al. Lymphatic mapping in the treatment of breast cancer. *Oncology* 1998;12:1283–1298.

Krag D, Weaver D, Ashikaga T, et al. The sentinel node in breast cancer—a multicenter validation study. *N Engl J Med* 1998;339:941–946.

Kroll SS, Khoo A, Singletary SE, et al. Local recurrence risk after skin-sparing and conventional mastectomy: a 6-year follow-up. *Plast Reconst Surg* 1999;104:421–425.

Kroll SS, Miller MJ, Schusterman MA, Reece GP, Singletary SE, Ames F. Rationale for elective contralateral mastectomy with immediate bilateral reconstruction. *Ann Surg Oncol* 1994;1:457–461.

Lind DS, Minter R, Steinbach B, et al. Stereotactic core biopsy reduces the reexcision rate and the cost of mammographically detected cancer. *J Surg Res* 1998;78:23–26.

Peoples GE, Quan R, Heaton KM, et al. Breast conservation therapy for large primary and locally advanced breast cancers after induction chemotherapy. *Ann Surg Oncol.* In press.

Schrag D, Kuntz KM, Garber JE, Weeks JC. Decision analysis—effects of prophylactic mastectomy and oophorectomy on life expectency among women with BRCA1 or BRCA2 mutations. *N Engl J Med* 1997;336:1465–1471.

Schrag D, Kuntz KM, Garber JE, Weeks JC. Life expectancy gains from cancer prevention strategies for women with breast cancer and BRCA1 or BRCA2 mutations. *JAMA* 2000;283:617–632.

Silverstein MJ, Lagios MD, Groshen S, et al. The influence of margin width on local control of ductal carcinoma in situ of the breast. *N Engl J Med* 1999;340:1455–1461.

Singletary SE, McNeese MD, Hortobagyi GN. Feasibility of breast-conservation surgery after induction chemotherapy for locally advanced breast carcinoma. *Cancer* 1992;69:2849–2852.

Sneige N, Zachariah S, Fanning TV, Dekmezian RH, Ordonez NG. Fine-needle aspiration cytology of metastatic neoplasms in the breast. *Am J Clin Pathol* 1989;92:27–35.

Winchester DP, Strom EA. Standards for diagnosis and management of ductal carcinoma in situ (DCIS) of the breast. *CA Cancer J Clin* 1998;48:108–128.

8 RECONSTRUCTIVE SURGERY

Geoffrey L. Robb

CHAPTER OVERVIEW

Breast reconstruction is available today to almost any woman undergoing surgery for breast cancer. Several methods are available for reconstructing the breast either at the same time as breast cancer surgery (immediate reconstruction) or months or even years later, when the patient chooses (delayed reconstruction). These options include using autologous soft tissues from areas such as the abdomen, hips, back, or buttock and using a prosthetic implant to create a new breast mound. The new skin-sparing approach to mastectomy has facilitated immediate breast reconstruction and resulted in improved cosmetic outcomes. The risk of recurrence with this new approach has recently been determined to be no different from the risk of recurrence with standard mastectomy. Both immediate reconstruction (as opposed to delayed reconstruction) and use of the patient's own tissues (as opposed to use of an implant) have certain advantages. Adjuvant radiation therapy or chemotherapy can affect the breast reconstruction adversely, so careful preoperative planning is essential for the best cosmetic outcome. For the patient who has just learned of her breast cancer diagnosis and is confused about what outcome lies ahead, reassurance that her breast can be restored esthetically so that she can wear the same clothes she wore before surgery, including her bathing suit, and have essentially the same personal body image and level of self-esteem allows the patient to be confident that she can return to her family and workplace after treatment feeling whole and restored.

INTRODUCTION

Breast reconstruction after surgery for breast cancer is one of the most satisfying surgical procedures in practice today. Because of conceptual and technical advances in breast reconstructive surgery over the past decade, surgeons can now create a very natural-appearing breast after a complete or partial mastectomy, effectively restoring the natural form, shape, color, texture, and feel of the breast. Today, many patients with breast cancer choose to have breast reconstruction instead of living with a flat or depressed chest wall or, in the case of partial mastectomy, with a defect in the breast.

CURRENT STATUS OF BREAST RECONSTRUCTION
IN THE UNITED STATES

Over the past decade, there has been a gradual but significant shift in breast cancer treatment such that restoration of the patient's psychological and physical well-being is now considered an important part of her overall treatment.

The use of breast reconstruction in the United States has increased dramatically over the past decade. A total of 69,685 breast reconstructions were performed in 1998. This represents an increase of 64% over the number of breast reconstructions performed in 1996 and an increase of 135% over the number of breast reconstructions performed in 1992. In 1998, 30% of breast reconstructions in the United States were performed using autologous tissues. Forty-nine percent of breast reconstructions were performed in women aged 35 to 50 years, and 36% were performed in women aged 51 to 64 years. Immediate breast reconstructions made up 39% of the total. Our experience at M. D. Anderson Cancer Center reflects these national trends. We performed 32 breast reconstructions in 1986. In 1997, we performed more than 200 immediate breast reconstructions, approximately 1 for every 2 mastectomies performed that year.

The importance of breast reconstruction has recently been acknowledged at the federal and state levels in the form of laws requiring insurance companies to cover the costs of breast reconstruction. The Omnibus Budget Bill passed by the House of Representatives and the Senate in 1998 includes a requirement that insurance companies cover not only breast reconstruction for women undergoing breast cancer surgery but also the procedures necessary to restore symmetry between the reconstructed breast and the opposite, normal breast. In recent years, 29 states have also passed laws requiring insurance coverage for breast reconstruction, and the Omnibus Budget Bill will not preempt the state laws that already provide for at least the same level of coverage.

During the 1980s and 1990s, lawsuits were brought against implant manufacturers alleging that implants caused autoimmune disorders, and the plaintiffs were successful in a number of cases. However, in 1998, an independent National Science Panel appointed by Federal District Judge Sam C. Pointer, Jr., Coordinating Judge for the Federal Breast Implant Multi-District Litigation, made public a report that indicated there was no evidence to link silicone breast implants to systemic disease. This report included data from several studies supporting the conclusion that silicone implants do not alter the risk or severity of autoimmune disease. The report indicated no overt association between breast implants and specific connective tissue diseases, and it concluded that numerous rheumatologic symptoms in women with breast implants are also common in the general population of women. However, despite the lack of scientific evidence, implants have developed a reputation outside the medical community for potentially causing autoimmune or degenerative diseases, and as a result, many patients now distrust foreign-body devices and prefer reconstruction with autologous tissues.

TIMING OF RECONSTRUCTION

Breast reconstruction can be performed at the same time as breast cancer surgery (immediate reconstruction) or months or even years later, when the patient chooses (delayed reconstruction).

Until recent years, there was a misconception that breast reconstruction must be delayed for several years after mastectomy because reconstruction might prevent or delay detection of a local recurrence. If no recurrence was detected after 2 or more years of close follow-up, the patient was considered eligible for reconstruction. Of course, breast cancer can recur at any time after a mastectomy, regardless of reconstructive status, so patient self-examination and careful postoperative follow-up are strongly urged. However, there is no evidence to indicate that reconstruction delays or prevents detection of tumor recurrence, and several longer-term follow-up studies at M. D. Anderson actually indicate a lower incidence of local recurrence after reconstruction. Nevertheless, because of the historical concerns about immediate reconstruction, many patients with breast cancer who are facing surgery today are unaware that their breasts can be reconstructed at the same time as the mastectomy.

At M. D. Anderson, we recommend immediate reconstruction to eligible patients as often as possible because it is more labor-effective, is more cost-effective, is more convenient for the patient, and generally provides more cosmetically pleasing results than those typically achieved with delayed reconstruction. Both autogenous tissues and implants are available to patients who are considering immediate reconstruction. We have also shown that there is no difference in the rates of cancer recurrence between patients who undergo reconstruction and those who do not.

Advantages of Immediate Reconstruction

One of the most compelling advantages of immediate reconstruction is the superior cosmetic appearance of the reconstructed breast (Figure 8–1). The superior cosmetic results are due in large part to use of the skin-sparing approach to mastectomy, in which as much of the patient's own skin is preserved as is oncologically safe. The skin-sparing technique, first described by Toth and Lappert in 1991, is designed to facilitate and simplify breast reconstruction after modified radical mastectomy. During immediate reconstruction, the preserved breast skin guides restoration of the overall size and shape of the breast and, especially, the position of the breast on the chest wall relative to that of the normal breast.

The skin-sparing approach reduces visible scarring and reduces the color and texture mismatch that can occur with delayed reconstruction, especially when the immediate reconstruction is done with autologous tissues. Even in the case of reconstruction with implants, immediate reconstruction generally results in better cosmetic outcomes because the extra skin preserved with the skin-sparing approach facilitates subsequent expansion of the skin for placement of the permanent implant. In delayed reconstruction, expansion of the flat and foreshortened chest wall skin and muscle can be challenging because of the scarring of the chest wall and soft tissues.

Patients undergoing immediate reconstruction also have a reduced risk of anesthesia-related complications because anesthesia is induced only

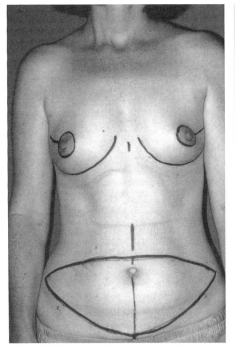 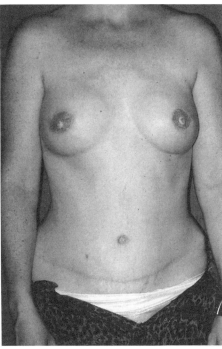

A   B

Figure 8–1. Bilateral skin-sparing mastectomy and immediate free transverse rectus abdominis myocutaneous flap breast reconstruction. A, Preoperative markings. B, Postoperative result after reconstruction including nipple reconstruction and areolar tattooing.

once, not twice, and patients have the added convenience of 1 hospitalization instead of 2. Many patients who undergo immediate reconstruction state that they would not likely have come back for reconstruction at a later time because the experience would have been too strong a reminder of their original cancer ordeal and the recovery would have seemed too great a challenge once they had recovered from the mastectomy.

Immediate reconstruction also has psychological benefits for the patient. With immediate reconstruction, the patient awakens from breast surgery with an intact breast. Thus the patient never has to live with chest wall deformity. In the past, breast reconstruction was sometimes delayed with the goal of making the patient more anxious for and appreciative of breast reconstruction. This practice is now considered outmoded and unacceptable. Many studies have confirmed that immediate reconstruction preserves normal body image, self-esteem, and sexual functioning.

The resource savings possible with immediate reconstruction in comparison with delayed reconstruction are significant. One recent study from

M. D. Anderson's Department of Plastic Surgery compared hospital charges for patients who underwent immediate ($n = 221$) or delayed ($n = 55$) reconstruction with autologous tissues. The mean total corrected resource cost of mastectomy with delayed reconstruction was 62% higher than the cost of mastectomy with an immediate plastic surgery procedure. The savings came primarily from less total operating time and fewer days of inpatient hospitalization.

Immediate Reconstruction in Patients with Locally Advanced Breast Cancer

Immediate reconstruction is possible even in patients with locally advanced breast cancer. A study at M. D. Anderson compared 50 patients with locally advanced breast cancer who had undergone modified radical mastectomy and immediate breast reconstruction between 1990 and 1993 with 72 patients with locally advanced breast cancer who underwent modified radical mastectomy without reconstruction during the same time period. All the patients were treated on a standard protocol for locally advanced breast cancer, including preoperative chemotherapy, postoperative chemotherapy, and radiation therapy. Among patients who underwent immediate breast reconstruction, 70% had reconstruction with autologous tissue flaps, and 30% had reconstruction with implants. There were 2 partial flap losses but no complete flap losses. Seven of the 15 patients who had reconstruction with implants required removal of the implants because of infection, severe internal scarring, or capsule problems after radiation therapy. The time to postoperative chemotherapy was marginally better in the patients who did not undergo reconstruction. No significant differences in local or distant relapse rates were observed between the 2 groups over the 58-month mean follow-up period. This study suggests that immediate breast reconstruction can be performed in patients with locally advanced breast cancer with acceptable morbidity and suggests that these patients have a risk of relapse similar to that of patients who do not undergo reconstruction. An important insight from this study was that outcomes of reconstruction in patients with locally advanced breast cancer are better when the reconstruction is accomplished using autologous tissues. The reason for this finding is that a high percentage of these patients need radiation therapy, which may cause implant problems and eventual loss of the implant.

OPTIONS FOR RECONSTRUCTION

Breast reconstruction can be performed with prosthetic implants, autologous tissues, or both materials in combination. Although each method of reconstruction has both advantages and disadvantages, reconstruction with autologous tissues tends to produce consistently superior outcomes. Use of the patient's own tissues tends to provide the most natural-appearing breast in terms of shape, contour, fullness of the upper breast, and, especially, softness of the breast. Use of implants generally cannot reproduce the natural appearance and feel of the breast as well as use of the patient's own tissues can. Another factor to consider in the use of the patient's own tissues is the long-term costs of the reconstruction. Initially, the implant approach costs less than the autologous-tissue approach. Thus reconstruction with implants is attractive to health maintenance organizations and third-party payers. However, M. D. Anderson statistics show that within 4 years after reconstruction, the cost of reconstruction with implants begins to overtake the cost of reconstruction with autologous tissues.

Today, many candidates for breast reconstruction are focused on obtaining the best possible long-term functional and cosmetic results and minimizing the potential for additional surgery to correct complications. Reconstruction with autologous tissues generally provides the best chance of achieving these goals. The majority of patients at M. D. Anderson who elect to have reconstruction with implants do so because of the relative simplicity of the procedure and the shorter operating time.

Reconstruction with Implants

Breast implants are filled with either saline or silicone, and they are available in a variety of shapes—round, oval, or anatomic. Regardless of their internal composition, all implants have an outer vulcanized silicone shell. The shell can be smooth or "textured," which means that the outer silicone shell has an irregular surface.

In most cases, reconstruction with implants—whether immediate or delayed—requires several stages because the chest wall skin and underlying muscle must be expanded to create a space large enough for the permanent implant. This expansion is accomplished with the use of a tissue expander, which looks and feels very much like an implant but has a slightly thicker vulcanized silicone outer shell. This outer shell contains a small metal port into which saline solution is injected, usually on a weekly basis. The chest wall skin and underlying muscle are expanded over several months to a size somewhat larger than that necessary for the reconstruction. Then the expander is reduced to the appropriate size and exchanged for the permanent saline or silicone implant. The size and location of the implant are planned with the goal of achieving symmetry with the opposite breast (Figure 8–2).

If the patient wishes to avoid multiple operations with a tissue expander, reconstruction with an implant in combination with autologous tissues may be an option. The most common application of this option is the use of the latissimus dorsi myocutaneous flap with an implant. The

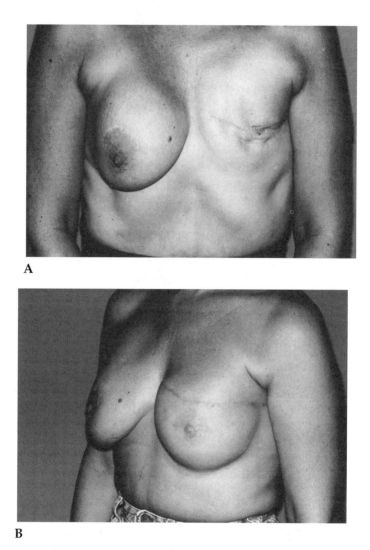

Figure 8–2.   Implant-based reconstruction. A, Patient with left mastectomy defect and augmented right breast. B, Same patient after tissue expansion and placement of an implant.

implant defines the drape and projection of the breast, while the muscle provides an insulating and protective cover for the implant.

In general, reconstruction with an implant results in a breast with the same color and texture as the normal breast whether the procedure is done on an immediate or delayed basis. The advantage of the immediate skin-sparing approach is that the additional skin available facilitates the expansion of the skin shell and underlying muscle to an appropriate size for the permanent implant. The redundant breast skin can drape over the subpectoral first-stage expander with minimal skin tension, minimizing the potential for mastectomy flap necrosis.

Especially in nonirradiated patients, good results and a high level of patient satisfaction can generally be achieved with implants. However, good patient selection is necessary to ensure successful outcomes. Patients with small, firm breasts are the best candidates for breast reconstruction with implants because these patients have the highest likelihood of long-term symmetry between the reconstructed and the natural breast. In any patient, the breast with the implant will always remain more erect and projecting than the natural breast. The reconstructed breast will not become ptotic and may in fact rise higher on the chest wall because of tightening of the internal capsule. Furthermore, the asymmetry may become more pronounced over time as the normal breast continues to droop because of the natural attenuation of Cooper's ligaments. In patients with small breasts, the breasts will be symmetrical after several months if the implant is positioned carefully. Breast symmetry is more difficult to achieve in patients with larger breasts unless the normal breast is lifted or reduced in size to match the position and projection of the reconstructed breast. (When the patient wears a bra, however, the symmetry often appears better because the normal breast is lifted up to match the higher projection of the reconstructed breast.) Of course, in patients who have bilateral reconstruction, the final size of the breasts can be determined by factors such as the chest size and width in proportion to the patient's height.

Although reconstruction with implants can produce good cosmetic outcomes, complication rates for implant-based reconstruction can run as high as 40%. Problems such as cellulitis and infection, implant exposure, chronic capsular contracture, chronic seroma, and rupture or deflation of the implant can occur and can adversely affect the cosmetic outcome and increase the long-term costs because of further surgery and hospitalization.

One significant disadvantage of reconstruction with implants is that the implant capsule may become tighter over time, making the reconstructed breast feel somewhat firmer and stiffer than the normal breast. This condition is known as capsular contracture (Figure 8–3). If the implant capsule tightens, the patient will frequently complain of chronic chest wall discomfort and possibly restricted range of motion of her shoulder or arm. The patient will often describe difficulty sleeping on the affected side because of the chest discomfort. If these clinical symptoms develop, many patients decide to have the constricting scar capsule around the implant released. This procedure, which can be accomplished on an outpatient basis, usually relieves many of the symptoms, but in a

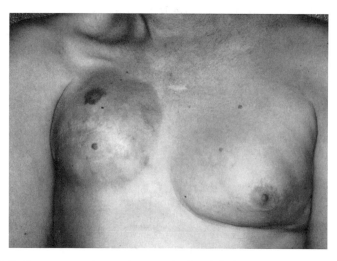

Figure 8–3. Severe capsular contracture in the right breast.

moderate percentage of patients, the same or similar problems may recur within 1 or 2 years.

Another prevalent concern about the long-term outcome of reconstruction with implants is the potential for deflation of saline implants or rupture of silicone implants. Deflation of saline implants can be caused by "fold failure," which refers to creasing or folding in the shell of an implant that has been underfilled, often in an attempt to create a softer reconstructed breast. This creasing or folding results in breakdown of the integrity of the implant's silicone shell and leakage of the saline contents into the surrounding soft tissues. Rupture of silicone implants has been associated with strong manual efforts to rupture the constricting capsule around the implant in an effort to soften the feel of the breast and, in some cases, improve the appearance. Older silicone implants (10–15 years old) are now known to be susceptible to shell fatigue and spontaneous rupture. Silicone rupture into the surrounding soft tissues can cause the development of small silicone granulomas and local chest wall pain but can just as often be completely asymptomatic.

Another concern associated with the use of implants is the potential for calcification of the implant capsule. Calcification of the capsule can occur with both saline and silicone implants and seems to be related to the generation of the implant, the duration of implantation, and the integrity of the implant shell. An obvious concern about calcifications is that they will make tumor detection difficult; another concern is that the hardened capsule can cause focal areas of unusual implant firmness and discomfort for the patient.

Reconstruction with Autologous Tissues

In breast reconstruction, autologous tissues can be used alone or in combination with an implant. At M. D. Anderson, the gold standard for reconstruction of the breast, especially since the innovation of the skin-sparing mastectomy, is the transverse rectus abdominis myocutaneous (TRAM) flap. However, a variety of other flaps can also be used for breast reconstruction and are described in this section.

Reconstruction with the Transverse Rectus Abdominis Myocutaneous Flap

The TRAM flap, which is taken from the lower abdomen, is the most convenient and expendable tissue flap used for breast reconstruction. The TRAM flap is considered ideal for breast reconstruction because the donor scar is well camouflaged in the lower abdomen along normal cosmetic unit lines and the donor area is easily accessible, such that the patient does not have to be repositioned during surgery. The TRAM flap is ideal if the patient has enough redundant skin and subcutaneous fat in the lower abdominal or midabdominal region, ideally just below the umbilicus. In the TRAM flap procedure, often referred to as a tummy tuck, this redundant skin and fat is removed, leaving a flatter and more youthful-appearing abdomen. This extra tissue is then used to create and shape the breast.

Two main versions of the TRAM flap are used: the pedicled TRAM flap and the free TRAM flap. Use of the pedicled TRAM flap relies on the intrinsic blood supply of the rectus muscle, which has to traverse a narrowed watershed area of perfusion within the muscle; this narrow area of perfusion also limits the quantity of tissue that can be transferred by tunneling under the abdominal flap to the chest area. The pedicled TRAM flap procedure also requires sacrifice of the whole rectus abdominis muscle, which may weaken the abdominal wall.

To minimize problems with blood supply to the flaps and abdominal wall weakness, many surgeons experienced in microvascular surgery have turned to the free TRAM flap based on the deep inferior epigastric vascular system, which is the predominant blood supply to the lower abdominal skin. The free flap is transferred to the breast area, and then an anastomosis is created between the flap vessels and, typically, the thoracodorsal or internal mammary vessels. Free flaps require more operative time, are more labor-intensive, and are associated with a risk of total flap loss secondary to vessel thrombosis, particularly during the first few days after surgery. However, in the hands of experienced microsurgeons, these drawbacks are thought to be outweighed by the advantages of free flaps: first, the increased vascular supply to these flaps typically maximizes the amount of flap tissue usable for the reconstruction, reducing the risk of partial flap loss and fat necrosis, and second, compared with the pedicled TRAM flap procedure, there is less interference with the abdominal wall and breast inframammary fold, which often results in a more esthetic breast reconstruction.

Sometimes the surgeon chooses to use both of the lower abdominal muscles in the pedicled TRAM flap manner so that the blood supply for the transferred skin and fat is improved. The flap with both muscles attached is referred to as a bipedicled TRAM flap. The main disadvantage of this approach is the loss of both lower abdominal muscles, which can weaken abdominal strength and aggravate any existing back trouble.

In some cases, if large vessels penetrate the soft tissue through the rectus abdominis muscle, this muscle can be completely spared and left in place. The skin, fat, and isolated pedicle vessels are then referred to as a perforator flap. The perforator flap can be used to reconstruct small to medium-sized breasts but is usually not suitable for reconstruction of large breasts. This is because the number of blood vessels supplying the soft tissues used to reconstruct the breast is usually less with the perforator flap than with the TRAM flap.

All the TRAM flap techniques described here can produce excellent outcomes. The free TRAM flap has some advantages in terms of cosmesis, ease of shaping of the reconstructed breast (Figure 8–4), and avoidance of excess abdominal muscle sacrifice. A bulge or hernia can develop in the abdomen after any TRAM flap procedure, but this complication is not common. Of course, a number of other problems, such as infections, partial or total loss of the transferred tissues, scarring, asymmetry, and loss of the "belly button," can also occur, but major problems are unusual. Any of these complications may require another relatively minor operation to revise or repair the problem.

Adequate vascularization of the tissue flap is critical. If more tissue is used in the breast reconstruction than can be adequately vascularized, the risk increases that a large portion of the fat making up the reconstructed breast will become firm and fibrotic during healing. This complication is referred to as a partial flap loss. Firm areas found in the reconstructed breast are usually small and sometimes resolve on their own without direct excision. However, all firm masses occurring after reconstruction require careful physical examination and possibly sonographic or mammographic scrutiny for documentation and treatment-planning purposes. Smaller masses (<2 cm) may require needle biopsy for confirmation of fat necrosis; areas larger than 2 to 3 cm are usually excised because complete resolution of the fibrotic fat is unlikely. If a portion of the reconstructed breast does not survive, a breast revision is usually necessary, the extent of which is directly related to how much of the flap is lost. If the entire flap is lost, another free tissue transfer can be considered, or an expander/implant option may be selected.

In most patients who undergo breast reconstruction with autologous tissues, a breast revision procedure is necessary to perfect the breast shape or size and breast symmetry. This procedure is usually performed no

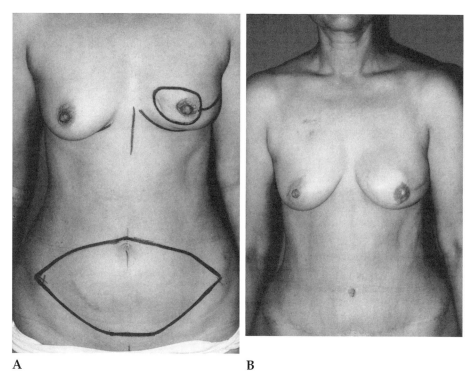

A   B

Figure 8–4.   Skin-sparing mastectomy and immediate TRAM flap breast reconstruction. A, Preoperative markings. B, Result after left breast reconstruction, including nipple reconstruction and areolar tattooing.

sooner than 2 to 3 months after the reconstruction. Limited liposuction, scar revision, and reduction of the reconstructed breast can be done as outpatient procedures. The next step, which can sometimes be done at the same time as the revision procedure, is reconstruction of the nipple. The nipple can be formed from the tissue over an implant or from the flap tissue itself. Small delicate flaps of tissue are raised from the front of the new breast and then shaped into a projecting nipple. After a period of about a month to allow healing of the nipple flaps, the nipple and the surrounding area can be tattooed with an appropriate color of pigment to create the appearance of an areola.

Recovery from TRAM flap reconstruction or a similar procedure usually takes about 6 to 8 weeks. Most patients are quite active during this period, focusing on nonstressful modes of exercise, like walking. Most patients are back to work within 6 to 8 weeks depending on the level of physical activity involved in their particular routine. The most important restriction is to avoid lifting, pulling, or pushing more than about 15 pounds during the first 6 months to minimize the strain on the abdomen. Persistent stress on the abdomen due to excessive physical effort during the early healing period can promote the development of laxity in the abdomen in the form of a bulge or hernia.

Reconstruction with the Latissimus Dorsi Flap and an Implant

Another common method of reconstructing the breast after mastectomy is use of the latissimus dorsi muscle in combination with an implant. The back muscle is transferred to the front of the chest to cover an implant, which provides the shape and projection of the new breast. The advantages of this reconstructive option are the relative ease of the operation and the shorter operating time; the disadvantage is that the cosmetic outcome is totally dependent on the esthetics of the implant shape and position. This technique, which was very popular in the late 1980s, can produce excellent long-term results in many patients (Figure 8–5). It is particularly applicable for patients with small to medium-sized breasts, in whom the implant can be of limited size. However, if a patient develops a significant capsular contracture around the implant, the breast may appear constricted and displaced superiorly, which will affect breast symmetry. Any symptomatic breast constriction will need to be corrected surgically to improve the appearance of the breast, the softness of the breast, and the position of the breast on the chest wall.

Reconstruction with the Latissimus Dorsi Flap Alone

For smaller breasts, the latissimus dorsi muscle can sometimes provide the volume of tissue necessary for the entire breast reconstruction. This "extended" application of the muscle usually involves including as much of the surrounding subcutaneous fat and overlying skin as is practical to provide a large volume of tissue with which to shape a projecting breast and provide for any missing external skin. The extended flap is most appropriate for patients with a higher percentage of body fat who have more subcutaneous fat and smaller breasts and who perhaps would also like to avoid using an implant (or who have had radiation therapy). For most patients, the recovery time for this procedure is limited to several weeks, with the most common restriction being the need for an extended back drain for up to 3 to 4 weeks.

Other Tissue Flaps Used in Breast Reconstruction

For patients in whom prior abdominal surgery prevents use of the TRAM flap, a few additional but lesser-used free muscle and perforator flaps are sometimes options. The gluteal or lateral thigh area is sometimes a good donor site provided that the patient does not object to the scarring and possible deformity (including asymmetry) that can result from harvesting these flaps. Other flaps that may be used for breast reconstruction include the Rueben's flap from the outer hip area (occasionally usable even after a TRAM flap procedure); the superior gluteal flap or perforator flap (no muscle included) from the upper buttock; and the inferior gluteal flap from the lower buttock region. These tissue flaps can provide a reasonable breast reconstruction, but dissection of these flaps is more difficult and time-consuming than dissection of the TRAM flap or latissimus dorsi flap, and the tissues are often more difficult to shape into a breast. Nonetheless, for the patient who prefers to avoid an implant and who is not a candidate for reconstruction with a TRAM flap or an abdominal perforator flap, these options can offer a practical solution.

Reconstruction After Mastectomy

In patients with early-stage breast cancer, reconstruction after mastectomy is usually done on an immediate basis. The reconstruction may be delayed for some patients with advanced-stage disease and patients who require postmastectomy radiation therapy.

Immediate Reconstruction

Immediate breast reconstruction after mastectomy—especially immediate reconstruction using autologous tissues—has become more established since the introduction of the skin-sparing mastectomy in the early 1990s. This approach to mastectomy minimizes the incisional scars on the breast, and the good esthetic outcome has convinced many breast cancer patients to view mastectomy with reconstruction as a viable and positive treatment choice.

Skin-sparing mastectomy requires more time and expertise on the part of the surgical oncologist than does conventional mastectomy. The delicate breast skin flaps must be elevated carefully, and even with very careful technique, the flap skin closest to the nipple-areola complex often becomes necrotic because of poor vascularity. Given the risk of skin loss, the plastic surgeon must carefully examine the skin flaps at the time of surgery to check for nonviable areas. Any such area that is detected should be excised before the breast reconstruction is completed. Ensuring the viability of the skin flaps is especially important when reconstruction is accomplished with the use of an implant. In this situation, the implant or tissue expander will have to remain covered by muscle, skin, and subcutaneous tissue. If the implant or expander becomes exposed, it usually must be removed.

When patients have had radiation therapy before mastectomy, as in the case of previous breast conservation therapy, more than the usual amount of the breast skin must be removed in the skin-sparing mastectomy because the viability of this skin is predictably poor. The abdominal skin on the autologous tissue flap is then used to replace any skin excised from

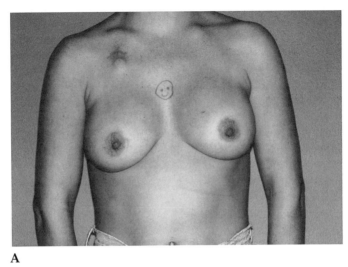

A

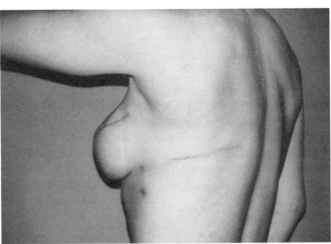

B

Figure 8–5. Skin-sparing mastectomy and immediate breast reconstruction with a latissimus dorsi muscle flap plus an implant. A, Appearance before surgery. B, Postoperative result with donor scar within bra line.

the breast shell. Thus, in the breast reconstructed after radiation therapy, much of the external shape and contour of the breast is formed by abdominal skin and tissue.

Concerns have been raised about the long-term risk of tumor recurrence after skin-sparing mastectomy. At M. D. Anderson, a study was recently completed on the incidence of local recurrence and distant me-

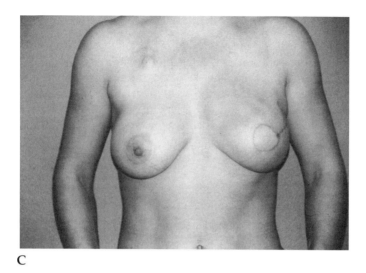

C

Figure 8–5. *(continued)* C, Postoperative result without nipple reconstruction. Reprinted with permission from Robb GL. Skin-sparing mastectomy and immediate reconstruction. In: Singletary SE, Robb GL, editors. *Advanced Therapy of Breast Disease.* Hamilton: BC Decker Inc; 2000:197–209.

tastases and survival in patients with early breast cancer (T1 or T2) who had undergone skin-sparing or non-skin-sparing mastectomy and reconstruction. The median follow-up time was 6 years. There was no significant difference in the incidence of local recurrence between the skin-sparing mastectomy and non-skin-sparing mastectomy groups. Distant metastases were less common in patients who had skin-sparing mastectomy ($P = 0.0867$), with 99.1% of the patients still alive. Although patients were not randomly assigned to skin-sparing or non-skin-sparing mastectomy, the results suggest that the skin-sparing mastectomy is oncologically safe.

At M. D. Anderson, in selected patients with small (T1 or T2) peripherally located tumors treated with skin-sparing mastectomy, the nipple-areola complex has been saved on the inferior mastectomy flap. In these cases, frozen sections have been examined intraoperatively to ensure negative margins at the subareolar location. In all cases to date, the preserved nipple-areola complexes have healed completely with the mastectomy flaps without loss of tissue. In most cases, the lower mastectomy flap is closer than the upper flap to the better blood supply of the chest wall, so the nipple-areola complex has a better chance of surviving on the lower flap. Naturally, in patients in whom the nipple-areola complex can be safely preserved, the cosmetic result will be far superior because of the enhanced appearance and projection of the normal nipple complex, especially when reconstruction is accomplished with the use of autologous tissues (Figure 8–6).

A retrospective study was recently undertaken at M. D. Anderson to determine the incidence of occult nipple-areola involvement in patients treated with skin-sparing mastectomy and to determine whether occult nipple-areola involvement affected local recurrence, distant metastasis, or survival. The study included 326 patients who had mastectomy between 1993 and 1996. Occult tumor involvement was found in 5.6% of mastectomy specimens. Of 18 local recurrences in the group, only a single recurrence within 1 cm of the circumareolar incision was documented. These findings suggested that the incidence of nipple-areola involvement is low and is not specifically related to local recurrence, distant metastasis, or survival. Further careful follow-up and study are planned. We hope that findings will indicate that preservation of the nipple-areola complex in association with the skin-sparing technique is not associated with increased risk of recurrence.

Delayed Reconstruction

When the plastic surgeon performs delayed postmastectomy reconstruction with an implant, the same measures must be taken to maintain sterile protection of the implant as are taken with immediate reconstruction. The main clinical differences between immediate and delayed reconstruction with implants are the tightness of the chest wall skin and soft tissue at

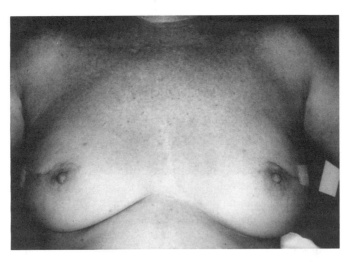

Figure 8–6. Result after bilateral skin- and areola-sparing mastectomies and immediate TRAM flap reconstructions.

the beginning of the expansion. In the case of delayed reconstruction, the soft tissue scarring caused by the prior mastectomy somewhat inhibits the expansion process.

The main disadvantage of delayed reconstruction after mastectomy is that no extra skin is spared. Instead, the majority of the skin is removed so that the chest wall tissues will heal smoothly. As healing progresses, of course, the chest wall becomes flat. In the delayed reconstruction, if the patient's own tissues are used, the back or abdominal skin is used to replace much of the breast or chest wall skin, predominantly on the lower half to two thirds of the reconstructed breast mound. The back or abdominal skin is naturally different in color, texture, and feel from the normal chest wall and breast skin, and this contrast is usually readily visible on the reconstructed breast (Figure 8–7).

RECONSTRUCTION AFTER LUMPECTOMY OR PARTIAL MASTECTOMY

Today, many women diagnosed with breast cancer are good candidates for breast-conserving surgery—i.e., lumpectomy or partial mastectomy. Women who elect conservative surgery wish to retain as much of their breast form and as much of their natural superficial skin sensation as possible. Patients may believe that by selecting breast conservation therapy instead of mastectomy they will completely avoid breast deformity. However, depending on the amount of skin and breast tissue excised, some permanent visible irregularity or deformity causing asymmetry will most likely occur after a period of healing and wound contraction. The breast contour may have depressions or irregularities. Nipple-areola distortions are especially common because of the collapse of the internal tissues with healing and tissue contraction. Additional patient tissues are often necessary to fill in the contracted areas and thus reestablish the normal contour of the breast and, especially important, repair the position and orientation of the nipple so that it is symmetrical with the nipple of the normal breast.

At M. D. Anderson, when the amount of tissue to be removed in a lumpectomy or partial mastectomy is likely to cause long-term deformity and breast asymmetry after radiation therapy, the present standard of care is to proactively refer the patient to a plastic surgeon for consultation about immediate breast reconstruction. Of course, before any planned repair procedure is undertaken in a woman undergoing conservative breast surgery, the surgical specimen is examined thoroughly to ensure that the margins are negative. At M. D. Anderson, these specimens are routinely examined with whole-specimen radiography in conjunction with painstaking pathologic examination of frozen sections.

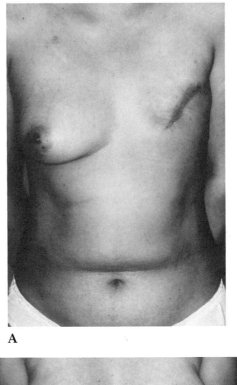

A

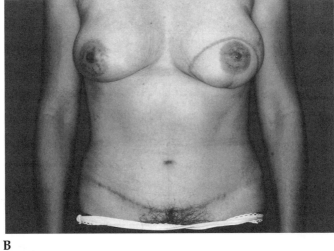

B

Figure 8–7.   Delayed TRAM flap reconstruction of the left breast after mastectomy. A, Result after mastectomy. B, Result after reconstruction.

Timing

Plastic surgeons usually prefer to complete any planned reconstructive procedure at the same time as the lumpectomy or partial mastectomy because the tissue is better vascularized and no scarring or contractures are present. If repair of a defect resulting from lumpectomy or partial mastectomy is delayed until after the patient's breast and axillary areas have been irradiated, the repair is much more difficult because of the additional internal scarring and fibrosis that occur secondary to the radiation treatments. After irradiation, the breast tissues are often more stiff and less vascular, which decreases the optimal healing potential of any subsequent revisionary procedure.

Repair of Defects Resulting from Lumpectomy

Small lumpectomy defects in large breasts usually do not necessitate a reconstructive procedure. In a small to medium-sized breast, if less than 25% of the breast volume is removed, repair of the defect may require only some rearrangement of the local breast tissue itself. The best local tissue to use for this purpose is tissue from the lateral lower breast, which is the fullest part of the breast and the most expendable. This tissue can be rotated or advanced into the breast defect along incision lines camouflaged by the inframammary and anterior axillary folds.

Repair of Defects Resulting from Partial Mastectomy

When a partial mastectomy is required, this procedure is usually approached as a definitive plastic surgery breast reduction procedure, which is a common operation that results in a smaller, pleasingly shaped breast with modest scarring. The same type of procedure is performed at the same time on the opposite breast to achieve breast symmetry.

If the defect from the partial mastectomy will be too large to permit the breast-reduction approach, there are 2 options for reconstruction. The first is complete mastectomy followed by breast reconstruction with autologous tissues or an implant; the second is partial mastectomy followed by repair using soft tissues from near the breast.

The latissimus dorsi muscle, a thin, broad muscle from the mid to low back, can carry a significant amount of subcutaneous fat and overlying skin that can contribute the extra amount of soft tissue necessary for repair of the partial-mastectomy defect in the larger breast. The muscle tissue is taken from the same side as the affected breast. The tissue can be harvested through a short incision in the back. If no external skin is required, the muscle can be removed endoscopically. Once separated from its origin along the midback and posterior iliac crest, the muscle is tunneled through the same area of the axilla where the lymphadenectomy was performed and is then positioned in the area of the breast defect. The muscle flap is inset so that it eliminates the dead space created by the partial mastectomy and restores the contour of the external aspect of the breast as much as possible. Sometimes additional external skin is required to complete the reconstruction and maintain the breast shape and contour; in this case, the skin left on the muscle during its elevation and transfer is simply retained as necessary. Use of the latissimus dorsi flap can generally produce excellent cosmetic results in the repair of large defects resulting from partial mastectomy.

The skin of the muscle donor site in the back is simply re-approximated to restore the normal back contour. If an incision is used to harvest the flap, this incision is frequently made along the bra line to minimize the visibility of the scar. Although the side where the muscle is removed becomes thinner than the normal side of the back, there is no overt depression in the area of the harvested muscle. Often, however, the scarring that can occur is hypertrophic or wide and erythematous. The single long-term advantage of the latissimus dorsi flap is that the scar is not readily apparent to the patient since it is behind her and it thus tends to be more acceptable.

A final option for repair of larger defects (>25% of the breast volume) resulting from partial mastectomy is use of the TRAM flap. This flap is generally not used for repair of partial-mastectomy defects in small to medium-sized breasts because other options, such as the latissimus dorsi flap, can provide a better solution in terms of cosmetic outcome and ease of the surgery. Harvesting the TRAM flap takes longer and is more difficult than harvesting other flaps, and patients who undergo TRAM flap reconstruction require longer to return to normal activity. Another disadvantage of using the TRAM flap for repair of defects resulting from partial mastectomy is that if the patient were to need a completion mastectomy in the future, the TRAM flap, the best reconstructive option, would not be available. This disadvantage is especially important because reconstruction with an implant would not be recommended in this situation owing to the previous radiation therapy associated with the partial mastectomy.

Delayed breast reconstruction is an important option in dealing with larger defects resulting from partial mastectomy (Figure 8–8). The main goal of this approach is to avoid irradiation of the muscle flap itself. In some cases, assessment of the breast defect may be more accurate after the initial healing is complete and the changes induced by radiation therapy have occurred. However, the primary disadvantage of delayed reconstruction in this setting is the difficulty usually encountered in operating on irradiated tissues, including the axillary area, which the latissimus dorsi muscle must be tunneled through before being inset into the breast defect. Healing problems due to radiation can occur in this setting and pose a significant hazard for the patient. Lymphedema in the arm on the side of the mastectomy, one of the breast cancer patient's worst fears, can also be aggravated by tunneling through the axilla a second time after radiation therapy and the initial breast healing.

Delayed breast reconstruction with a TRAM flap can be an excellent option for the patient with a medium-sized to large breast who has undergone breast-conserving surgery and radiation therapy without breast reconstruction and then develops a significant breast scar contracture or other deformity during the postoperative healing process (Figure 8–9). In this case, often the original incision must be released to re-create the operative defect, and then enough well-vascularized tissue and extra skin

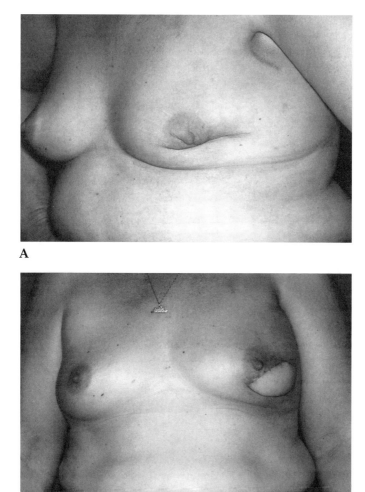

A

B

Figure 8–8. Repair of nipple-areola defect following partial mastectomy. A, Result after partial mastectomy. B, Early result after pedicled latissimus dorsi myocutaneous flap reconstruction of the breast contour.

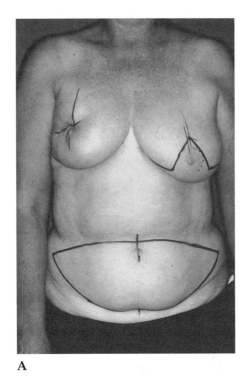

A

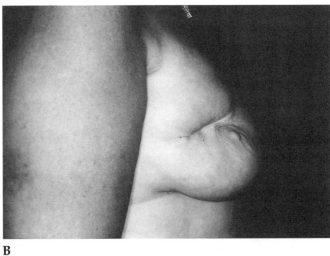

B

Figure 8–9.   Delayed reconstruction with a free TRAM flap to correct deformity following breast conservation therapy. A, Preoperative markings. A left breast lift was planned. B, Marked deformity of the right breast after partial mastectomy.

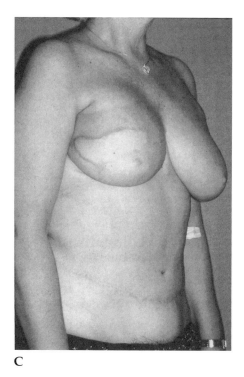

C

Figure 8–9. *(continued)* C, Early postoperative result after recontouring with a free TRAM flap. The left breast lift was not performed since symmetry was achieved with use of the TRAM flap.

must be placed to restore a more normal shape and projection of the breast and improve the healing potential that has been adversely affected by the radiation therapy.

PLANNING THE BREAST RECONSTRUCTION

Breast reconstruction is a complex procedure, and careful patient counseling and patient selection are essential for a successful outcome.

Patient Counseling

Breast cancer patients often have their initial consultation with a plastic surgeon just after learning of their cancer diagnosis. At this initial consultation, patients are often overwhelmed with anxiety and confused about their surgical treatment options. Having to make important decisions about more complex reconstructive surgery increases the patient's stress.

Before the initial consultation with the plastic surgeon, the patient has usually been offered several treatment options by her surgical oncologist.

Depending on the stage of disease, these options may include breast-conserving surgery with postoperative radiation therapy or mastectomy with or without reconstruction. The plastic surgeon must determine whether the patient is medically and psychologically a candidate for breast reconstruction. If so, the plastic surgeon must help the woman decide which type of reconstruction is best given her expectations and lifestyle. The plastic surgeon elaborates all the options available to the patient on the basis of her past medical and surgical history, the results of her physical examination, her body shape and size, and the natural appearance of her breasts before surgery. The plastic surgeon details all aspects of the reconstructive surgery, including the length of hospitalization; the risks, benefits, and possible complications, including the potential effects of radiation therapy and chemotherapy on the reconstructive outcome; and the potential need for delayed outpatient surgeries for "touch-ups" of the reconstructed breast. The plastic surgeon attempts to make this information as clear and easily understandable as possible.

Family visibility and support during the preoperative period are very important, and the plastic surgeon facilitates education for both the patient and her family. When family members are present during meetings with the plastic surgeon, they can help the patient remember specific details discussed with the surgeon and provide the always necessary moral support.

For some patients, several meetings with the plastic surgeon are required before patient and surgeon reach a mutually satisfactory decision about breast reconstruction. Both the surgical oncologist and the plastic surgeon must assess the patient's suitability for a particular procedure and must help the patient develop realistic expectations about the reconstructive outcome. Sometimes the patient does not seem to completely understand the reconstructive options or the potential risks and complications of breast reconstruction or expresses unrealistic expectations after the surgical counseling sessions. When the patient has unrealistic expectations, the role of the plastic surgeon can be very difficult. The problem can sometimes be resolved by having the patient see a psychologist, who can better determine the patient's motivation and emotional state. In these situations, the patient is encouraged to understand that the plastic surgeon is truly interested in doing what is best for her, both physically and emotionally.

M. D. Anderson has developed an educational videotape about breast reconstruction for breast cancer patients and their families. The videotape, which gives basic information about breast reconstruction, seems to be especially helpful for patients with no prior exposure to the concept of breast reconstruction who want additional information to aid in decision-making regarding treatment options. After the patient has viewed the videotape and discussed reconstruction with one of the plastic surgeons, she also has the opportunity to talk individually with a woman who has already undergone breast reconstruction at M. D. Anderson and has volunteered to talk with other breast cancer patients about her own personal experience. These volunteers are often even willing to show their reconstructed breast to the patient if she so requests.

Some patients feel overwhelmed by their breast cancer diagnosis and are unwilling to accept the further stress associated with making additional difficult decisions about breast reconstruction. These patients may be tempted to complete their cancer treatment first before turning their full attention to the very important issue of breast reconstruction. Occasionally, the patient's surgical oncologist may recommend that the patient wait some time after the breast cancer surgery before even consulting with a plastic surgeon about the possibility of breast reconstruction. However, delaying consultation with the plastic surgeon is not standard practice because most patients who are interested in either immediate or delayed reconstruction would benefit from seeing a plastic surgeon as soon as possible after the diagnosis of breast cancer. At M. D. Anderson, there is a strong sentiment that once a patient has been counseled to her satisfaction about her particular options for the ablative and reconstructive surgery, she is better informed and less anxious.

Patient Selection

Several factors must be taken into account in determining whether a patient is a suitable candidate for breast reconstruction and, if so, which reconstructive options are appropriate. These factors include disease stage, comorbid conditions, the use of adjuvant therapy, and the presence of preexisting cosmetic breast implants.

Disease Stage

Patients with early breast cancer are often good candidates for breast reconstruction. Such patients can choose from many different types of breast reconstruction best suited to the specific surgery recommended for their breast cancer.

In some circumstances, patients with advanced breast cancer may be candidates for breast reconstruction if they so desire. The reconstructive effort, however, should not be counterproductive in terms of the patient's cancer treatment. The patient's primary medical and surgical oncologists must assist the plastic surgeon in determining whether the patient can tolerate the additional stress and healing time necessary for the breast reconstruction.

Comorbid Conditions

For women with medical conditions such as high blood pressure, diabetes, or vascular or connective-tissue disease, counseling regarding breast reconstruction is tailored to the individual. If a woman with one of these conditions is considered to be a candidate for breast reconstruction, a simpler reconstructive procedure (e.g., reconstruction with an implant) may be most appropriate. Patients who are obese or who smoke have a higher risk of complications with breast reconstruction, so these patients, under the guidance of the plastic surgeon, must carefully consider these possible outcomes and the associated risks versus the expected benefits.

Older age, by itself, is not a strict barrier to reconstruction. Older patients in good general health often desire breast reconstruction and are sometimes found to be good candidates for even the more strenuous types of breast reconstruction. Often, however, older patients are better candidates for the simpler, shorter procedures.

Radiation Therapy

One of the most important considerations affecting the feasibility of breast reconstruction and the method chosen is the role of radiation therapy in the patient's treatment plan. If either preoperative or postoperative radiation therapy is planned, the use of an implant in the reconstruction is strongly discouraged because radiation therapy increases the risk of capsular contracture, a contracting scar process around the implant. Capsular contracture not only can deform the appearance of the reconstructed breast but also can cause chronic localized chest wall pain and tightness. This not uncommon complication of implant placement occurs when the patient's body, recognizing the breast implant as a foreign body, creates an isolating scar around the implant that then constricts to minimize the volume occupied by the implant.

Radiation therapy also affects reconstructions done with well-vascularized autologous tissues. After radiation therapy, the shape of the reconstructed breast may become distorted, and the breast may contract upward in relation to its former position on the chest wall. These changes are especially noticeable in smaller breasts. However, even in larger breasts, the reconstructed breast is generally firmer and stiffer than the normal breast because of increased fibrosis present throughout the irradiated autologous tissues. The net adverse effect that is usually most bothersome to patients is the resulting breast asymmetry, which is difficult to correct. Improvement or restoration of symmetry may require transfer of tissue to the reconstructed breast to open secondary contractures or to realign the inframammary fold so that it is symmetrical with the opposite side. Occasionally, the reconstructive tissues only need to be reshaped or moved with local geometric flaps to accomplish the necessary improvement in contour or shape. However, even these relatively minor procedures can still be hazardous because the internal scarring and decrease in vascularity in the irradiated areas affect the quality of the healing. There is often a resulting chronic induration of the operated tissues or frank skin and fat necrosis that necessitate further excision. If the reconstructed breast is initially larger than the normal breast, which is not unusual,

KEY PRACTICE POINTS

- Breast reconstruction (if the patient desires it) is considered vital to the patient's rehabilitation and is an intrinsic part of her breast cancer treatment.

- Immediate breast reconstruction is available to most candidates for breast reconstruction.

- Skin-sparing mastectomy has proven to be a safe and effective surgical approach that also facilitates the most esthetic breast reconstruction.

- Adjuvant therapy can complicate breast reconstruction; therefore, in patients scheduled to receive adjuvant radiation therapy or chemotherapy, precautions and thorough patient counseling are of major importance.

- Reconstruction with autologous tissues tends to produce the most natural-looking and natural-feeling breasts.

- The most common source of autologous tissue for breast reconstruction, especially at M. D. Anderson, is the TRAM flap, from the lower abdomen. The redundant skin and fat of this flap permit excellent restoration of the breast.

- Reconstruction with implants is less complicated than reconstruction with autologous tissues and can produce excellent results, especially in patients with smaller breasts. However, implants are generally not compatible with irradiated tissues.

many of these changes or revisions may then facilitate a reasonable symmetry between the breasts.

Chemotherapy

Chemotherapy can also adversely affect the healing of the reconstructed breast. Because of the additional blood supply brought in by the patient's own tissue, breasts reconstructed using autologous tissue can generally withstand the slower healing or wound infections that can occur after chemotherapy. However, in breasts reconstructed using implants, poor or incomplete healing due to chemotherapy can have a more dramatic effect. For example, patients receiving postoperative chemotherapy may develop systemic infections at any time, and these infections can involve the implant. In these circumstances, intravenous antibiotics are required to help salvage the reconstructed breast. The earlier the infection is recognized and the patient is treated, the better the chance that the implant can be saved. Unfortunately, the outcome is unpredictable in many cases, and control of the infection often requires removal of the implant. If the implant is removed, the patient must wait 4 to 6 weeks after resolution of the infection before the implant (or more commonly the first-stage tissue expander, which prepares the ultimate space for the permanent implant) can be replaced. Although more local chest wall scarring will be present because of the infection, good results from the reconstruction are still commonly obtained, even with secondary tissue expansion and implant placement.

Preexisting Cosmetic Implant

If a patient has a preexisting cosmetic implant in place and requires breast cancer surgery, the preoperative consultation will often focus on reconstruction with implants because most patients who already have an implant in place are comfortable with the concept of breast implants. If the implant is in the submammary position, it must be removed as part of the breast cancer surgery because the implant is directly under the breast itself, over the pectoralis major muscle. In contrast, if the implant is in the subpectoral space, it may be retained if the position and shape of the implant will allow creation of a satisfactory reconstructed breast. In many cases, however, the subpectoral implant will need to be exchanged for a tissue expander placed under the pectoralis major muscle to create a larger implant space and thus allow for a better reconstructed breast. If the patient needs adjuvant radiation therapy after her cancer surgery, the implant will need to be removed.

Suggested Readings

Blondeel PN, Boeckx WD. Refinements in free flap breast reconstruction: the free bilateral deep inferior epigastric perforator flap anastomosed to the internal mammary artery. *Br J Plast Surg* 1994;47:495–501.

Carlson GW. Skin sparing mastectomy: anatomic and technical considerations. *Am Surg* 1996;62:151–155.

Carlson GW, Bostwick J III, Styblo TM, et al. Skin-sparing mastectomy. Oncologic and reconstructive considerations. *Ann Surg* 1997;225:570–575.

Dean C, Chetty U, Forrest AP. Effects of immediate breast reconstruction on psychosocial morbidity after mastectomy. *Lancet* 1983;1(8322):459–462.

Elliot D, Lewis-Smith PA, Piggot TA. The expanded latissimus dorsi flap. *Br J Plast Surg* 1988;41:319–321.

Federal Breast Implant Multidistrict Litigation Web site. Available at: http://www.fjc.gov/BREIMLIT/md1926.htm. Accessed February 1, 1999.

Godfrey PM, Godfrey NV, Romita MC. Immediate autogenous breast reconstruction in clinically advanced disease. *Plast Reconstr Surg* 1995;95:1039–1044.

Hartrampf CR Jr, Noel RT, Drazan L, Elliott FL, Bennett GK, Beegle PH. Ruben's fat pad for breast reconstruction: a peri-iliac soft-tissue free flap. *Plast Reconstr Surg* 1994;93:402–407.

Khoo A, Kroll SS, Reece G, et al. A comparison of resource costs of immediate and delayed breast reconstruction. *Plast Reconstr Surg* 1998;101:964–968.

Kroll SS. The value of skin-sparing mastectomy [letter]. *Ann Surg Oncol* 1998;5:660–662.

Kroll SS, Ames F, Singletary SE, Schusterman MA. The oncologic risks of skin preservation at mastectomy when combined with immediate reconstruction of the breast. *Surg Gynecol Obstet* 1991;172:17–20.

Kroll SS, Baldwin B. A comparison of outcomes using three different methods of breast reconstruction. *Plast Reconstr Surg* 1992;90:455–462.

Kroll SS, Coffey JA Jr, Winn RJ, Schusterman MA. A comparison of factors affecting aesthetic outcomes of TRAM flap breast reconstructions. *Plast Reconstr Surg* 1995;96:860–864.

Kroll S, Khoo A, Singletary SE, et al. Local recurrence risk after skin-sparing and conventional mastectomy: a 6-year follow-up. *Plast Reconstr Surg* 1999;104:421–425.

Laronga C, Robb GL, Singletary SE. The feasibility of skin-sparing mastectomy with preservation of the nipple-areola complex. *Breast Diseases: A Year Book Quarterly* 1998;9:125–127.

Miller MJ. Immediate breast reconstruction. *Clin Plast Surg* 1998;25:145–156.

Miller MJ, Rock CS, Robb GL. Aesthetic breast reconstruction using a combination of free transverse rectus abdominis musculocutaneous flaps and breast implants. *Ann Plast Surg* 1996;37:258–264.

Newman L, Kuerer H, Hunt K, et al. Feasibility of immediate breast reconstruction for locally advanced breast cancer. *Ann Surg Oncol* 1999; 6:671–675.

Paulson RL, Chang FC, Helmer SD. Kansas surgeons' attitudes toward immediate breast reconstruction: a statewide survey. *Am J Surg* 1994;168:543–546.

Peters W, Pritzker K, Smith D, et al. Capsular calcification associated with silicone breast implants: incidence, determinants, and characterization. *Ann Plast Surg* 1998;41:348–360.

Plastic Surgery Information Service. National Clearing House of Plastic Surgery Statistics. Vol. 1999. Available: at http://www.plasticsurgery.org. Accessed July 17, 2000.

Robb GL, Miller MJ. Muscle harvest. In: Ramirez D, Daniel RK, eds. *Endoscopic Plastic Surgery.* New York: Springer Verlag; 1995.

Schover LR, Yetman RJ, Tuason LJ, et al. Partial mastectomy and breast reconstruction. A comparison of their effects on psychosocial adjustment, body image, and sexuality. *Cancer* 1995;75:54–64.

Shaw W, Ahn C. Free flap breast reconstruction. In: Habal M, ed. *Advances in Plastic and Reconstructive Surgery.* Vol 9. St. Louis: Mosby Year Book; 1993:221–241.

Spear SL, Majidian A. Immediate breast reconstruction in two stages using textured, integrated-valve tissue expanders and breast implants: a retrospective review of 171 consecutive breast reconstructions from 1989 to 1996. *Plast Reconstr Surg* 1998;101:53–62.

Teimourian B, Adham MN. Louis Ombredanne and the origin of muscle flap use for immediate breast mound reconstruction. *Plast Reconstr Surg* 1983;72:905–910.

Toth BA, Lappert P. Modified skin incisions for mastectomy: the need for plastic surgical input in preoperative planning. *Plast Reconstr Surg* 1991;87:1048–1053.

Wellisch DK, Schain WS, Noone RB, Little JJ III. Psychosocial correlates of immediate versus delayed reconstruction of the breast. *Plast Reconstr Surg* 1985;76:713–718.

9 RADIATION THERAPY FOR EARLY AND ADVANCED BREAST DISEASE

Eric A. Strom

CHAPTER OVERVIEW

Radiation therapy is an important tool in the treatment of women with breast cancer. For patients with in situ carcinoma and early invasive carcinoma, radiation therapy plays a central role in breast conservation therapy. For many patients with intermediate and locally advanced disease, the use of radiation therapy after mastectomy results in a two-thirds reduction in local-regional recurrence rates. In patients at high risk for recurrence, this improved local-regional control contributes substantially to improved disease-free survival, as shown by large prospective trials. Radiation therapy also plays an important role in the treatment of inflammatory carcinoma, local-regionally recurrent carcinoma, and unknown primary carcinomas involving the axillary nodes. Finally, the judicious use of radiation therapy in patients with symptomatic metastases materially improves the patients' quality of life and helps them maintain a high level of function.

INTRODUCTION

Radiation therapy has an important role in the management of every stage of breast cancer. The following chapter will begin with a brief review of the relevant anatomy, which is central to understanding the choice of treatment targets and techniques. The next section will review the use and indications for radiation therapy in breast conservation therapy for women with ductal carcinoma in situ (DCIS) and early-stage invasive carcinoma of the breast. A brief discussion of treatment planning and delivery is also included. The next section reviews postmastectomy irradiation for primary treatment and treatment of local recurrences. Finally, the approach to patients with unidentified primary tumors in axillary lymph nodes (presumed to be breast in origin) and the use of radiation therapy for palliative care are reviewed.

PERTINENT ANATOMY

A clear understanding of the anatomy of the breast and its draining lymphatics is required by the radiation oncologist for both initial assessment and subsequent treatment planning. While the majority of glandular breast tissue is located in the protuberant breast mound, thin layers of mammary parenchyma can be found extending medially to the midsternum, laterally to the latissimus dorsi muscle, superiorly to the clavicle, and inferiorly to the lower costal margin. The greatest bulk of active mammary parenchyma is located in the upper outer quadrant of the breast, and in some individuals, the adjacent tail of Spence can contain substantial amounts of breast tissue and even have the appearance of an accessory breast.

The first-echelon lymph nodes that drain the majority of the breast are located in the ipsilateral axilla. These nodes are divided into 3 levels on the basis of their position in relation to the pectoralis major muscle: level I (proximal), level II (middle), and level III (distal). Generally, the level I nodes are the first to be involved by metastatic tumor deposits, and level

I is the most common location in which sentinel lymph nodes are identified during lymphatic mapping. As the axillary tumor burden increases, the incidence of involvement of the more distal nodes also increases (Danforth et al, 1986; Veronesi et al, 1987; Rosen et al, 1983). With further increases in the axillary tumor burden, involvement of the interpectoral nodes (Rotter's nodes) and infraclavicular nodes can occur. Ultimately, the nodes of the supraclavicular fossa become involved. Located at the confluence of the internal jugular and subclavian veins, these nodes are generally appreciated lateral to the clavicular head of the sternocleidomastoid muscle.

An alternative lymphatic drainage system exists for portions of the medial and central breast. The internal mammary nodes, located in the first 3 to 5 intercostal spaces at the lateral sternal margin, are loose aggregates of lymphatic tissue that lie in close association with the internal mammary vessels. Metastatic deposits in these nodes can rarely be detected clinically; generally detection of such metastases requires the use of sonography, computed tomography, or magnetic resonance imaging. Historical studies of extended radical mastectomy indicate that for central and medially located tumors with evident axillary metastases, the probability of histologic involvement of the internal mammary nodes ranges from 20% to 50% (Handley, 1975; Bucalossi et al, 1971; Deemarski and Seleznev, 1984; Lacour et al, 1976, 1987; Urban and Marjani, 1971). This is one of the primary rationales for inclusion of the internal mammary chain in the radiation target volume during treatment planning for node-positive breast cancer.

ROLE OF RADIATION THERAPY IN BREAST CONSERVATION THERAPY

Breast conservation therapy (breast-conserving surgery plus radiation therapy) is now considered a mainstay of treatment for early-stage invasive carcinoma of the breast. In addition, breast conservation therapy is appropriate for many patients with DCIS.

Treatment of Ductal Carcinoma In Situ

The optimum management of DCIS is a rapidly evolving area of study. The uncertainty about the optimum treatment for DCIS is in large measure due to the fact that DCIS includes a heterogeneous group of pathological findings with variable malignant potential. Clearly, some DCIS lesions, if left untreated, will become invasive carcinomas. Thus DCIS is viewed as an opportunity to treat a premalignant lesion before it becomes a risk to the patient's life. However, it is likely that some lesions classified as DCIS would never become malignant lesions, at least not in the patient's lifetime. Fundamentally, it is this difficulty in predicting the behavior of DCIS that is the root cause for conflicting opinions on the role of radiation therapy for DCIS.

The dramatic increase in the detection of DCIS is primarily due to the routine use of screening mammography. In the premammography era, DCIS was an uncommon finding, and DCIS lesions were generally detected on physical examination as large, palpable areas of comedo-subtype disease. In the modern era, most cases of DCIS are small, nonpalpable lesions revealed by screening mammography, and frequently these lesions are of noncomedo subtypes. The small tumor burden and presumably lower malignant potential of lesions found on screening mammography means that the results of older series, in which clinically detected lesions predominate, are of little clinical value today.

Mastectomy is nearly always curative for patients with DCIS. After total mastectomy, local recurrence rates are probably 1% or less (Betsill et al, 1978; Fentiman, 1989; Sunshine et al, 1985). Patients with extensive DCIS manifesting as diffuse microcalcifications throughout the breast can be offered no reasonable alternatives and should be treated with mastectomy. However, for patients with smaller, focal lesions (the majority of DCIS lesions), breast conservation therapy has a high probability of success and should routinely be presented as an alternative option. The use of breast conservation therapy for DCIS was based initially on extrapolation of data from prospective, randomized trials showing that mastectomy and breast conservation therapy produced similar outcomes in patients with invasive cancer. Subsequently, retrospective studies of patients with DCIS confirmed that mastectomy and breast conservation therapy produce similar outcomes in these patients.

Successful treatment of DCIS must begin with complete excision of all malignant-appearing micocalcifications. This makes mastectomy the only reasonable treatment option for patients with extensive DCIS. Incomplete excision of malignant-appearing microcalcifications with breast conservation therapy results in local recurrence rates of nearly 100% (Sneige et al, 1995). On the basis of these observations, breast conservation should be contemplated only for patients in whom the entire mammographic abnormality can be completely excised with an acceptable cosmetic outcome. Although some investigators have reported that young age (< 40 years), comedo subtype, high nuclear grade, the presence of necrosis, and DCIS presenting as a bloody nipple discharge appear to predict for a high risk of local recurrence, other investigators have not been able to confirm these associations.

In the best of hands, conservative surgery and radiation therapy for mammographically detected DCIS generally results in a 5-year actuarial risk of breast recurrence of less than 10%. Additional breast recurrences are seen between 5 and 10 years after treatment, resulting in 10-year actuarial breast recurrence rates ranging from 6% to 23%, with breast cancer–specific mortality rates ranging from 0% to 4% (Table 9–1) (Solin et al, 1993, 1996; Fowble et al, 1997; Vicini et al, 1997; Hiramatsu et al, 1995; Kuske et al, 1993; Silverstein et al, 1995a,b; Sneige et al, 1995). Although the reported series of breast conservation therapy for DCIS differ from one another with respect to patient selection, the extent of resection, and the degree of mammographic and pathologic correlation, they all point out the necessity of long-term follow-up in this disease, especially in the case of low-grade lesions.

Two prospective, randomized trials are available that permit assessment of the incremental benefit of radiation therapy for DCIS: the National Surgical Adjuvant Breast and Bowel Project (NSABP) B-17 trial and the European Organization for Research and Treatment of Cancer (EORTC) 10853 trial (Table 9–2). The NSABP trial enrolled a total of 814 patients with clinically or radiographically detected DCIS between 1985 and 1990. Eighty-three percent of the tumors were detected by screening mammography and were not palpable; however, there were no limits on the size of the area of DCIS (Fisher et al, 1998). After complete surgical excision, defined by the NSABP as no visible DCIS at the inked margins, patients were randomly assigned to receive postoperative irradiation or observation. No additional therapy was permitted. At a median follow-up time of 8 years, patients treated with excision plus irradiation had a significantly decreased risk of ipsilateral breast recurrence (12.1% vs 26.8%). Even more striking was the reduction in the risk of invasive recurrences (3.9% vs 13.4%). The risks of distant metastases and death from ipsilateral breast cancer did not differ significantly between the 2 groups.

The EORTC 10853 trial (Julien et al, 2000) began recruiting patients in 1986. Its design was very similar to that of the NSABP B-17 trial. A total of 1010 patients were randomly assigned to excision or excision plus radiation therapy, and at a median follow-up time of 4 years, 1002 patients were available for analysis. Seventy-one percent of the lesions were detectable by mammography only, and the mean diameter of the mammographic abnormality was 20 mm. Tumor-free surgical margins were required, but the extent of the margins was not specified other than that DCIS should not be present at the margin of the specimen. In patients who received radiation therapy, the whole breast was treated to 50 Gy at 2 Gy per fraction. Only 5% of patients received a radiation boost. At a median follow-up time of 4 years, the local relapse-free survival rate was significantly increased by radiation therapy (91% vs 84%; $P = .005$).

Recently, a few vocal advocates have championed wide excision alone without radiation therapy for some patients with DCIS (Lagios and Silverstein, 1997; Silverstein et al, 1995a,b). Although these investigators have reported 10-year actuarial risks of local recurrence of 20% to 25% and although half to one third of these recurrences are invasive, these investigators point out that the large majority of patients are adequately

Table 9–1. Results of Conservative Surgery and Radiation Therapy for Mammographically Detected Ductal Carcinoma In Situ

First Author, Year	No. of Patients	Recurrence Rate at 5 Years (%)	Annual Hazard (%)	Recurrence Rate at 10 Years (%)	Annual Hazard (%)
Solin, 1993, 1996 (Collaborative Group)	172	7	1.4	14	1.4
Fowble, 1997	110	1	0.2	15	1.5
Vicini, 1997	102	4	0.8	6	0.6
Hiramatsu, 1995	54	2	0.4	23	2.3
Kuske, 1993	44	7	1.4	—	—
Silverstein, 1995a,b	33	7	1.4	19	1.9
Sneige, 1995	31	0	0	8	0.8
Weighted Average		6.7	1.4	14.5	1.5

Table 9–2. Ipsilateral Breast Recurrence in Randomized Trials of Excision with and without Breast Irradiation for Ductal Carcinoma In Situ

Study	No. of Patients	Follow-up Time	Risk of Ipsilateral Breast Recurrence	
			Excision Alone	Excision and Irradiation
NSABP B-17 (Fisher et al, 1998)	814	8 years (mean)	26.8% (all) 13.4% (invasive)	12.1% (all) 3.9% (invasive)
EORTC 10853 (Julien et al, 2000)	1002	4 years (median)	16% (all) 8% (invasive)	9% (all) 4% (invasive)

EORTC, European Organization for Research and Treatment of Cancer; NSABP, National Surgical Adjuvant Breast and Bowel Project.

managed with surgery. It is clear from the 2 prospective trials discussed earlier in this chapter that wide local excision alone is associated with higher local recurrence rates than excision plus radiation therapy. Nonetheless, the incremental benefit from radiation therapy may be small in certain patient groups, and regardless of the type of local treatment, the risk of death from breast cancer in patients with DCIS is negligible.

Because of the limitations of the available data, at M. D. Anderson Cancer Center, patients with "good risk" DCIS are enrolled in an intergroup trial sponsored by the Radiation Therapy Oncology Group. This phase III trial compares the results of treatment with tamoxifen alone versus tamoxifen plus radiation therapy for good-risk DCIS. To be eligible, patients must have unicentric, mammographically detected DCIS measuring up to 2.5 cm in greatest dimension on mammograms. Histologically, the lesions must be classified as low or intermediate grade and must have been excised with inked margins measuring 3 mm or more. Patients may be started on tamoxifen 20 mg daily and are randomly assigned to whole-breast irradiation or observation. It is estimated that nearly 1000 patients will need to be assigned to each arm of the study to permit detection of a 40% reduction in the 5-year local recurrence rate with radiation therapy.

At M. D. Anderson, patients with intermediate- to high-risk DCIS (defined as close margins of resection, lesion size >1 cm, the presence of necrosis, or high nuclear grade) who are not eligible for or choose not to participate in the intergroup trial are routinely offered radiation therapy. The techniques and doses used are similar to those for invasive carcinoma of the breast, discussed in detail below. The whole breast mound is encompassed in a pair of tangential fields (usually 6-MV photons), and 50 Gy is delivered in 25 fractions over 5 weeks. Subsequently, the operative bed is boosted with an additional 10 to 14 Gy, the higher dose being used in the case of close margins.

Treatment of Early-Stage Invasive Cancer

Numerous prospective randomized trials have established the role of breast conservation therapy as an alternative to mastectomy for early-stage invasive breast cancer (van Dongen et al, 1992; Blichert-Toft et al, 1992; Fisher et al, 1998). In the aggregate, these studies enrolled more than 3000 patients and have reported follow-up times ranging from 3.3 to 18 years. While there are subtle yet important differences between the trials with respect to surgical and radiation therapy techniques, none of these trials demonstrated significant differences in disease-specific or overall survival between the 2 treatment arms. In 5 of the 6 trials, local-regional recurrence rates were equivalent between the 2 arms, with local recurrence rates in the treated breast or chest wall ranging from 3% to 19%. As a result of these compelling studies, breast conservation therapy is considered a mainstay of treatment for early-stage invasive carcinoma of the breast.

Investigators have attempted to identify subsets of patients with early-stage invasive breast cancer for whom radiation therapy is not required after limited surgery. Seven prospective trials have been reported that compare excision and radiation therapy with conservative surgery alone (Fisher et al, 1995; Clark et al, 1996; Veronesi et al, 1993; Forrest et al, 1996; Renton et al, 1996; Liljegren et al, 1994, 1997; Schnitt et al, 1996) (Table 9–3). As a group, the trials show that radiation therapy results in a 2.2- to 9-fold reduction in ipsilateral breast tumor recurrence. Studies with shorter follow-up demonstrate a smaller absolute magnitude of benefit. However, when their annual hazard rate is projected to 10 years, a minimum 35% breast failure rate is anticipated for excision alone. At this time, no group of patients has been identified who should not routinely receive breast irradiation as a component of breast conservation therapy.

The most rigorous attempt to prospectively identify patients with early-stage breast cancer who may not require radiation therapy was a study performed at Harvard (Schnitt et al, 1996). This study had a sequential design and eventually accrued 87 patients. All patients with unicentric, clinically T1 carcinomas of ductal, mucinous, or tubular histologic subtype without an extensive intraductal component or lymphatic vessel invasion were eligible. All patients underwent an axillary dissection and had histologically negative lymph nodes, and all patients underwent a wide excision and had pathologically documented negative margins of at least 1 cm. The majority (76%) of the lesions were detected by mammography alone. The median pathologic tumor size was 9 mm.

The protocol was closed before the target accrual was reached because at a median follow-up time of 56 months, the investigators crossed a pre-defined stopping boundary: an average annual local recurrence rate of 4.2% (cumulative recurrence rate at closing, 16%). The authors noted that 11 of the 14 recurrences were in the vicinity of the initial tumor, despite the fact that re-excision immediately after the initial excision had revealed no residual tumor. The authors concluded that even in this highly selected group of patients, the risk of local recurrence after wide excision alone was substantial. They further concluded that even if a subset of patients was identified in whom radiation therapy could be omitted after conservative surgery, such patients would most likely account for only a small proportion of women with breast cancer.

Some authors have concluded that older patients and those with very small, low-grade lesions may be adequately treated without radiation therapy (Liljegren et al, 1997). The number of patients in these studies has been small, the follow-up time has been short, and these patient subgroups were only recognized retrospectively using subset analyses. A prospective trial to assess the role of radiation therapy in elderly patients, sponsored by the Cancer and Leukemia Group B and conducted through

Table 9–3. Local Recurrence in Randomized Trials of Conservative Surgery with and without Radiation Therapy for Invasive Breast Cancer

Trial	No. of Patients	Conservative Surgery Alone		Conservative Surgery Plus Radiation Therapy		Interval Reported (years)
		Recurrence Rate	Annual Hazard (% per year)	Recurrence Rate	Annual Hazard (% per year)	
NSABP (Fisher et al, 1995)	1265	35	2.9	10	0.8	12
Ontario (Clark et al, 1996)	837	40	4.0	18	1.8	10
Milan III (Veronesi et al, 1993)	601	18	3.6	2	0.4	5
Scottish (Forrest et al, 1996)	556	28	5.6	6	1.2	5
British (Renton et al, 1996)	399	35	7.0	13	2.6	5
Uppsala-Örebro (Liljegren et al, 1994, 1997)	381	18	3.6	2	0.4	5
Harvard (Schnitt et al, 1996)	87	16	3.4	NA	NA	4.7

NA, not available; NSABP, National Surgical Adjuvant Breast and Bowel Project.

the intergroup mechanism, has recently finished accrual. The trial enrolled women at least 70 years of age with T1 N0 breast cancers. All women underwent breast-conserving surgery and were placed on tamoxifen. They were subsequently randomly assigned to radiation therapy or observation. The results of this strategy have not been reported at this time.

Treatment Parameters

The goal of breast irradiation after breast conservation therapy is to deliver tumoricidal doses of radiation to the remaining breast tissue. At the same time, it is necessary to avoid adjacent normal tissue not at risk for harboring residual tumor cells. The technical aspects of breast radiation therapy are central to its success and should not be minimized. Customized treatment planning with attention to variations in anatomy, location of the tumor bed, and protection of intrathoracic contents is necessary for complication-free, successful outcomes.

During treatment planning, the glandular breast is encompassed in a pair of tangential megavoltage photon (x-ray) beams. Excess exposure of the lung (usually considered more than 2 to 3 cm in chordal dimension) or left ventricle is to be avoided. The use of individualized patient immobilization devices, beam-shaping blocks, wedge or compensating filters, and advanced dosimetric techniques may be useful in improving the therapeutic index. At M. D. Anderson, most patients are treated at 2 Gy per fraction to a total dose of 50 Gy in 5 weeks. Subsequently, an additional 10 Gy is delivered to the volume of breast surrounding the excision site (boost dose) in 5 fractions. Patients with close or positive margins of resection may receive a higher boost dose. For patients with DCIS and most patients with early-stage invasive carcinoma of the breast, usually no additional treatment fields are indicated (Figure 9–1).

In patients with locally advanced breast carcinoma who are offered breast conservation therapy, the volume at risk also includes the regional lymph node basins. The radiation therapy fields are appropriately modified to encompass these areas in addition to the glandular breast. This frequently involves the use of multiple adjacent treatment portals, which must be precisely matched to avoid the consequences of double treatment or geographic miss. Double-treated junctions develop late fibrosis, telangiectasia, decreased range of motion, and possibly even necrosis. Conversely, in the case of a geographic miss, an area of tissue containing residual tumor receives less than the appropriate dose of radiation. Geographic miss can result in local-regional recurrence of disease after radiation therapy. In patients with advanced breast cancers downstaged with neoadjuvant (preoperative) chemotherapy, our current practice is to design treatment fields based on the original extent of disease. In these circumstances, the treatment volume may be expanded to include the ipsilateral supraclavicular fossa, axilla, or internal mammary nodes or any combination of these areas in addition to the glandular breast.

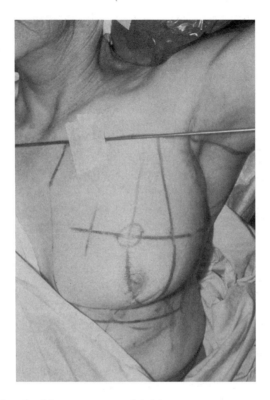

Figure 9–1.   Standard breast tangential fields.

Side Effects

The side effects of radiation therapy are well studied and quite predict-able. They are a function of the volume treated, the techniques used, and the total dose and fractionation schedule employed. Acute side effects of breast irradiation include mild to moderate redness of the treated skin and areas of patchy dry desquamation. While moist desquamation can occur in skin folds, moist desquamation is unusual in other parts of the breast. Most patients notice itching of the treated skin but rarely complain of a true "burning" sensation. During the first 6 months after completion of radiation therapy, mild to moderate breast edema and thickening of the breast skin ensues. This is particularly true in the dependent portions of the breast. A faint pink cast accompanied by skin edema (peau d'orange and ridging) may be present during the posttreatment period. These nor-mal effects may need to be differentiated from an inflammatory-type tu-mor recurrence by an experienced clinician. In most cases, breast edema disappears by 12 to 18 months after completion of radiation therapy; only in rare patients are late effects from radiation apparent. These may include telangiectases (dilated blood vessels due to injury of the reticular dermis) and tenderness in the region.

Pneumonitis (defined as a nonproductive cough accompanied by radiographic infiltrate in the area of the lung conforming to the radiation volume) is a subacute phenomenon seen occasionally. In patients treated with breast conservation therapy, pneumonitis usually occurs between 6 weeks and 6 months after the radiation therapy is completed and is uncommon thereafter. The risk of pneumonitis is directly related to the aggregate volume of lung included in the radiation portals as well as the use of any radiation-sensitizing agents, especially chemotherapy (Lingos et al, 1991). The risk of pneumonitis is generally less than 1% for patients who undergo irradiation of the breast alone without chemotherapy. The risk of pneumonitis may be as high as 10% for patients treated with comprehensive breast and lymph node irradiation and concurrent or high-dose chemotherapy.

There is compelling evidence that certain radiation therapy techniques can result in late cardiac mortality (Gyenes et al, 1996; Rutqvist et al, 1992). After a long latency period, possibly as much as 15 to 20 years, radiation techniques that include significant amounts of myocardium can lead to an increased risk of ischemic heart disease. The highest-risk techniques include large amounts of the left ventricle and the coronary arteries within deep tangential fields or use appositional photon fields to treat the internal mammary chain, which results in excess exit into the heart (Janjan et al, 1989). Avoidance of these high-risk techniques should reduce any excessive cardiovascular mortality from breast irradiation.

Patients and clinicians alike express great concern about the risks of radiation-induced carcinogenesis. Sarcomas in the radiation portals are a rare complication of breast irradiation. Risk factors related to the development of sarcomas are not fully defined, but it is likely that beam energy, total radiation dose, and the development of regional edema are contributing factors. On the basis of large retrospective studies of thousands of patients, the frequency of radiation-induced sarcoma at 10 years is estimated to be 0.2% (Taghian et al, 1991; Karlsson et al, 1996). Among randomized controlled trials comparing mastectomy with lumpectomy plus radiation therapy, no trial detected a significant increase in second malignant neoplasms in patients receiving radiation therapy. These results suggest that the risk of carcinogenic effects from breast irradiation is clinically insignificant.

Special Case: Treatment of Advanced-Stage Disease

One of the most exciting developments in recent years in the field of breast cancer treatment is the use of combined-modality therapy with neoadjuvant chemotherapy to permit breast conservation therapy in patients with advanced disease at presentation (Hortobagyi et al, 1988, 1991, 1995; Jacquillat et al, 1988; Danforth et al, 1986; Mauriac et al, 1991). Patients with large tumor size, advanced nodal presentation, or breast/tumor ratios that make primary surgery impossible or ill advised can have their disease "downstaged" using neoadjuvant chemotherapy. Patients are first assessed by a multidisciplinary team that includes the surgeon, the medical oncologist, the diagnostic radiologist, and the radiation oncologist. Patients then undergo neoadjuvant chemotherapy, which typically includes doxorubicin or a taxane. While the majority of patients have objective responses to neoadjuvant chemotherapy, only one quarter of patients meet all the requirements for breast conservation therapy, which are as follows (Singletary et al, 1992):

- Complete resolution of skin edema
- Residual tumor size of less than 5 cm, including suspicious microcalcifications
- Absence of known tumor multicentricity or extensive intramammary lymphatic invasion

If the tumor response to neoadjuvant chemotherapy is sufficient to fulfill these criteria for breast conservation, the surgeon attempts a wide local excision of the residual abnormality as well as an axillary dissection. All mammographically abnormal tissue must be removed, and histologically clear margins are required. After surgery, patients are given any additional planned chemotherapy, followed by radiation therapy to the breast and regional lymphatics.

The radiation therapy technique used for breast conservation in patients with locally advanced breast cancer can be challenging. In contrast to the situation in patients with early-stage breast cancer, the target volume in patients with locally advanced breast cancer extends beyond the intact breast to include the regional lymphatics. These may include lymph nodes of the axilla, the interpectoral (or Rotter's) nodes, and the nodes of the supraclavicular and internal mammary chains. Classically, irradiation of this target volume involves the use of multiple adjacent fields, resulting in greater complexity of set-up and reproducibility. Imprecise matching of adjacent fields can result in either underdose in this region or areas of dose excess with resulting normal tissue complications. Ideally, the use of noncoplanar beams with precise matching techniques such as those recommended by Chu et al (1990) are used when photon fields abut one another. Use of adjacent electron beam fields with shaped, matching field edges may be useful when part of the target area (such as the internal mammary chain) can be adequately covered with electrons. An example of a typical field arrangement is shown in Figure 9–2. Typically, the breast and undissected lymphatics will be treated to a dose of 50 Gy in 25 fractions over 5 weeks, followed by a 10-Gy boost to the tumor bed (Strom et al, 1993).

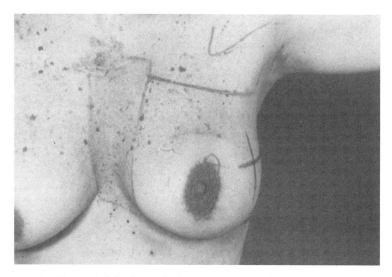

Figure 9–2.   Expanded fields used after neoadjuvant chemotherapy for advanced presentations.

An analysis of the first patients treated in this manner at M. D. Anderson revealed encouraging results (Vlastos et al, 2000). Between 1982 and 1994, a total of 93 patients underwent breast conservation therapy after neoadjuvant chemotherapy. The stage distribution at presentation for these patients was as follows: IIA, 24%; IIB, 28%; IIIA, 33%; IIIB, 12%; and IV (supraclavicular nodes only), 3%. The majority of patients (93%) had invasive ductal carcinoma not otherwise specified. With a median follow-up of 59 months, the crude local recurrence rate was 7.5%, and the rate of freedom from distant metastasis was 94%. The overall survival rate for the group at 5 years was 89%. The local control and survival rates for this highly selected patient group are very encouraging and warrant further study of breast conservation therapy after neoadjuvant chemotherapy for large primary and locally advanced breast cancers.

POSTMASTECTOMY IRRADIATION

In properly selected patients, radiation therapy after mastectomy significantly reduces the risk of local-regional recurrence and thereby improves both quality of life and survival.

Rationale and Choice of Targets

Postmastectomy irradiation is most effective when it is used to treat subclinical tumor in the remaining tissue of the anterior chest wall and the regional lymphatic basins. Since this subclinical disease is by definition undetectable, the probability of its presence and its likely distribution must be inferred from a variety of data sources. These include data from histologic analysis of surgical specimens, pattern-of-failure analyses, and prospective trials in which individuals or specific target volumes are allotted to treatment versus observation. Most patients with early-stage breast cancer are at low risk for local-regional recurrence after treatment with modified radical mastectomy and are unlikely to benefit from radiation therapy. Patients without residual viable tumor in the chest wall or regional nodes cannot be expected to benefit from postmastectomy irradiation.

Three recent prospective, randomized clinical trials have shown that when radiation therapy is appropriately utilized in patients with a high risk of persistent local-regional disease, the resulting improvement in local-regional control contributes to improved survival. Since the routine use of radiation therapy in low-risk patients has not been shown to produce a similar survival benefit, it is likely that there is a threshold phenomenon. On the basis of this assumption, radiation therapy is not routinely offered to patients at M. D. Anderson unless their cumulative risk of local-regional recurrence exceeds 20%. Therefore, only patients assessed as having an intermediate to high risk of persistent local-regional disease after mastectomy should be considered for treatment. The difficulty is defining which clinical parameters will accurately predict an intermediate to high risk of local-regional recurrence. Most authors would agree that these factors include locally advanced primary breast cancer, extensive lymph node involvement, and incomplete surgery. The factors predicting low risk of local-regional recurrence are less well defined.

Two recent retrospective studies at M. D. Anderson have been designed to assess which factors in our practice predict for an intermediate to high risk of local-regional recurrence after mastectomy (Katz et al, 2000). These studies included a cohort of 1031 patients who were treated with mastectomy and doxorubicin-based chemotherapy without irradiation in 5 prospective clinical trials. The median follow-up time was nearly 10 years. Patients with 4 or more involved nodes were found have local-regional recurrence rates in excess of 20% (Table 9–4). Within the group of patients with 1 to 3 involved nodes, those who had tumors measuring 4 cm or larger, gross extranodal extension, or inadequate axillary dissection also experienced higher rates of local-regional recurrence. The majority of patients with stage II breast cancer and 1 to 3 involved nodes had a substantially lower risk of local-regional recurrence and would be unlikely to benefit from radiation therapy.

The pattern of local-regional recurrence was also instructive. The vast majority of local-regional recurrences had a chest wall component (Table 9–5). The second most common location for recurrences was the anterior structures of the undissected (level III) axilla, infraclavicular fossa, or supraclavicular fossa. These findings are consistent with those of numerous other reports. Recurrence in the dissected portion of the axilla

Table 9–4. Ten-Year Risk (%) of Local-Regional Recurrence (LRR) after Mastectomy and Doxorubicin-Containing Chemotherapy at M. D. Anderson According to Tumor Size and Number of Involved Lymph Nodes*

Tumor Stage	Number of Involved Nodes			
	0	1–3	4–9	≥10
Isolated LRR				
T1	6	7	9	17
T2	11	12	23	17
T3	29	9	31	29
Cumulative LRR				
T1	11	9	17	17
T2	14	16	27	34
T3	29	23	40	29

*Isolated LRR indicates LRR alone as the first site of failure. Cumulative LRR indicates LRR at any time.
Adapted from Katz et al, 2000.

Table 9–5. Patterns of Local-Regional Recurrence (LRR) after Mastectomy and Doxorubicin-Containing Chemotherapy at M. D. Anderson*

Location of Recurrence	Isolated LRR**		Cumulative LRR	
	No.	%	No.	%
Chest wall	122	98	122	68
Supraclavicular nodes	41	33	71	40
Axilla	21	17	25	14
Infraclavicular nodes	10	8	12	7
Internal mammary chain	—	—	15	8
Any site	124	100	179	100

*Some patients experienced more than 1 site of failure, resulting in cumulative percentages greater than 100%.
**Isolated LRR indicates LRR alone as the first site of failure. Cumulative LRR indicates LRR at any time.
Adapted from Katz et al, 2000.

(level I and II) was very rare (3%). The risk of failure in the midaxilla was not significantly higher for patients with higher number of involved nodes, higher percentage of involved nodes, larger nodal size, or gross extranodal extension. These data suggest that specific irradiation of the axilla is rarely indicated if the axilla has been adequately dissected.

Treatment of the internal mammary chain continues to be hotly debated. This controversy arises because the data on this issue are confusing and seemingly contradictory. Histologic sampling of the internal mammary chain in patients with node-positive breast cancer reveals clinically occult disease in 20% to 50% of cases. In contrast, clinical recurrence in the internal mammary chain is rare. Further complicating this apparent paradox, the randomized trials showing survival advantages for post-mastectomy irradiation included the internal mammary chain in their intended treatment volume. The basic philosophy at M. D. Anderson is to attempt to include the internal mammary chain in the treatment volume provided that it does not compromise other aspects of the treatment. A more complete exploration of this issue has been published elsewhere (Strom and McNeese, 1999).

Radiation Therapy Technique

At M. D. Anderson, the choice of radiation therapy techniques and volumes is the result of the synthesis of our own experience with important studies from other institutions. A substantial portion of our patient population has locally advanced breast cancer, and this clearly has an impact on our perceptions about breast cancer and, in particular, our postmastectomy radiation therapy techniques for patients with intermediate-stage disease. In our practice, metastases to the internal mammary chain, interpectoral region, and supraclavicular nodes are commonly seen. This results in a treatment philosophy in which we usually strive to include all local-regional volumes at risk, even if encompassing these volumes is technically difficult. Multiple adjacent fields are commonly employed to optimize treatment and minimize irradiation of uninvolved adjacent structures.

Chest Wall

The chest wall is always treated when postmastectomy irradiation is delivered. Tangential 6-MV photons are most commonly employed; occasionally higher-energy photons are used. An adjacent, matching electron beam field is routinely added to treat the most medial chest wall and encompass the lymph nodes of the ipsilateral internal mammary chain. In addition to covering both targets, this treatment plan has the added benefit of broad coverage of the chest wall while avoiding excessive amounts of the intrathoracic contents. With this technique, the left ventricle can be completely excluded from the treatment volume in the case of left-sided cancers. Generally, inclusion of a maximum of 2 to 3 cm of lung in the treatment volume is acceptable (Figures 9–3 and 9–4).

Alternatively, electrons can be used to treat the chest wall and internal mammary nodes. Although this technique has the advantage of improved conformation of the treatment volume to the target volume, there is a greater risk of geographic miss of tumor or excess transmission into lung. Variations in tissue thickness make treatment planning difficult, particularly in patients with irregular surface contours.

Regardless of the technique employed, the entire volume of the mastectomy flaps must be included in the treatment volume. This includes the entire length of the mastectomy scar as well as any clips and drain

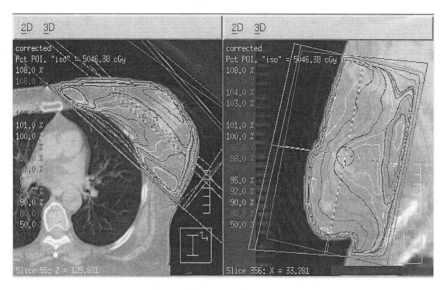

Figure 9–3. Treatment plan and isodose distribution for breast tangents. The routine use of computed tomography–based treatment planning permits more precise delineation of the volume encompassed in the high-dose region. In this patient, an additional cardiac block was subsequently added to avoid treatment of the epicardial vessels.

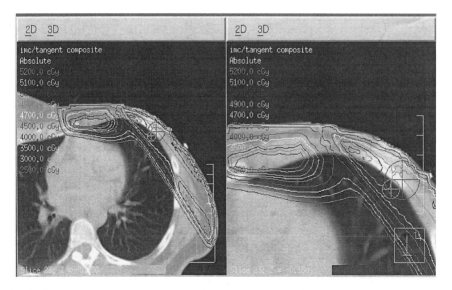

Figure 9–4. Treatment plan and isodose distribution for postmastectomy irradiation.

sites. Typically, the fields extend from midsternum to at least the midaxillary line. Depending on the extent of original disease and patient anatomy, the fields may need to extend even to the posterior axillary line. A common error in treatment planning is to skimp on the inferior border. This border should be placed approximately 2 cm caudad to the previous location of the inframammary sulcus.

The superior border of the chest wall fields abuts the supraclavicular field. To avoid junctional hot spots, one of several techniques must be employed to eliminate a divergent edge. We routinely use the "rod and chain" technique described by Chu et al (1990). This technique has several advantages: the border can be placed in any desired orientation, the full length of the tangential beam can be utilized, and the match line can be confirmed visually during treatment. The other alternative, using a mono-isocentric technique, has the disadvantage that only half of the available length (usually 20 cm) can be used for chest wall treatment. In patients with long torsos, this results in an excessively large supraclavicular field, and as a consequence, treatment of a larger volume of lung.

Computed tomography–based treatment planning is important since it permits precise visualization of the intrathoracic contents encompassed by the proposed treatment fields. Treatment of any cardiac volume should be actively avoided since such treatment is associated with late morbidity and mortality. Although most reports evaluating the cardiac morbidity of breast irradiation have studied the treated portion of the myocardium, it is likely that the sensitive target structures are the epicardial vessels. The implication is that there is no safe volume of heart that can be included in the high-dose volume.

We routinely utilize tissue heterogeneity correction in our planning process to minimize the hot spots caused by increased lung transmission. The dose of 50 Gy in 25 fractions is specified at an isodose that encompasses the entire target; thus it represents the target minimum dose. Moderate bolus schedules permit the completion of treatment without interruption. Typically, 3-mm or 5-mm bolus is used every other day for the first 2 to 3 weeks. Additional bolus can be used during the boost if the patient's skin reaction permits. Moderate erythema and dry desquamation are the desired end results

All patients receive a boost to the chest wall flaps. These fields represent only a moderate reduction in the field size as compared to the initial chest wall fields. Using electrons (2 fields are often required), the skin and subcutaneous tissues are the primary targets and are included within the distal 90% line. For patients with negative margins, 10 Gy in 5 fractions is given. For patients with close or positive margins, 14 to 16 Gy is the usual boost dose. Electron doses are all specified at the 100% isodose line, consistent with the recommendations of the International Commission on Radiation Units and Measurements (ICRU, 1978, 1993).

Supraclavicular Fossa

The second obligate treatment target of postmastectomy radiation therapy is the lymphatics of the supraclavicular fossa and undissected axillary apex. After a classic level I and II axillary dissection, the undissected portion of the axillary apex lies directly beneath the pectoralis major muscle. Therefore, the supraclavicular field extends from the jugular groove medially to the lateral edge of the pectoralis muscle. Careful placement of the inferior border (which is also the superior border of the chest wall fields) to ensure that it is as cephalad as possible can substantially reduce the volume of lung included in the aggregate treatment fields. Although photons are most commonly used to treat the supraclavicular and axillary apical nodes, the use of electrons may be considered in thin patients since all the structures are anterior. The dose for microscopic disease is 50 Gy in 25 fractions.

Internal Mammary Nodes

When the decision has been made to treat the internal mammary nodes (see the section Rationale and Choice of Targets earlier in this chapter), one of 2 techniques may be employed. The preferred technique uses a separate electron beam field on the most medial chest wall. Since the nodes typically lie 3 to 3.5 cm from the midline, this field must extend even further laterally to compensate for beam constriction. The field usually extends 5 to 6 cm away from the midline and is shaped to precisely match the edge of the tangent fields. Frequently, a small lateral tilt results in better field matching at depth. Computed tomography–based treatment planning with heterogeneity correction is mandatory to select an electron beam that covers the nodes without excess exit into the lung. Ideally, the nodes will be located within the distal 90% line, and the dose of 50 Gy in 25 fractions is specified at the 100% isodose line.

Some anatomic conformations are unfavorable for the use of a separate electron beam field to treat the internal mammary nodes. This is especially true in obese patients, patients with an intact breast, and patients who underwent breast reconstruction after mastectomy. The use of a "half wide" tangent field can be considered in these cases. The tangent fields are made extra deep at the superior border to encompass the first 3 intercostal spaces. Additional field blocking is placed on the lower portion of the tangents, similar to that used in a standard conformation. This technique has a number of disadvantages. The volume of lung treated is substantially increased compared to the volume treated with other techniques. In addition, the upper field edges frequently extend well beyond the midline, resulting in treatment of part of the contralateral breast. For these reasons, immediate reconstruction is strongly discouraged if postoperative irradiation is planned.

Axilla

Specific treatment of the dissected axilla is rarely required (see the section Rationale and Choice of Targets earlier in this chapter). In those circumstances in which irradiation of the axilla is desired, the majority of the axillary dose is delivered via the anterior supraclavicular field using photons. It is important to verify that all operative clips left by the surgeon in the axilla are included in either the chest wall fields or the lateral portion of the supraclavicular field. In the typical patient, delivering 50 Gy to the supraclavicular field results in 35 to 37 Gy at the midline axillary structures. A posterior photon field is then used to supplement the midaxilla to the desired target dose. Because of the morbidity of axillary irradiation and the infrequency of axillary failure, the usual dose is 40 Gy. Higher doses are employed only in patients with extensive axillary soft-tissue disease or an undissected axilla.

Treatment of Inflammatory Breast Cancer

Inflammatory carcinoma of the breast remains a most challenging entity for the oncology team. Patients with this uncommon type of locally advanced breast cancer present with the clinical triad of erythema, ridging, and peau d'orange, along with a clinical history consistent with a rapid growth pattern. The rapid doubling time of inflammatory breast cancer and its facility for hematogenous and local-regional spread necessitate precise coordination of systemic and local modalities.

Typically, treatment is initiated using cytotoxic agents. In most cases, initial local therapy with either surgery or radiation therapy is inappropriate. If the clinical response to the initial chemotherapy is inadequate, definitive local-regional therapy may begin. As a result of the clinical experience gained through serial prospective trials, our current approach to local-regional therapy for inflammatory breast cancer includes mastectomy followed by comprehensive radiation therapy (Hortobagyi, 1994; Singletary et al, 1994). This strategy permits the highest probability of local-regional disease control possible while minimizing the likelihood of late morbidity. Surgery is contemplated only when major resolution of the inflammatory change is seen, when it is anticipated that negative surgical margins can be achieved.

A series of prospective investigations at M. D. Anderson has demonstrated the usefulness of twice-daily fractionation and dose escalation in radiation therapy for inflammatory carcinoma. Radiation alone or combined with surgery resulted in local-regional failure rates of 50% with conventional fractionation (Barker et al, 1980). The introduction of twice-daily fractionation improved local control rates, but 27% of patients still did not have permanent local-regional control. Even with the use of tri-modality therapy (surgery, radiation therapy, and chemotherapy), 25% of patients had a local-regional recurrence as the first site of failure. In 1989, our study of twice-daily fractionation showed relatively few complications, and it was concluded that dose escalation could be performed safely (Thoms et al, 1989). Therefore, the dose given to the entire chest wall and regional nodes was increased from 45 Gy to 51 Gy. The boost dose to the chest wall remained at 15 Gy (for patients with negative surgical margins), for a total of 66 Gy instead of the previous 60 Gy.

At 5 years, these patients who received the higher dose of twice-daily fractionation had significant improvement in the rate of local-regional control compared with patients in the historical, lower-dose group (84% vs 58%) (Liao et al, 2000). Rates of long-term complications of radiation, such as severe arm edema, rib fractures, fibrosis, and symptomatic pneumonitis, were similar in the 2 groups. Better overall survival rates were also seen in the group that received the higher dose in spite of the fact that the chemotherapy regimens did not change significantly during this time.

The basic field selection parameters for inflammatory carcinoma are similar to those used for other forms of locally advanced breast cancer. Since inflammatory carcinoma typically spreads by dermal lymphatic channels, very broad margins on the chest wall flaps are required. The skin of the anterior chest is treated from slightly across the midline laterally to the posterior axillary line. The inferior border of the treatment fields is carried several centimeters beyond the location of the previous inframammary sulcus. The regional nodal fields are tailored to the volume of disease encountered at initial presentation. Extensive use of bolus is employed so as to achieve a brisk erythema and dry desquamation at completion of therapy. Patchy areas of moist desquamation are common and should not deter the clinician from an aggressive course. Ultimately, local-regional recurrence of disease is far more morbid than these temporary treatment-related symptoms.

TREATMENT OF LOCAL-REGIONALLY RECURRENT CANCER

Local-regionally recurrent breast cancer after mastectomy represents a heterogeneous mix of entities resulting from inadequate initial treatment or virulent tumor biology. The patient with an isolated chest wall nodule after a long disease-free interval has a different prognosis from the patient with an extensive, inflammatory-type recurrence involving the entire chest wall. Nonetheless, a few basic principles may be applied.

Patients with local-regional recurrence should not be treated with palliative intent as though they had visceral metastases. Although up to half of patients with local-regional recurrence will also manifest visceral metastases at presentation, a substantial portion of patients will be free of documented metastasis and can be long-term survivors when treated with curative intent. Aggressive systemic and local-regional therapy is indicated. Occasionally, local-regionally recurrent breast cancer can be completely resected with clear margins. In these circumstances, systemic therapy and local-regional irradiation can be delivered in the adjuvant setting. More commonly, neoadjuvant chemotherapy is required to render the disease resectable, and radiation therapy is delivered after surgery. With the use of these strategies, 4 of 5 patients treated at M. D. Anderson will have long-term local-regional control of disease.

Patients with local-regionally recurrent disease that does not respond to neoadjuvant chemotherapy have a guarded prognosis. The treatment of macroscopic recurrences with radiation therapy alone is unlikely to be successful. In our series of patients treated with multimodal therapy (Ballo et al, 1999), the actuarial local-regional control rate at 5 years in patients with gross disease present at initiation of radiation therapy was 36%. Inevitably, these individuals also developed distant metastases. Because typically a massive amount of tumor is present, it is not surprising that reasonable doses of radiation failed to control the disease. Although dose escalation may have some value in this population, we are currently investigating concurrent chemotherapy and radiation therapy as an alternative.

The appropriate treatment volume for local-regionally recurrent breast cancer is similar to that in the postmastectomy setting. The entire chest wall and the undissected lymphatics of the axillary apex and supraclavicular fossa comprise the minimum treatment volume. Commonly, the internal mammary chain and the midaxilla will also be treated. Because of the substantial number of treatment failures seen with the use of doses similar to those used in the postmastectomy setting, we currently use a 10% escalated dose (compared with the dose used in other postmastectomy settings) when treating local-regionally recurrent disease. All areas being treated prophylactically are treated to 54 Gy in 27 fractions, and all areas to be boosted for microscopic disease receive an additional 12 Gy in 6 fractions.

TREATMENT OF ADENOCARCINOMA IN AXILLARY NODES WITH UNKNOWN PRIMARY TUMOR

Although adenocarcinoma presenting in axillary lymph nodes without an identifiable primary tumor is an uncommon clinical entity, the oncologist must be aware of its predictable clinical course. Most commonly the cause of the metastases is an occult primary breast tumor, although carcinomas of the thyroid, lung, stomach, and colorectum may also metastasize to axillary nodes. Once initial investigation (including mammography, breast sonography, and breast magnetic resonance imaging) has failed to disclose an obvious primary lesion, the subsequent therapeutic plan is based on the assumption that a microscopic cancer is present in the ipsilateral breast.

In most cases, axillary lymph nodes must reach a substantial size before the patient notices any abnormality. Thus axillary disease without a known primary tumor is most commonly staged T0 N2 (stage IIIA). After careful assessment of the extent and distribution of the regional disease— usually by a combination of physical and ultrasound examinations of the axilla, infraclavicular fossa, and supraclavicular fossa—treatment is initiated in a manner consistent with the treatment of any other stage III breast cancer. Neoadjuvant chemotherapy is the norm, and typically 6 to 8 cycles are given preoperatively.

Local therapy consists of surgical excision of all gross disease followed by radiation therapy to the breast and regional lymphatics. In most cases, surgical removal of the apparently normal breast has no therapeutic advantage since in any case comprehensive irradiation will be required. In a recent analysis of 27 patients who had adenocarcinoma in axillary nodes and an unknown primary tumor and were treated with breast conservation therapy, high rates of local and regional control were achieved (Read et al, 1996). The 5-year actuarial local control rate in the breast was 100%, and the regional control rate was 92.6%.

The ipsilateral breast is treated with tangential fields of megavoltage photons to a dose of 50 Gy in 25 fractions. The supraclavicular fossa and axillary apex are also treated to 50 Gy in 25 fractions, and the midaxilla is frequently supplemented using a posterior field.

RADIATION THERAPY FOR PALLIATION

Radiation therapy is an effective palliative tool for patients with symptomatic tumor. The clinical indications that call for local palliative therapy fall into 2 broad groups: relief of symptoms such as pain or malodorous discharge, and cessation of local tumor growth to prevent symptoms. These symptoms can be due to increasing pressure or structural compromise, such as impending paralysis or extensive cortical destruction of a weight-bearing bone.

Optimal palliation is achieved by balancing the potential benefits of local treatment with the side effects, costs, and inconvenience that the patient must bear. Various schemes are employed, depending upon the volume to be irradiated, the tolerance of the surrounding tissues, and comorbid conditions. Generally, higher cumulative doses and smaller fractions are utilized for patients with a relatively good long-term prognosis, while ultrarapid schedules are preferred for patients with rapidly growing disease.

Bone metastases respond particularly well to radiation therapy. Relief of pain and reversal of disability can be expected in the majority of patients. While some pain relief can be expected during the radiation therapy course, the majority of benefit occurs after completion of treatment. It is after treatment that restoration of bone can be expected, although normalization of radiographs is uncommon. It is important to keep patients physically moving even though they have metastasis. Effective use of nonsteroidal antiinflammatory drugs and narcotic analgesics along with physical therapy support is crucial to good long-term function.

Since breast cancer patients with bone-only disease are likely to live for years or even decades, careful treatment planning requires the minimization of late effects and the anticipation of future courses of therapy. The careful selection of field borders and the use of an appropriate fractionation scheme are both factors that contribute to these goals. Typically, 30 Gy is delivered in 10 fractions over 2 weeks, although higher doses may be appropriate in patients with indolent disease and 8 Gy in a single fraction can be used for patients with limited life expectancy.

Patients with extensive soft-tissue disease involving the breast, chest wall, or brachial plexus frequently require intensive radiation therapy to minimize pain, neuropathy, and wound care problems. Patients with unresectable disease that is unresponsive to systemic agents may experience substantial palliation after irradiation. Because of the large volume of disease, high doses are required to achieve the desired effect. At a minimum, the region is treated to 45 Gy in 15 fractions with vigorous use of bolus over cutaneous nodules. Since it is common to see confluent moist desquamation and exfoliation of thin layers of normal skin overlying bulk tumor, a treatment break is usually required after this initial therapy. An additional 15 to 30 Gy can be delivered to residual tumor when treatment resumes (presuming no dose-limiting structures reside in the boost volume). Recent pilot studies using concurrent radiation therapy and chemosensitizing agents, such as paclitaxel, docetaxel, and capecitabine, have resulted in encouraging response rates. Additional study is required before this approach can be recommended outside the context of a clinical trial.

The development of brain metastases usually represents the beginning of an accelerated phase of breast cancer. Whenever possible, symptomatic brain lesions should be excised to achieve the most rapid response. While whole-brain irradiation is probably effective in controlling microscopic and small-volume macroscopic disease, it is important to balance these benefits against the potential late morbid effects on normal brain parenchyma. Both total dose and fraction size contribute to the potential risk of late effects in this setting. Use of 2-Gy or 2.5-Gy fractions is preferable to use of larger fractions. A dose of 30 Gy is commonly delivered to the whole brain, and boosts may be directed at individual tumor nodules, using either reduced-field or radiosurgical techniques.

Spinal cord compression represents a true radiotherapeutic emergency. After initiation of high-dose steroids, patients with symptomatic com-

---

KEY PRACTICE POINTS

- Ideal treatment of DCIS is evolving. Whenever possible, patients with favorable characteristics should be enrolled in cooperative-group trials.

- All patients with invasive carcinoma should receive radiation therapy as part of breast conservation therapy. In patients with implants, collagen vascular disorders, very large breast size, or large tumors downstaged by neoadjuvant chemotherapy, it is helpful to have the radiation oncologist see the patient before surgery.

- Postoperative irradiation is appropriate for all patients with stage III breast cancer and patients with stage II breast cancer and at least 4 positive lymph nodes. For patients with stage II disease with 1 to 3 nodes containing tumor, the data are conflicting. The preferred option is to enroll these patients in the intergroup randomized clinical trial.

- Locally advanced and local-regionally recurrent breast cancer are curable diseases but require particularly careful integration of treatment modalities. Ideally, all the potential care services should see the patient before therapy is begun.

- Patients with symptomatic metastases should be considered for appropriate local therapy in addition to being given adequate analgesia. Bone metastases, spinal cord compression, brain metastases, and extensive soft tissue disease are particularly suited for palliative irradiation.

---

pression of the cord by tumor should undergo irradiation as quickly as possible to prevent irreversible myelopathy. The diagnostic dilemma is to differentiate this clinical scenario from cord impingement by retropulsed bony fragments from a collapsed vertebra. In this latter setting, surgical intervention is preferred since radiation therapy cannot reverse the mechanical abnormality. Typically, 30 to 45 Gy is delivered using parallel opposed fields using 3-Gy fractions.

SUGGESTED READINGS

Ballo MT, Strom EA, Prost H, et al. Local-regional control of recurrent breast carcinoma after mastectomy: does hyperfractionated accelerated radiotherapy improve local control? *Int J Radiat Oncol Biol Phys* 1999;44:105–112.

Barker JL, Montague ED, Peters LJ. Clinical experience with irradiation of inflammatory carcinoma of the breast with and without elective chemotherapy. *Cancer* 1980;45:625–629.

Betsill WL Jr, Rosen PP, Lieberman PH, Robbins GF. Intraductal carcinoma. Long-term follow-up after treatment by biopsy alone. *JAMA* 1978;239:1863–1867.

Blichert-Toft M, Rose C, Andersen JA, et al. Danish randomized trial comparing breast conservation therapy with mastectomy: six years of life-table analysis. Danish Breast Cancer Cooperative Group. *NCI Monogr* 1992;11:19–25.

Bucalossi P, Veronesi U, Zingo L, Cantu C. Enlarged mastectomy for breast cancer. Review of 1,213 cases. *Am J Roentgenol Radium Ther Nucl Med* 1971;111:119–122.

Chu JC, Solin LJ, Hwang CC, Fowble B, Hanks GE, Goodman RL. A nondivergent three field matching technique for breast irradiation. *Int J Radiat Oncol Biol Phys* 1990;19:1037–1040.

Clark RM, Whelan T, Levine M, et al. Randomized clinical trial of breast irradiation following lumpectomy and axillary dissection for node-negative breast cancer: an update. Ontario Clinical Oncology Group. *J Natl Cancer Inst* 1996;88:1659–1664.

Danforth DJ, Findlay PA, McDonald HD, et al. Complete axillary lymph node dissection for stage I–II carcinoma of the breast. *J Clin Oncol* 1986;4:655–662.

Deemarski L, Seleznev IK. Extended radical operations on breast cancer of medial or central location. *Surgery* 1984;96:73–77.

Fentiman IS. The treatment of in situ breast cancer. *Acta Oncol* 1989;28:923–926.

Fisher B, Anderson S, Redmond CK, Wolmark N, Wickerham DL, Cronin WM. Reanalysis and results after 12 years of follow-up in a randomized clinical trial comparing total mastectomy with lumpectomy with or without irradiation in the treatment of breast cancer. *N Engl J Med* 1995;333:1456–1461.

Fisher B, Dignam J, Wolmark N, et al. Lumpectomy and radiation therapy for the treatment of intraductal breast cancer: findings from National Surgical Adjuvant Breast and Bowel Project B-17. *J Clin Oncol* 1998;16:441–452.

Forrest AP, Stewart HJ, Everington D, et al. Randomised controlled trial of conservation therapy for breast cancer: 6-year analysis of the Scottish trial. Scottish Cancer Trials Breast Group. *Lancet* 1996;348:708–713.

Fowble B, Hanlon AL, Fein DA, et al. Results of conservative surgery and radiation for mammographically detected ductal carcinoma in situ (DCIS). *Int J Radiat Oncol Biol Phys* 1997;38:949–957.

Gyenes G, Fornander T, Carlens P, Glas U, Rutqvist LE. Myocardial damage in breast cancer patients treated with adjuvant radiotherapy: a prospective study. *Int J Radiat Oncol Biol Phys* 1996;36:899–905.

Handley RS. Carcinoma of the breast. *Ann R Coll Surg Engl* 1975;57:59–66.

Hiramatsu H, Bornstein BA, Recht A, et al. Local recurrence after conservative surgery and radiation therapy for ductal carcinoma in situ. *Cancer J Sci Am* 1995;1:55.

Hortobagyi GN. Multidisciplinary management of advanced primary and metastatic breast cancer. *Cancer* 1994;74:416–423.

Hortobagyi GN, Ames FC, Buzdar AU, et al. Management of stage III primary breast cancer with primary chemotherapy, surgery, and radiation therapy. *Cancer* 1988;62:2507–2516.

Hortobagyi GN, et al. Primary chemotherapy (PCT) for breast cancer (BCa). M. D. Anderson experience. In: Third International Congress on Neo-Adjuvant Chemotherapy. New York: Springer-Verlag; 1991.

Hortobagyi GN, Buzdar AU, Strom EA, Ames FC, Singletary SE. Primary chemotherapy for early and advanced breast cancer. *Cancer Lett* 1995;90:103–109.

International Commission on Radiation Units and Measurements. ICRU Report 29: Dose Specification for Reporting External Beam Therapy with Photons and Electrons. Washington: ICRU; 1978.

International Commission on Radiation Units and Measurements. ICRU Report 50: Prescribing, Recording, and Reporting Photon Beam Therapy. Bethesda: ICRU, 1993.

Jacquillat C, Baillet F, Weil M, et al. Results of a conservative treatment combining induction (neoadjuvant) and consolidation chemotherapy, hormonotherapy, and external and interstitial irradiation in 98 patients with locally advanced breast cancer (IIA-IIIB). *Cancer* 1988;15:1977–1982.

Janjan NA, Gillin MT, Prows J, et al. Dose to the cardiac vascular and conduction systems in primary breast irradiation [published erratum appears in Med Dosim 1989;14:305]. *Med Dosim* 1989;14:81–87.

Julien JP, Bijker N, Fentiman IS, et al. Radiotherapy in breast-conserving treatment for ductal carcinoma in situ: first results of the EORTC randomised phase III trial 10853. EORTC Breast Cancer Cooperative Group and EORTC Radiotherapy Group. *Lancet* 2000;355:528–533.

Karlsson P, Holmberg E, Johansson KA, Kindblom LG, Carstensen J, Wallgren A. Soft tissue sarcoma after treatment for breast cancer. *Radiother Oncol* 1996;38: 25–31.

Katz A, Strom EA, Buchholz TA, et al. Locoregional recurrence patterns after mastectomy and doxorubicin-based chemotherapy: implications for postoperative irradiation. *J Clin Oncol* 2000;18:2817–2827.

Kuske RR, Bean JM, Garcia DM, et al. Breast conservation therapy for intraductal carcinoma of the breast. *Int J Radiat Oncol Biol Phys* 1993;26:391–396.

Lacour J, Bucalossi P, Cacers E, et al. Radical mastectomy versus radical mastectomy plus internal mammary dissection. Five-year results of an international cooperative study. *Cancer* 1976;37:206–214.

Lacour J, Le MG, Hill C, Kramar A, Contesso G, Sarrazin D. Is it useful to remove internal mammary nodes in operable breast cancer? *Eur J Surg Oncol* 1987;13:309–314.

Lagios MD, Silverstein MJ. Ductal carcinoma in situ. The success of breast conservation therapy: a shared experience of two single institutional nonrandomized prospective studies. *Surg Oncol Clin N Am* 1997;6:385–392.

Liao Z, Strom EA, Buzdar AU, et al. Locoregional irradiation for inflammatory breast cancer: effectiveness of dose escalation in decreasing recurrence. *Int J Radiat Oncol Biol Phys* 2000;47:1191–1200.

Liljegren G, Holmberg L, Adami HO, Westman G, Graffman S, Bergh J. Sector resection with or without postoperative radiotherapy for stage I breast cancer: five-year results of a randomized trial. Uppsala-Orebro Breast Cancer Study Group. *J Natl Cancer Inst* 1994;86:717–722.

Liljegren G, Lindgren A, Bergh J, Nordgren H, Tabar L, Holmberg L. Risk factors for local recurrence after conservative treatment in stage I breast cancer. Definition of a subgroup not requiring radiotherapy. *Ann Oncol* 1997;8:235–241.

Lingos TI, Recht A, Vicini F, Abner A, Silver B, Harris JR. Radiation pneumonitis in breast cancer patients treated with conservative surgery and radiation therapy. *Int J Radiat Oncol Biol Phys* 1991;21:355–360.

Mauriac L, Durand M, Avril A, Dilhuydy JM. Effects of primary chemotherapy in conservative treatment of breast cancer patients with operable tumors larger than 3 cm. Results of a randomized trial in a single centre. *Ann Oncol* 1991;2:347–354.

Overgaard M. Overview of randomized trials in high risk breast cancer patients treated with adjuvant systemic therapy with or without postmastectomy irradiation. *Semin Radiat Oncol* 1999;9:292–299.

Overgaard M, Christensen JJ, Johansen RA, et al. Postmastectomy irradiation in high-risk breast cancer patients. Present status of the Danish Breast Cancer Cooperative Group trials. *Acta Oncol* 1988;27:707–714.

Overgaard M, Hansen PS, Overgaard C, et al. Postoperative radiotherapy in high-risk premenopausal women with breast cancer who receive adjuvant chemotherapy. Danish Breast Cancer Cooperative Group 82b trial. *N Engl J Med* 1997;337:949–955.

Overgaard M, Jensen MB, Overgaard PS, et al. Postoperative radiotherapy in high-risk postmenopausal breast-cancer patients given adjuvant tamoxifen: Danish Breast Cancer Cooperative Group DBCG 82c randomised trial. *Lancet* 1999;353:1641–1648.

Ragaz J, Jackson SM, Le N, et al. Adjuvant radiotherapy and chemotherapy in node-positive premenopausal women with breast cancer. *N Engl J Med* 1997;337:956–962.

Read NE, Strom EA, McNeese MD. Carcinoma in axillary nodes in women with unknown primary site—results of breast-conserving therapy. *Breast J* 1996;2:403–409.

Renton SC, Gazet JC, Ford HT, Corbishley C, Sutcliffe R. The importance of the resection margin in conservative surgery for breast cancer. *Eur J Surg Oncol* 1996;22:17–22.

Rosen PP, Lesser ML, Kinne DW, Beattie EJ. Discontinuous or "skip" metastases in breast carcinoma. Analysis of 1228 axillary dissections. *Ann Surg* 1983;197:276–283.

Rutqvist LE, Lax I, Fornander T, Johansson H. Cardiovascular mortality in a randomized trial of adjuvant radiation therapy versus surgery alone in primary breast cancer. *Int J Radiat Oncol Biol Phys* 1992;22:887–896.

Schnitt SJ, Hayman J, Gelman R, et al. A prospective study of conservative surgery alone in the treatment of selected patients with stage I breast cancer. *Cancer* 1996;77:1094–1100.

Silverstein MJ, Barth A, Poller DN, et al. Ten-year results comparing mastectomy to excision and radiation therapy for ductal carcinoma in situ of the breast. *Eur J Cancer* 1995a;9:1425–1427.

Silverstein MJ, Poller DN, Waisman JR, et al. Prognostic classification of breast ductal carcinoma-in-situ. *Lancet* 1995b;345:1154–1157.

Singletary S, Ames F, Buzdar A. Management of inflammatory breast cancer. *World J Surg* 1994;18:87–92.

Singletary SE, McNeese MD, Hortobagyi GN. Feasibility of breast-conservation surgery after induction chemotherapy for locally advanced breast carcinoma. *Cancer* 1992;69:2849–2852.

Sneige N, McNeese MD, Atkinson EN, et al. Ductal carcinoma in situ treated with lumpectomy and irradiation: histopathological analysis of 49 specimens with emphasis on risk factors and long term results. *Hum Pathol* 1995;26:642–649.

Solin LJ, Kurtz J, Fourquet A, et al. Fifteen-year results of breast-conserving surgery and definitive breast irradiation for the treatment of ductal carcinoma in situ of the breast. *J Clin Oncol* 1996;14:754–763.

Solin LJ, Yeh IT, Kurtz J, et al. Ductal carcinoma in situ (intraductal carcinoma) of the breast treated with breast-conserving surgery and definitive irradiation. Correlation of pathologic parameters with outcome of treatment. *Cancer* 1993;71:2532–2542.

Strom EA, McNeese MD, Fletcher GH. Treatment of the peripheral lymphatics: rationale, indications, and techniques. In: Fletcher GH, Levitt SH, eds. *Controversial Issues in the Management of Breast Cancer.* New York: Springer-Verlag; 1993:57–72.

Strom EA, McNeese MD. Postmastectomy irradiation: rationale for treatment field selection. *Semin Radiat Oncol* 1999;9:247–253.

Sunshine JA, Moseley HS, Fletcher WS, Krippaehne WW. Breast carcinoma in situ. A retrospective review of 112 cases with a minimum 10 year follow-up. *Am J Surg* 1985;150:44–51.

Taghian A, de Vathaire F, Terrier P, et al. Long-term risk of sarcoma following radiation treatment for breast cancer. *Int J Radiat Oncol Biol Phys* 1991;21:361–367.

Thoms WJ, McNeese MD, Fletcher GH, Buzdar AU, Singletary SE, Oswald MJ. Multimodal treatment for inflammatory breast cancer. *Int J Radiat Oncol Biol Phys* 1989;17:739–745.

Urban JA, Marjani MA. Significance of internal mammary lymph node metastases in breast cancer. *Am J Roentgenol Radium Ther Nucl Med* 1971;111:130–136.

van Dongen JA, Bartelink H, Fentiman IS, et al. Randomized clinical trial to assess the value of breast-conserving therapy in stage I and II breast cancer, EORTC 10801 trial. *Monogr Natl Cancer Inst* 1992;11:15–18.

Veronesi U, Luini A, Del Vecchio M, et al. Radiotherapy after breast-preserving surgery in women with localized cancer of the breast. *N Engl J Med* 1993; 328:1587–1591.

Veronesi U, Rilke F, Luini A, et al. Distribution of axillary node metastases by level of invasion: an analysis of 539 cases. *Cancer* 1987;59:682–687.

Vicini FA, Lacerna MD, Goldstein NS, et al. Ductal carcinoma in situ detected in the mammographic era: an analysis of clinical, pathologic, and treatment-related factors affecting outcome with breast-conserving therapy. *Int J Radiat Oncol Biol Phys* 1997;39:627–635.

Vlastos G, Mirza NQ, Lenert JT, et al. The feasibility of minimally invasive surgery for stage IIA, IIB, and IIIA breast carcinoma patients after tumor downstaging with induction chemotherapy. *Cancer* 2000;88:1417–1424.

10   Serum and Tissue Markers for Breast Cancer

Francisco J. Esteva and Herbert A. Fritsche, Jr.

Chapter Overview

The use of tumor markers for assessing prognosis and treatment response in breast cancer has been investigated in clinical trials. Carcinoembryonic antigen, the *MUC-1* gene product, and the HER-2/*neu* extracellular domain are serum markers that have been found to be useful in assessing response to hormonal therapy and chemotherapy in patients with metastatic breast cancer. Likewise, tissue markers such as Ki-67, the estrogen and progesterone receptors, and HER-2/*neu* have been found to be useful in assessing prognosis in patients with breast cancer. A variety of other tissue markers, including oncogenes, tumor suppressor genes, markers of angiogenesis, and proteins associated with the invasive phenotype, are under investigation for their potential utility in assessing prognosis and treatment response in breast cancer. Similar applications can be envisioned for assays that detect cancer cells in the peripheral circulation and micrometastases in the bone marrow. Tumor markers are also being used to detect micrometastases in bone marrow and cancer cells in circulating blood.

INTRODUCTION

Tumor markers can be broadly defined as biochemical substances that are overproduced by cancer tissue or by the host in response to the presence of cancer. Tumor markers can be produced by normal genes that are amplified and overexpressed in tumors. These normal-gene products are not specific to cancer; rather, they represent 1 or more of the biochemical events that facilitate the process of neoplasia. Tumor markers may also be produced by mutated genes that give rise to uncontrolled signaling mechanisms and that are key factors in the initiation, development, and progression of cancer.

Both serum and tissue measurements of tumor markers can be used as differential diagnostic aids in patients with symptoms of cancer. Tumor markers found in serum, urine, and other body fluids are also useful in the early detection of cancer, especially in asymptomatic people who are at high risk for cancer development. Tumor markers found in tissue can provide prognostic information and information useful for the selection of the optimal drugs or a specific therapeutic plan for systemic treatment. Serial measurements of serum tumor markers can provide an early assessment of treatment response. In addition, in patients who have a partial or complete response to treatment, serial monitoring with tumor markers can provide an early indication of recurrent or progressive disease (Robertson et al, 1999).

In breast cancer, tumor markers have been successfully used for some but not all of these clinical applications. The steroid and growth factor receptor proteins that are sometimes overexpressed in breast tumor tissue guide the selection of agents for hormonal therapy and chemotherapy, respectively. These tumor markers also provide prognostic information with regard to disease recurrence and survival. Serum assays for carcinoembryonic antigen (CEA) and the *MUC-1* gene product are useful in monitoring patients' response to treatment. New serum markers currently under investigation may prove useful in the early detection of breast cancer. Future applications for tumor markers include their use in (1) the detection of breast cancer cells in the blood and the bone marrow, which may improve staging of breast cancer, and (2) new-drug selection tests, which may identify the optimal chemotherapy regimen for some patients.

SERUM MARKERS

Serum markers, including CEA, the *MUC-1* gene product, and the HER-2/*neu* oncogene product, are useful in the clinical management of patients with breast cancer. These markers have been studied for assessing whether hormonal therapy is appropriate for individual patients, to select optimal chemotherapy agents for individual patients, and to monitor response to both hormonal therapy and chemotherapy. Several novel serum markers are under investigation for use in these applications.

Carcinoembryonic Antigen

Carcinoembryonic antigen was first described by Gold and Freedman (1965) as an oncofetal antigen present in tumors of the digestive tract. It is now recognized that CEA is normally expressed in many adult tissues, including epithelial cells of the colon, ovary, and prostate; small cells of the lung; squamous cells of the esophagus and cervix; and duct cells of sweat glands. The antigen is also expressed in tumors arising from these tissues and in breast and pancreatic cancers.

Carcinoembryonic antigen is a 200-kDa glycoprotein. Considerable variability exists in the carbohydrate portion of CEA molecules, which results in significant molecular heterogeneity among them. Because of their biochemical differences in molecular makeup, CEA molecules are not equally detected by the immunoassay systems that are currently available; thus, there can be considerable test-value discordance between assay methods. The structural properties of CEA suggest that it is a cell adhesion molecule, but its specific biological role in normal and cancer tissues is not yet established.

The clinical use of serum CEA testing in breast cancer was pioneered by investigators at M. D. Anderson Cancer Center (Mughal et al, 1983). The early studies demonstrated that decreasing serum CEA values accurately reflected response to chemotherapy in patients with metastatic disease and that increasing CEA values reflected progressive disease. Changes in serum CEA values usually precede clinical evidence of treatment response or disease progression. A typical CEA pattern reflecting the clinical course of a patient with breast cancer is shown in Figure 10–1.

Several guidelines must be followed to ensure the effectiveness of patient monitoring with serial measurements of CEA or other serum tumor markers. First, the baseline value of the marker must be established. In

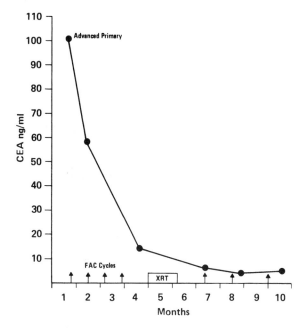

Figure 10–1. Serial serum CEA pattern of a patient with breast cancer who is responding to chemotherapy. The CEA pattern reflects the clinical course of disease. CEA, carcinoembryonic antigen; FAC, 5-fluorouracil, doxorubicin, and cyclophosphamide; XRT, radiation therapy.

some patients, baseline marker values vary considerably; thus, at least 2 values should be used to establish the baseline value. Second, serial serum testing should be performed on a regular and frequent basis. Serum tumor marker values should be determined at all clinic visits to assess response to treatment and, after treatment is finished, to monitor recurrent disease. Third, objective criteria should be used to determine when a change in the serum CEA value is clinically significant. A sustained increase in the CEA value to 2 times the upper limit of normal (6.0 ng/mL) may indicate disease recurrence in a patient who is in complete remission. The test should be repeated in several weeks to determine whether the increase in CEA value has been sustained. A 20% increase or decrease in an elevated serum CEA value is generally accepted to be a substantial change from the previous value; 20% is about 2 times the analytical test precision obtained in the laboratory.

Transient increases in the CEA value may be caused by inflammatory, nonneoplastic diseases. In such cases, the CEA value will return to normal after the acute phase of the disease. Paradoxical increases of CEA and other tumor markers may occur in some patients shortly after the initiation of chemotherapy (Figure 10–2). An increasing CEA value observed

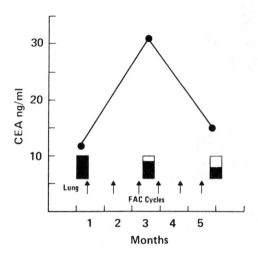

Figure 10–2. Paradoxical increase of CEA in a patient with breast cancer with lung metastasis who is responding to chemotherapy as demonstrated by x-ray assessment of the metastatic site. The borderline elevated pretreatment CEA value rises with response to treatment and returns to the pretreatment baseline value at the end of 6 cycles of chemotherapy. CEA, carcinoembryonic antigen; FAC, 5-fluorouracil, doxorubicin, and cyclophosphamide.

in a patient responding to chemotherapy is probably caused by tumor cell death and the resulting release of CEA into the circulation. A paradoxical increase in CEA is frequently observed in patients with breast cancer, with pretreatment CEA values ranging from 5.0 to 30.0 ng/mL. This increase is transient, however, and the value will return to baseline or lower in 3 to 6 months (Fritsche, 1993).

MUC-1 Gene Product

The *MUC-1* gene, located on chromosome 1q21–24, encodes a 160- to 230-kDa glycoprotein. The glycoprotein is a membrane protein, the extracellular portion of which consists of a variable number of tandem repeats containing 20 amino acid residues. The tandem repeats contain serine and threonine glycosylation sites. The number of repeats and the degree of glycosylation are responsible for the various molecular forms of the glycoprotein. The transmembrane region and a 72-amino-acid cytoplasmic region comprise the remainder of the molecule. The extracellular portion of the *MUC-1* gene product is present in serum, and it can be measured with the CA15.3 dual-monoclonal immunometric assay and the CA27.29 competitive inhibition immunoassay.

Hayes and coworkers were among the first to demonstrate the clinical utility of the CA15.3 test for the serial monitoring of patients with metastatic breast cancer (Hayes et al, 1986). It is now generally accepted that the CA15.3 and CA27.29 tests produce equivalent clinical correlations; that is, both tests produce serial serum patterns of the *MUC-1* gene product that reflect the clinical course of the disease. However, because of their technical differences, such as calibration standards and incubation times, the 2 assays do not always produce equivalent test results. Thus, the values of the 2 assays should not be used interchangeably.

The half-life of the *MUC-1* gene product in the circulation is equivalent to that of CEA: both range from 2 to 10 days. This variation in half-life is related to the production and clearance factors of the molecule. Most clinicians suggest that CA15.3 and CA27.29 tests be done at all clinic visits, as is the case with CEA. A 30% increase or decrease on a CA15.3 test is considered clinically significant. Most reports show CA15.3 and CA27.29 test values to be elevated in 80% to 90% of patients with metastatic breast cancer. CA15.3 reflects the disease course as accurately as does CEA, and it is elevated more frequently than CEA in patients with metastatic breast cancer.

Recent evidence suggests that the CA15.3 and CA27.29 tests for the *MUC-1* gene product are useful for the early detection of recurrence in patients with early-stage breast cancer. In a 2-year prospective study of 166 patients with breast cancer who had stage II or III disease, postoperative serial measurements of the *MUC-1* gene product revealed disease recurrence before there was clinical evidence of recurrence (Chan et al, 1997). Almost 60% (15 of 26 cases) of the recurrences were detected by 2 serial CA27.29 measurements showing increases above the upper limit of normal (38.0 units/mL). There were 11 false-positive results. The positive predictive value of CA27.29 was 83.3%, and the negative predictive value was 92.6%.

Studies of the *MUC-1* gene product currently in progress at M. D. Anderson are aimed at improving the early detection of recurrence. In 1 study, patients with early-stage breast cancer who have postoperative CA27.29 values below the upper limit of normal are being monitored to determine whether serial increases of more than 100% (twice the baseline value) can identify early those patients who have recurrent disease. Almost 60% of cases of recurrence are detected on the basis of this criterion. In this study, only 13 of 268 patients have had false-positive findings on CA27.29 testing. Some of the patients with false-positive findings have had documented disease recurrence, and the others are being followed to determine their outcome. However, there are some cases in which CA27.29 production is low or nonexistent; in these cases, the results can be false negative.

The goal of early detection of recurrence is to initiate early treatment that will result in increased survival duration and an improvement in quality of life (Fritsche and Liu, 2000). Thus, there is a need for new tumor markers for breast cancer that can improve the detection rate and permit earlier detection of disease recurrence.

HER-2/*neu* Oncogene Product

The HER-2/*neu* gene, also known as c-*erb*B-2, which is located on chromosome 17q11–12, encodes a membrane receptor protein with tyrosine kinase activity. Amplification of the HER-2/*neu* gene is associated with poor prognosis, tumor recurrence, and decreased survival duration in patients with breast cancer (Ross and Fletcher, 1999). Overexpression of the gene is observed in the tumor tissues of 20% to 30% of patients with breast cancer. In these cases, the extracellular domain of the cell membrane receptor protein can be clipped, and the 105-kDa protein is detected in the circulation. Enzyme-linked immunosorbent assays are now available for measuring the HER-2/*neu* protein in serum, and these assays are being investigated for their use in selecting systemic hormonal therapy and chemotherapy regimens for patients with breast cancer (Seidman et al, 1995).

Harris et al studied 188 patients with metastatic breast cancer who were treated with either cyclosphosphamide, doxorubicin, and 5-fluorouracil (CAF) or cyclophosphamide, methotrexate, and 5-fluorouracil (CMF). Although there was no difference in overall survival between patients with high serum levels of HER-2/*neu* extracellular domain and those with low serum levels of HER-2/*neu*, a significant improvement in disease-free survival and overall survival was observed in premenopausal patients with detectable levels of HER-2/*neu* extracellular domain who had received CAF chemotherapy compared with patients who received CMF (Harris et al, 1996).

The serum HER-2/*neu* extracellular domain assay is also being investigated for use in selecting patients with metastatic breast cancer for treatment with trastuzumab (Herceptin; Genentech Inc., San Francisco, CA), a monoclonal antibody to the HER-2/*neu* protein. This assay is also being investigated for use in assessing response to trastuzumab therapy. It has been known for some time that serial measurements of HER-2/*neu* in serum correlate with the clinical course of metastatic breast cancer, as do measurements of the *MUC-1* gene product and CEA. However, it remains to be determined how serum HER-2/*neu* testing can be added to CA27.29 or CEA in terms of providing a serum tumor marker for patients whose tumors do not produce the *MUC-1* gene product or CEA or for permitting earlier detection of recurrence in this subgroup of patients.

New Serum Tumor Markers

A number of new analytes have been proposed for use as tumor markers for breast cancer (Fritsche and Liu, 2000). The urokinase plasminogen activator (uPA) and its major enzyme inhibitor, the plasminogen activation inhibitor 1 (PAI-1), are produced by tumor tissues and have been established as independent indicators of prognosis in breast cancer. Urokinase plasminogen activator and PAI-1 play a major role in the metastatic process by converting plasminogen to plasmin, which degrades the basement membrane. Both of these tumor products are released into the circulation, and the enzyme inhibitor complex can be measured. In a preliminary report by Pedersen et al (1999), the uPA:PAI-1 complex was present in much higher quantities in the plasma of patients with advanced breast cancer than in patients with localized breast cancer and healthy women. It is not clear whether the concentration of this complex correlates with tumor burden or whether it is reflective of tumor aggressiveness and metastatic potential. Similarly, the uPA receptor has been detected in the circulation and may also have a role as a tumor marker.

Lysophosphatidic acid (LPA) and lysophosphatidyl choline (LPC) both function as extracellular signals via membrane receptors to activate cell proliferation and function. These phospholipids also appear to enhance production of uPA. Preliminary reports indicate that serum LPC is elevated in 90% of patients with early-stage breast cancer. Thus, serum LPA and serum LPC may be important new tumor markers for breast cancer.

RAK antigens are proteins of 25, 42, and 120 kDa that exhibit molecular and immunologic reactivity with proteins encoded by the human immunodeficiency virus type 1. In a recent study, more than 95% of breast tumors were demonstrated to contain these proteins, whereas only 10% (7 of 70) of normal breast tissues were positive for these proteins by immunohistochemical detection. If these data hold up, RAK proteins may also have potential as new tumor markers for breast cancer.

Finally, as new cancer-associated genes are discovered, many new tumor-marker gene products are being identified that offer promise for use in the early detection and staging of breast cancer and the determination of breast cancer prognosis.

TISSUE MARKERS

Interest in tissue markers as prognostic indicators has been stimulated by the success of adjuvant systemic therapy for early-stage, operable breast cancer (Esteva and Hortobagyi, 1999). In recent years, a number of tissue markers have become available for use in evaluating the prognosis of patients with breast cancer (Porter-Jordan and Lippman, 1994). However, most of these markers have not been validated in large prospective clinical trials and thus remain investigational. The tissue markers obtained routinely at M. D. Anderson include the proliferation marker Ki-67, the estrogen receptor (ER), the progesterone receptor (PR), and the HER-2/*neu* oncogene. These markers, along with the size of the tumor and the axillary lymph node status, allow oncologists to assess a patient's risk of recurrence and death, which is the first step in determining whether a patient is likely to benefit from adjuvant systemic therapy.

Ki-67

Ki-67 is a monoclonal antibody that identifies a nuclear antigen found in cells in the proliferative phases of the cell cycle (i.e., the G_1, S, G_2, and M phases) but not cells in the resting phase (i.e., G_0). Until recently, only fresh or frozen tissues could be used in Ki-67 assays, but new antibodies permit the use of immunohistochemical assays on fixed tissues. A study conducted at M. D. Anderson showed a strong correlation between the Ki-67 staining percentage and nuclear grade, patient age, and mitotic rate (Sahin et al, 1991). In nuclear grade 1 tumors (the most anaplastic grade), a significantly higher median percentage of cells were stained compared with the percentage of cells that were stained in nuclear grade 3 tumors. On univariate analysis, both 5-year disease-free survival rates and overall survival rates were strongly associated with the percentage of cells stained with Ki-67 antibody. Other studies have confirmed the prognostic value of Ki-67 staining in larger patient samples (Veronese et al, 1993).

Hormone Receptors

The ER and PR status are routinely assessed in patients with breast cancer. These proteins have been extensively studied over the past 2 decades and remain the best predictors of response to hormonal therapy. Most breast cancers express measurable amounts of ER. The frequency with which tumors contain ER and the concentration of ER increase with patient age, both reaching their highest levels in postmenopausal patients. Concentrations of 10 fmol/mg or more of cytosol protein are generally considered positive for clinical purposes, and upper levels can reach more than 1000 fmol/mg.

The PR is expressed only after transcriptional activation of its gene by a functional ER-estrogen complex. The presence of PR indicates that the ER pathway is intact, even if the tumor is reported as ER negative. The clinical importance of ER relates principally to the fact that its presence identifies hormone-sensitive tumors. About 50% to 60% of patients with tumors that express significant amounts of ER experience favorable response to hormonal therapy. A higher percentage experience response if the ER levels of their tumors are high and if their tumors are positive for both ER and PR.

Patients with ER-positive tumors have prolonged disease-free survival after primary treatment, longer overall survival, and longer survival duration after recurrence compared with patients with ER-negative tumors. This advantage is independent of axillary lymph node status. Estrogen receptor–positive tumors generally exhibit low-grade histology, favorable nuclear grade, low S-phase fraction, normal complement to DNA, low proliferative index, and low thymidine labeling index (Donegan, 1997). However, the value of ER status as an independent prognostic variable is diminished by its association with other established indicators of favorable prognosis and by its relationship to successful hormonal therapy.

The influence of therapy on prognosis is difficult to exclude because patients with ER-positive tumors regularly undergo and benefit from either adjuvant or palliative hormonal therapy. In some studies, longer disease-free survival and overall survival in patients with ER-positive tumors are seen only in the presence of hormonal therapy. Often the effect of ER-positive status as a discriminant between patients with better and worse prognosis is lost after several years, further suggesting a temporary influence of treatment (Shek and Godolphin, 1989; Hahnel et al, 1979). When patients with negative lymph nodes who were not receiving adjuvant hormonal therapy were studied, the 5-year disease-free survival rate was 20% higher for patients with ER-positive tumors than for patients with ER-negative tumors. However, the 5-year disease-free survival rate of the most favorable subgroup, patients with 1 to 3 positive lymph nodes and ER-positive tumors, did not exceed 60% (Thorpe et al, 1986). In a multivariate analysis of more than 3000 patients with breast cancer, McGuire et al (1990) studied prognostic factors, including ER and PR status. Estrogen receptor status was shown to be a more important prognostic factor than tumor size in node-negative cases but not in node-positive cases. In 1 study, ER status was shown to be less predictive of disease-free survival or overall survival than number of positive lymph nodes and nuclear grade (Fisher et al, 1986).

Enzyme immunoassay and immunohistochemical methods of measuring ER in tissues depend on colorimetric reactions or on scoring systems based on visual estimates of the number and intensity of stained cells. These semiquantitative methods show high correlations with the results of biochemical ligand-binding assays (Holmes et al, 1990). Similar correlations have been demonstrated with response to hormonal therapy and with prognosis (Allred et al, 1998). At M. D. Anderson, ER and PR status are assessed by immunohistochemistry.

The pS2 protein appears to identify a subset of ER-positive tumors with a particularly favorable outlook. The pS2 protein is an estrogen-regulated secretory protein of unknown function, but it probably indicates a more intact cellular estrogen-processing mechanism. It is expressed predominantly by ER-positive tumors. When found in ER-negative tumors, it is in much lower concentrations. The pS2 protein is not expressed in other normal human tissue except stomach. Values above 11 ng/mg are associated with increases in disease free survival duration and overall survival duration in patients with ER-positive tumors. After adjustment for tumor size, lymph node status, and ER status, negative pS2 status is still associated with early recurrence and death. Positive pS2 status in patients with ER-positive breast tumors indicates improved prognosis in patients with both negative and positive lymph nodes. In a study by Foekens and colleagues (1994) in patients with ER-positive and PR-positive tumors, positive pS2 status was associated with a 5-year overall survival rate of 97%, compared with an overall survival rate of 54% for negative pS2 status. In patients with breast cancer and negative lymph nodes, positive and negative pS2 status correlated with overall survival rates of 89% and 58%, respectively, whereas in patients with positive lymph nodes, positive and negative pS2 status correlated with overall survival rates of 88% and 34%, respectively. It has been suggested that pS2 status may be an even stronger predictor than ER status of response to adjuvant hormonal therapy (Predine et al, 1992). However, until this is conclusively proven, treatment decisions regarding hormonal therapy are based on the ER and PR status of the primary or metastatic tumor.

HER-2/*neu*

The available evidence indicates that abnormalities leading to HER-2/*neu* protein overexpression occur very early in the pathogenesis of breast cancer. In experimental systems, overexpression of the HER-2/*neu* gene profoundly affects cell phenotype. NIH 3T3 cells can be induced to the malignant phenotype by overexpression of a normal human HER-2/*neu* coding sequence. Transgenic mice engineered to overexpress the normal (unactivated) *neu* gene under the MMTV promoter develop mammary adenocarcinomas after a long latency, and these tumors have a tendency to metastasize. Introduction of the point-mutated (activated) *neu* gene in mice embryos by homologous recombination results in the rapid development of breast carcinomas. In humans, the HER-2/*neu* protein is not overexpressed in normal hyperplastic or dysplastic lesions of ductal breast epithelium. In contrast, the HER-2/*neu* gene is amplified, overexpressed, or both in 60% of cases of ductal carcinoma in situ (most of which are of the comedo type) and in almost 100% of cases of Paget's disease. HER-2/*neu* is amplified and overexpressed in 20% to 30% of infiltrating ductal carcinomas of the breast. Amplification or overexpression of the HER-2/*neu* gene has been associated with a poor prognosis in patients with breast cancer and both positive and negative lymph nodes (Esteva-Lorenzo et al, 1998). Measurement of the HER-2/*neu* protein by immunohistochemistry or fluorescence in situ hybridization is used to assess prognosis and to select patients for treatment with trastuzumab (Ross and Fletcher, 1999).

Recent reports have suggested that patients whose tumors overexpress the HER-2/*neu* gene may be less responsive to chemotherapy and hormonal therapy. An interaction between HER-2/*neu* expression and response to cytotoxic agents was first observed in vitro. Overexpression of the HER-2/*neu* gene in fibroblasts confers resistance to tumor necrosis factor alpha (TNF-α). Transfection of the HER-2/*neu* gene into breast cancer cells results in resistance to cisplatin. Anti-HER-2/*neu* monoclonal antibodies can restore TNF-α sensitivity to resistant HER-2/*neu*– overexpressing cells and enhance cisplatin- and doxorubicin-induced cytotoxicity. Overexpression of HER-2/*neu* has now been shown to correlate with resistance to a variety of agents used in the treatment of breast cancer.

HER-2/*neu* overexpression in primary adenocarcinomas of the breast has been associated with resistance to adjuvant CMF, although this area remains controversial (Pegram and Slamon, 1999). In a study conducted by the International (Ludwig) Breast Cancer Study Group, patients with positive lymph nodes were randomly assigned to 1 cycle of perioperative CMF plus prednisone (CMFP) or to 6 cycles of postoperative CMFP. Patients with HER-2/*neu*-overexpressing tumors did not seem to benefit from adjuvant CMFP, although the confidence intervals for response in patients with HER-2/*neu*–positive and HER-2/*neu*–negative tumors overlapped (Gusterson et al, 1992). In the Intergroup 0011 study, patients with breast cancer and negative lymph nodes were randomly assigned to CMFP versus no adjuvant chemotherapy. The results from the 2 groups were similar. Both studies are limited by their retrospective analysis of HER-2/*neu* status, the low sensitivity of the antibodies used, and small sample size. More recently, data from the original adjuvant CMF study (Bonadonna et al, 1995) showed that patients with HER-2/*neu*–positive tumors derive a benefit from CMF compared with no adjuvant treatment (Menard et al, 1999).

Interestingly, HER-2/*neu* overexpression has been associated with improved response to doxorubicin-based chemotherapy. In a study conducted by the Cancer and Leukemia Group B (the CALGB 8541 study), HER-2/*neu* overexpression was associated with longer survival duration in patients with early-stage breast cancer and positive lymph nodes who were receiving increasing doses of doxorubicin. In this study, patients with stage II and III breast cancer were randomly assigned to 3 CAF regimens. The 3 regimens were identical except for the dose and schedule of doxorubicin. A significant improvement in survival was observed in patients whose tumors overexpressed HER-2/*neu* and who received full doses of chemotherapy but not in patients with minimal or no HER-2/*neu* expression (Thor et al, 1998). In a study conducted by the National Surgical Adjuvant Breast and Bowel Project (the NSABP B-11 study), patients with breast cancer and positive lymph nodes were randomly assigned to melphalan and 5-fluorouracil or to melphalan, doxorubicin, and 5-fluorouracil (PAF). The overall survival was the same for both groups of patients; however, patients with HER-2/*neu*–overexpressing tumors had an improved overall survival if they were treated with the PAF regimen. In a study conducted by the Southwest Oncology Group, 1470 postmenopausal women with ER-positive breast cancer and positive lymph nodes were randomly assigned to receive CAF plus tamoxifen or tamoxifen alone. Overall survival rates were modestly improved for patients treated with CAF plus tamoxifen. Although there was a trend toward improved overall survival for patients with HER-2/*neu*–positive tumors who were treated with CAF plus tamoxifen, the interaction was not statistically significant. One of the limitations of this analysis is that only 21 of the patients assigned to receive tamoxifen alone had a HER-2/*neu*–positive tumor (Ravdin et al, 1998). Taken together, these data suggest that patients whose tumors overexpress the HER-2/*neu* oncoprotein benefit from the use of doxorubicin-based chemotherapy in the adjuvant setting.

The association between HER-2/*neu* overexpression and response to hormonal therapy is controversial. In a study conducted by the Gruppo Universitario Napoletano (the GUN-1 trial), 308 patients with early-stage breast cancer were randomly assigned to receive tamoxifen 30 mg/day for 2 years or no hormonal therapy. HER-2/*neu* expression was evaluated retrospectively by immunohistochemistry on 245 paraffin-embedded tumors. Specimens were considered HER-2/*neu* positive if at least 10% of the cells stained with the anti-HER-2/*neu* antibody. At 20 years, tamoxifen improved overall survival in all patients compared with no treatment. Interestingly, only patients with HER-2/*neu*–negative tumors had an improved disease-free survival and overall survival if treated with tamoxifen, whereas overall survival was not improved with the use of tamoxifen for patients with HER-2/*neu*–positive tumors (Bianco et al, 1998). In the Cancer and Leukemia Group B 8541 study, patients with hormone receptor–positive tumors were treated with CAF plus tamoxifen. All patients with ER-positive tumors derived a survival benefit from tamoxifen treatment that was independent of HER-2/*neu* status. Another Southwest Oncology Group study evaluated specimens from 205 patients treated with tamoxifen for ER-positive, metastatic breast cancer. In this series, there was no difference in response rate, time to treatment failure, or overall survival rates between patients with HER-2/*neu*–positive and HER-2/*neu*–negative tumors.

Trastuzumab is a monoclonal antibody directed against the HER-2/*neu* protein. Trastuzumab has recently been approved by the Food and Drug Administration for patients with metastatic breast cancer whose tumors overexpress HER-2. Preliminary data indicate that only patients with high levels of expression (score 3+ by immunohistochemistry or positive by fluorescence in situ hybridization) benefit from trastuzumab therapy.

In summary, patients with HER-2/*neu*–overexpressing tumors appear to derive benefit from CMF and doxorubicin-based adjuvant chemotherapy. Because anthracycline-based therapy is superior to CMF, our practice at M. D. Anderson is to treat patients with 5-fluorouracil, doxorubicin, and cyclophosphamide (FAC) regardless of HER-2/*neu* status unless there is a contraindication for anthracycline-based therapy. Patients with involvement of the axillary lymph nodes are considered for paclitaxel in addition to FAC. Tamoxifen is recommended for patients with ER- and PR-positive tumors regardless of the HER-2/*neu* status of the primary tumor. Patients with metastatic breast cancer whose tumors overexpress the HER-2/*neu* protein are considered for trastuzumab-based therapy.

Novel Tissue Markers

A number of new markers are being investigated for their potential as tumor markers for breast cancer, including oncogenes, apoptosis-related genes, markers of angiogenesis, and the protease cathepsin D.

Oncogenes

A number of proto-oncogenes and oncogenes have been investigated for their prognostic value. Proto-oncogenes are normal genes involved with cell growth and proliferation whose altered forms promote neoplastic transformation. Examples include the epidermal growth factor receptor (*EGFR*), c-*ras*, and c-*myc*. Loss of tumor suppressor genes may also play an important role in prognosis. Examples include mutations involving *p53*, *nm23*, and the retinoblastoma (*Rb*) gene.

The EGFR is a large, transmembrane, tyrosine kinase, cell-surface receptor that binds epidermal growth factor and transforming growth factor alpha (TGF-α). The *EGFR* gene is expressed by more than 50% of breast cancers, and overexpression or overstimulation of *EGFR* could result in unrestrained cell proliferation. Although *EGFR* gene amplification is rare in breast cancers, correlations between *EGFR* expression and prognosis have been the subject of a number of studies. High levels of EGFR are associated with ER-negative tumors, suggesting that this receptor might identify tumors less likely to respond to hormonal therapy; however, this has not been shown convincingly. Although some researchers have reported an association between *EGFR* overexpression and poor outcome (Klijn et al, 1992), the data are inconsistent; a lack of routine assessment of this marker also rules this observation inconclusive. Less extensively studied proto-oncogenes in breast cancer include c-*ras* and c-*myc*. The c-*ras* gene is mutated in approximately 5% of breast cancers. In 1 study, high levels of the p21 ras protein were associated with nodal involvement, advanced anatomic stage, and recurrence, suggesting a role in tumor progression (Clair et al, 1987).

Apoptosis-Related Genes

Apoptosis, also known as programmed cell death, is an active process triggered by a variety of stimuli, including chemotherapy and radiation therapy. The *p53* tumor suppressor gene is a negative regulator of cell proliferation and plays an important role in the control of apoptosis. When the *p53* gene is mutated, *p53* proteins are altered, which results in a prolonged half-life that can be measured by immunohistochemistry. Approximately 50% of sporadic breast cancers overexpress the mutated p53 protein. Its overexpression has been associated with highly proliferating features (i.e., poor nuclear grade, HER-2/*neu* overexpression, and aneuploidy), but its overexpression seems to be independent of age, nodal status, and tumor size (Borresen et al, 1995).

In one study, *p53* overexpression was associated with a negative influence on disease-free survival and overall survival in patients with breast cancer and lymph node involvement (Silvestrini et al, 1993). In other reports, the disease-free survival of patients with breast cancer and negative lymph nodes without mutant p53 expression has been considerably lower. Allred et al (1993) found that 52% of the tumors of 700 patients with negative lymph nodes showed some nuclear staining for the mutant p53 protein. Increased staining correlated with progressive decreases in disease-free survival and overall survival. The disease-free survival rate at 5 years fell from 80% in patients with negative immunostaining to 58% in those with the most intense staining. In this study, the prognostic importance of positivity for the mutated p53 protein was independent of S-phase fraction, but this has not been found by other investigators (Isola et al, 1992).

Available data do not support the role of *p53* as an independent prognostic indicator, but overexpression of the mutated p53 protein is clearly associated with other established adverse prognostic indicators. Overexpression of the mutated p53 protein as a predictor of response to therapy is under investigation. In 1 study, patients with tumors overexpressing the mutated p53 protein did not respond well to doxorubicin-based neoadjuvant chemotherapy (Berruti et al, 1998), whereas another study showed that paclitaxel was more effective for patients whose tumors overexpressed the mutated p53 protein (Kandolier-Eckersberger et al, 1998). These associations are intriguing and merit further investigation.

The Bcl-2 protein is another important molecule in the control of apoptosis. Bcl-2 expression is associated with ER-positive status and low proliferation rates. Archer and colleagues (1998) showed that patients with Bcl-2–negative tumors were more likely to respond to anthracycline-based chemotherapy than patients with Bcl-2–positive tumors. The *Bcl-2* gene is being studied as a therapeutic target in patients with breast cancer and other solid tumors.

Markers of Angiogenesis

It is now accepted that solid tumors must develop a vascular network to grow beyond 1 cm^3, and they do so by stimulating the formation of new blood vessels through a process called angiogenesis. Interest in neovascularity as a prognostic factor was stimulated by the work of Judah Folkman on tumor angiogenesis and by the potential for treatment with antiangiogenic agents (Folkman, 1995). The prognostic relevance of tumor angiogenesis was first reported by Weidner et al (1991), who counted microvessels (veins and arteries) in the most densely vascularized areas of 49 invasive carcinomas and found that their number and density significantly increased in cases with nodal and distant metastasis. The frequency of distant metastasis increased with an increase in the microvessel count.

Subsequently, other investigators have produced varying results (Van Hoef et al, 1993). A blinded study of 220 cases of invasive breast carcinoma revealed considerable variability in microvessel count in different parts of the same tumor and between the readings of 2 evaluators. These investigators found no significant correlation between microvessel count and other tumor factors of prognostic value and no significant correlation between microvessel counts and survival or metastasis-free survival (Axelsson et al, 1995). The development and validation of angiogenesis assays is an area of active investigation.

Cathepsin D

Proteases are enzymes involved in tumor invasion and metastasis. Cathepsin D, one of the best characterized proteases in breast cancer, is synthesized in an estrogen-dependent manner by normal tissues and overexpressed and secreted by some breast cancers. Its secreted 52-kDa protein precursor (pro-CD) has mitogenic activity and is proteolytic for basement membranes.

Cathepsin D is suspected of facilitating invasion and metastasis of breast cancer, and indeed, levels of cathepsin D tend to be higher in women with breast cancer who have positive lymph nodes. The enzyme is measured by western blot analysis, radioimmunoassay, or immunohistochemistry. High levels are found in one third of breast cancers. Overexpression of cathepsin D in breast cancer is associated with high risk of recurrence and poor survival, largely because of its relationship with node status. Whether it has any further implication has not been determined because the results obtained by investigators have been inconsistent.

Most studies suggest that cathepsin D has some prognostic significance in patients with positive lymph nodes. Among patients with breast cancer and negative lymph nodes, results have been conflicting, even in studies by the same investigators (McGuire et al, 1990). In a multivariate analysis, Isola et al (1993) found that cathepsin D status, tumor size, and S-phase fraction were each independent predictors of disease-free survival in patients with breast cancer and negative lymph nodes. But early indications that cathepsin D may discriminate among patients with breast cancer and negative lymph nodes were not confirmed in a much larger study of 1489 patients at The University of Texas at San Antonio (Ravdin et al, 1994). The lack of uniform assay techniques among investigators may contribute to such inconsistencies. Because of strong linkage with node status and conflicting results of analyses, perhaps due to lack of standardization, the role of cathepsin D and its 52-kDa protein precursor as independent prognosticators remains uncertain.

MARKERS FOR SPECIAL CONSEQUENCES OF BREAST CANCER

Detection of bone marrow micrometastases and cancer cells in the circulating blood have been investigated for their potential use as prognostic indicators. Bone-related complications that occur as a consequence of breast cancer are a substantial clinical problem. Tumor markers could be useful in diagnosing and determining appropriate treatment for these problems.

Bone Marrow Micrometastases

Immunologic techniques used to detect bone marrow micrometastases in combination with traditional prognostic variables, such as axillary lymph node status and tumor diameter, may help identify patients at high risk for systemic disease who may benefit from adjuvant systemic chemotherapy. Immunofluorescent and immunohistochemical monoclonal antibody techniques can detect 1 cytokeratin-expressing (epithelial) cell among a million bone marrow mononuclear cells (Pantel et al, 1999).

A recent study showed that the presence of breast cancer micrometastases in the bone marrow at the time the primary disease is diagnosed may be predictive of early distant relapse (Braun et al, 2000). In this study, cancer cells were identified in bone marrow aspirates from patients with stage I, II, and III disease using an antibody directed against a common epitope on several cytokeratins (A45-B/B3). Patients with bone marrow involvement had a higher risk of developing distant metastases, independent of axillary lymph node status. Interestingly, the prognosis of patients with negative (uninvolved) lymph nodes and positive (involved) bone marrow was similar to that of patients with positive lymph nodes and negative bone marrow. Moreover, the survival rate of patients with negative lymph nodes and negative bone marrow was 99%.

This study sets the stage for ongoing prospective clinical trials of adjuvant systemic therapy using bone marrow involvement as one of the criteria for patient selection. However, until these data are available, bone marrow aspirations should not be performed routinely in patients with early-stage breast cancer.

Cancer Cells in the Circulating Blood

Cancer cells can also be detected in the peripheral circulation by antibody-based and molecular techniques, such as reverse transcriptase–polymerase chain reaction. Obtaining serial blood samples by this technique is much easier than the process involved in obtaining bone marrow aspirates; however, this approach is limited by the low frequency of occult tumor cells present in the circulation. This obstacle may be overcome by 1 of 2 methods of tumor enrichment: (1) removal of leukocytes via incubation with antihematopoietic, antibody-coated beads or positive selection with anticarcinoma, antibody-coated beads (Noga et al, 1997) or (2) immunomagnetic methods (Martin et al, 1998).

Despite clear improvements in methodology, the clinical relevance of circulating tumor cells is not well established (Pantel et al, 1999). Prospective studies are needed to determine whether the presence of cancer cells in circulating blood is an independent prognostic marker in patients with early-stage breast cancer.

Bone Disease

More than half of patients with metastatic breast cancer develop metastases to the bones. Bone metastases in breast cancer are associated with a substantial amount of morbidity, including multiple sites of fracture, frequent occurrence of bone pain, and special neurologic compromises such as base-of-skull syndrome with cranial nerve deficits and spinal cord or nerve root compression, which may result in radicular pain or paresis. Hypercalcemia may occur as a consequence of bone metastases but is a relatively infrequent observation at present.

Bone metastases develop in the background of actively and continuously remodeling bone. This process is driven by osteoblast-mediated bone formation and osteoclast-mediated bone destruction. Factors that may be involved in osteotropism of tumor metastases include mechanical/vascular factors; adhesion molecules, especially the integrin family; and a variety of osteoclast-activating factors, including prostaglandins and parathyroid hormone–like peptide. A number of factors can affect adherence of metastatic cells in the marrow matrix, including cell-cell and cell–extracellular matrix adhesion via integrins as well as nonintegrin-related adhesion factors such as laminin, proteoglycans, and cadherins. Tumor cells produce a number of degradative enzymes that can independently result in bone destruction, including serine proteases, cysteine proteases, metalloproteinases, and endoglucosidases. Tumor-derived osteoblast/osteoclast activators include colony-stimulating factor 1, macrophage colony-stimulating factor, TNF-α, TNF-β, TGF-α, TGF-β, interleukin (IL)-1, IL-6, prostaglandin E_2, vitamin D_3, the parathyroid hormone, and the parathyroid hormone–related protein. The latter is a protein that has multiple active fragments and an amino acid sequence the first 13 amino acids of which are the same as endogenous parathyroid hormone. Immunohistochemical studies have shown that the parathyroid hormone–related protein is localized in solid tumors and has increased expression in primary breast cancers, especially in breast cancers that have metastasized to the bone. However, none of these proteins are essential for osteoclast development in vivo (Theriault and Hortobagyi, 1992).

The osteoprotegerin ligand (OPGL) is a recently discovered glycoprotein from the TNF receptor superfamily that blocks osteoclastogenesis in vitro and osteoclast differentiation in vivo (Simonet et al, 1997). The OPGL, also known as osteoclast differentiation factor, is highly expressed in osteoblast/stromal cells, and its expression can be upregulated by the bone-resorbing factors vitamin D_3, IL-11, prostaglandin E_2, and parathyroid hormone in vitro. Knockout mice lacking the OPGL gene (OPGL$^{-/-}$ mice) develop severe osteopetrosis, stunted growth, and a defect in tooth

---

KEY PRACTICE POINTS

- Serum tumor markers (CEA, CA27.29, HER-2/*neu*) provide important information that is used to make treatment decisions for patients with metastatic breast cancer.

- The proliferation marker Ki-67 provides important prognostic information, particularly for patients with small tumors and no axillary lymph node involvement.

- Estrogen receptor and PR are excellent predictors of response to hormonal therapy in patients with early-stage and advanced-stage breast cancer.

- Overexpression of the HER-2/*neu* protein is associated with poor prognosis and can be used to select patients for trastuzumab-based therapy.

---

eruption, as well as defects in early differentiation of T and B lymphocytes. OPGL$^{-/-}$ mice maintain normal differentiation of monocytes and macrophages, indicating that OPGL is a specific and essential differentiation factor for osteoclast precursors. A clinical trial has been initiated to determine the safety of OPGL for patients with breast cancer that has metastasized to the bones.

CONCLUSIONS

Serum tumor markers are useful in the clinical management of breast cancer. The *MUC-1* gene product is elevated in as many as 80% of patients who have metastatic disease and can be measured in the serum using the CA15.3 and CA27.29 assays. Serial monitoring can supplement other clinical procedures that are used to assess response to therapy. Although CEA is also useful in monitoring for cancer recurrence, the greater sensitivity and specificity of the *MUC-1* antigen make it the preferred test for this clinical application.

Current practice guidelines from the American Society of Clinical Oncology and the European Group on Tumor Markers support the use of serum markers for this purpose. Patients who have early-stage disease and are treated surgically for cure may develop metastatic disease. Postoperative serial monitoring using the CA27.29 assay may identify as many as 60% of these patients with a lead time of up to 12 months. Unfortunately, this approach has not produced improvements in survival. New serum tumor markers are needed to facilitate the detection and treatment of minimal residual disease. It is generally recognized that as treatments for breast cancer are improved, serum and tissue tumor markers will become more important in the identification of patients who require adjuvant therapy, in the selection of the most effective treatments for individual patients, and for monitoring tumor response and patient status.

Suggested Readings

Allred DC, Clark GM, et al. Association of p53 protein expression with tumor cell proliferation rate and clinical outcome in node-negative breast cancer. *J Natl Cancer Inst* 1993;85:200–206.

Allred DC, Harvey JM, Berardo M, Clark GM. Prognostic and predictive factors in breast cancer by immunohistochemical analysis. *Mod Pathol* 1998;11:155–168.

Archer CD, Ashley S, Dowsett M, et al. Biomarkers for the prediction of complete clinical response to primary chemotherapy in early breast cancer. *Proceedings of the American Society of Clinical Oncology* 1998;17:484A.

Axelsson K, Ljung BE, Moore DH II, et al. Tumor angiogenesis as a prognostic assay for invasive ductal breast carcinoma. *J Natl Cancer Inst* 1995;87:997–1008.

Berruti A, Bottini A, Bersiga A, et al. p53 expression and reduction in kinetic cell activity in predicting clinical complete response to primary chemotherapy in breast cancer patients. *Proceedings of the American Society of Clinical Oncology* 1998;17:393A.

Bianco AR, Laurentiis MD, Carlomagno C, et al. 20 year update of the Naples GUN trial of adjuvant breast cancer therapy: evidence of interaction between c-erbB-2 expression and tamoxifen efficacy. *Proceedings of the American Society of Clinical Oncology* 1998;17:373A.

Bonadonna G, Valagussa P, Moliterni A, Zambetti M, Brambilla C. Adjuvant cyclophosphamide, methotrexate, and fluorouracil in node-positive breast cancer: the results of 20 years of follow-up. *N Engl J Med* 1995;332:901–906.

Borresen AL, Andersen TI, Eyfjord JE, et al. TP53 mutations and breast cancer prognosis: particularly poor survival rates for cases with mutations in the zinc-binding domains. *Genes Chromosomes Cancer* 1995;14:71–75.

Braun S, Pantel K, Muller P, et al. Cytokeratin-positive cells in the bone marrow and survival of patients with stage I, II, or III breast cancer. *N Engl J Med* 2000;342:525–533.

Chan DW, Beveridge RA, Muss H, et al. Use of Truquant BR radioimmunoassay for early detection of breast cancer recurrence in patients with stage II and stage III disease. *J Clin Oncol* 1997;15:2322–2328.

Clair T, Miller WR, Cho-Chung YS. Prognostic significance of the expression of a ras protein with a molecular weight of 21,000 by human breast cancer. *Cancer Res* 1987;47:5290–5293.

Donegan WL. Tumor-related prognostic factors for breast cancer. *CA Cancer J Clin* 1997;47:28–51.

Esteva-Lorenzo FJ, Sastry L, King CR. The *erb*B-2 gene: from research to application. In: Dickson RB, Salomon DS, eds. *Hormones and Growth Factors in Development and Neoplasia*. New York: John Wiley & Sons; 1998.

Esteva FJ, Hortobagyi GN. Adjuvant systemic therapy for primary breast cancer. *Surg Clin North Am* 1999;79:1075–1090.

Fisher B, Fisher ER, Redmond C, Brown A. Tumor nuclear grade, estrogen receptor, and progesterone receptor: their value alone or in combination as indicators of outcome following adjuvant therapy for breast cancer. *Breast Cancer Res Treat* 1986;7:147–160.

Foekens JA, Portengen H, Look MP, et al. Relationship of PS2 with response to tamoxifen therapy in patients with recurrent breast cancer. *Br J Cancer* 1994; 70:1217–1223.

Folkman J. Angiogenesis in cancer, vascular, rheumatoid and other disease. *Nat Med* 1995;1:27–31.

Fritsche HA. Serum tumor markers for patient monitoring: a case-oriented approach illustrated with carcinoembryonic antigen. *Clin Chem* 1993;39:2431–2434.

Fritsche HA, Liu FJ. Tumor markers at the millennium. Proceedings of Tumor Markers Conference (Santa Barbara, CA, 1999). *Journal Clinical Ligand* 2000;22:320.

Gold P, Freedman SO. Specific carcinoembryonic antigen of the human digestive system. *J Exp Med* 1965;122:467–481.

Gusterson BA, Gelber RD, Goldhirsch A, et al. Prognostic importance of c-erbB-2 expression in breast cancer. International Breast Cancer Study Group. *J Clin Oncol* 1992;10:1049–1056.

Hahnel R, Woodings T, Vivian AB. Prognostic value of estrogen receptors in primary breast cancer. *Cancer* 1979;44:671–675.

Hammarstrom S. The carcinoembryonic antigen (CEA) family: structures, suggested functions and expression in normal and malignant tissues. *Semin Cancer Biol* 1999;9:67–81.

Harris LN, Trock B, Berris M, Esteva-Lorenzo F, Paik S. The role of ERBB2 extracellular domain in predicting response to chemotherapy in breast cancer patients. *Proceedings of the American Society of Clinical Oncology* 1996;15:A96.

Hayes DF, Zurawski VR, Kufe DW. Comparison of circulating CA15–3 and carcinoembryonic antigen levels in patients with breast cancer. *J Clin Oncol* 1986;4:1542–1550.

Holmes FA, Fritsche HA, Loewy JW, et al. Measurement of estrogen and progesterone receptors in human breast tumors: enzyme immunoassay versus binding assay. *J Clin Oncol* 1990;8:1025–1035.

Isola J, Visakorpi T, Holli K, Kallioniemi OP. Association of overexpression of tumor suppressor protein p53 with rapid cell proliferation and poor prognosis in node-negative breast cancer patients. *J Natl Cancer Inst* 1992;84:1109.

Isola J, Weitz S, Visakorpi T, et al. Cathepsin D expression detected by immunohistochemistry has independent prognostic value in axillary node-negative breast cancer. *J Clin Oncol* 1993;11:36–43.

Kandolier-Eckersberger D, Taucher S, Steiner B, et al. P53 genotype and major response to anthracycline- or paclitaxel-based neoadjuvant treatment in breast cancer patients. *Proceedings of the American Society of Clinical Oncology* 1998;17:392A.

Klijn JG, Berns PM, Schmitz PI, Foekens JA. The clinical significance of epidermal growth factor receptor (EGF-R) in human breast cancer: a review on 5232 patients. *Endocr Rev* 1992;13:3–17.

Martin VM, Siewert C, Scharl A, et al. Immunomagnetic enrichment of disseminated epithelial tumor cells from peripheral blood by MACS. *Exp Hematol* 1998;26:252–264.

McGuire WL, Tandon AK, Allred DC, Chamness GC, Clark GM. How to use prognostic factors in axillary node-negative breast cancer patients. *J Natl Cancer Inst* 1990;82:1006–1015.

Menard S, Valagussa P, Pilotti S, et al. Benefit of CMF treatment in lymph-node positive breast cancer overexpressing HER2. *Proceedings of the American Society of Clinical Oncology* 1999;18:257.

Mughal AW, Hortobagyi GN, Fritsche HA, Buzdar AU, Yap HY, Blumenschein GR. Serial plasma carcinoembryonic antigen measurements during treatment of metastatic breast cancer. *JAMA* 1983;249:1881–1886.

Muss H, Berry D, Thor A, et al. Lack of interaction of tamoxifen use and erbB-2/HER-2/*neu* expression in CALGB 8541: a randomized adjuvant trial of three different doses of cyclophosphamide, doxorubicin and fluorouracil (CAF) in node-positive primary breast cancer. *Proceedings of the American Society of Clinical Oncology* 1999;18:256.

Noga SJ, Kennedy MJ, Valone F, Van Vlasselaer P, Moss TJ. Density adjusted cell sorting (DACS) combined with negative CD45 enrichment of hematopoietic stem cell (HSC) harvests increases the sensitivity of immunocytochemical (ICC) detection for breast cancer. *Proceedings of the American Society of Clinical Oncology* 1997;16:102A.

Pantel K, Cote RJ, Fodstad O. Detection and clinical importance of micrometastatic disease. *J Natl Cancer Inst* 1999;91:1113–1124.

Pedersen AN, Brunner N, Hoyer-Hansen G, et al. Determination of the complex between urokinase and its type-1 inhibitor in plasma from healthy donors and breast cancer patients. *Clin Chem* 1999;45:1206–1213.

Pegram M, Slamon DJ. Use of HER2 for predicting response to breast cancer therapy. *Diseases of the Breast Updates* 1999;3:1.

Porter-Jordan K, Lippman ME. Overview of the biologic markers of breast cancer. *Hematol Oncol Clin North Am* 1994;8:73–100.

Predine J, Spyratos F, Prud'homme JF, et al. Enzyme-linked immunosorbent assay of PS2 in breast cancers, benign tumors, and normal breast tissues. Correlation with prognosis and adjuvant hormone therapy. *Cancer* 1992;69:2116–2123.

Ravdin PM, Green S, Albain KS, et al. Initial report of the SWOG biological correlative study of c-erbB-2 expression as a predictor of outcome in a trial comparing adjuvant CAF T with tamoxifen (T) alone. *Proceedings of the American Society of Clinical Oncology* 1998;17:97A.

Ravdin PM, Tandon AK, Allred DC, et al. Cathepsin D by western blotting and immunohistochemistry: failure to confirm correlations with prognosis in node-negative breast cancer. *J Clin Oncol* 1994;12:467–474.

Robertson JF, Jaeger W, Syzmendera JJ, et al. The objective measurement of remission and progression in metastatic breast cancer by use of serum tumour markers. European Group for Serum Tumour Markers in Breast Cancer. *Eur J Cancer* 1999;35:47–53.

Ross JS, Fletcher JA. The HER-2/*neu* oncogene: prognostic factor, predictive factor and target for therapy. *Semin Cancer Biol* 1999;9:125–138.

Sahin AA, Ro J, Ro JY, et al. Ki-67 immunostaining in node-negative stage I/II breast carcinoma. Significant correlation with prognosis. *Cancer* 1991;68:549–567.

Seidman AD, Portenoy R, Yao TJ, et al. Quality of life in phase II trials: a study of methodology and predictive value in patients with advanced breast cancer treated with paclitaxel plus granulocyte colony-stimulating factor. *J Natl Cancer Inst* 1995;87:1316–1322.

Shek LL, Godolphin W. Survival with breast cancer: the importance of estrogen receptor quantity. *Eur J Cancer Clin Oncol* 1989;25:243–250.

Silvestrini R, Benini E, Daidone MG, et al. P53 as an independent prognostic marker in lymph node-negative breast cancer patients. *J Natl Cancer Inst* 1993;85:965–970.

Simonet WS, Lacey DL, Dunstan CR, et al. Osteoprotegerin: a novel secreted protein involved in the regulation of bone density. *Cell* 1997;89:309–319.

Theriault RL, Hortobagyi GN. Bone metastasis in breast cancer. *Anticancer Drugs* 1992;3:455–462.

Thor AD, Berry DA, Budman DR, et al. erbB-2, p53, and efficacy of adjuvant therapy in lymph node-positive breast cancer. *J Natl Cancer Inst* 1998;90:1346–1360.

Thorpe SM, Rose C, Rasmussen BB, et al. Steroid hormone receptors as prognostic indicators in primary breast cancer. *Breast Cancer Res Treat* 1986;7(suppl):91–96.

Van Hoef ME, Knox WF, Dhesi SS, Howell A, Schor AM. Assessment of tumour vascularity as a prognostic factor in lymph node negative invasive breast cancer. *Eur J Cancer* 1993;29A:1141–1145.

Veronese SM, Gambacorta M, Gottardi O, Scanzi F, Ferrari M, Lampertico P. Proliferation index as a prognostic marker in breast cancer. *Cancer* 1993;71:3926–3931.

Weidner N, Semple JP, Welch WR, Folkman J. Tumor angiogenesis and metastasis—correlation in invasive breast carcinoma. *N Engl J Med* 1991;324:1–8.

11 CHEMOTHERAPY FOR BREAST CANCER

Marjorie C. Green and Gabriel N. Hortobagyi

CHAPTER OVERVIEW

Over the past 30 years, numerous advances have contributed to improved survival for patients with breast cancer. Many of these advances involve the development and use of systemic chemotherapy in the adjuvant and metastatic settings. In terms of patient survival, anthracycline-containing regimens are superior to non-anthracycline-containing regimens. The optimal use of taxanes in the adjuvant setting is under continued investigation. In general, anthracyclines and taxanes are the cornerstones of the treatment paradigm employed at M. D. Anderson Cancer Center.

INTRODUCTION

Breast cancer has a long natural history, and local recurrence and distant metastases are the primary causes of breast cancer–related morbidity and mortality. Breast cancer remains a major cause of cancer-related death in women, second only to lung cancer. However, breast cancer mortality rates have been declining over the past 10 years. This reduction in mortality (approximately 1.8% per year) has been attributed both to early screening and detection and to advances in breast cancer treatment, including advances in systemic chemotherapy for breast cancer. In the past 10 years, new chemotherapeutic agents and regimens have emerged as active therapies for both operable and metastatic breast cancer. This chapter will describe many of these advances and M. D. Anderson Cancer Center's current approach to systemic chemotherapy for breast cancer.

ADJUVANT CHEMOTHERAPY

Adjuvant chemotherapy has been used at M. D. Anderson since 1973. Multiple studies have confirmed that adjuvant chemotherapy benefits all subgroups of women with operable breast cancer. However, the degree of benefit depends on patient and tumor characteristics, and the approach to each patient must be individualized. To ensure that each patient receives optimal care, a multidisciplinary approach should be utilized in the development of treatment plans. All patients should be educated about possible enrollment in clinical trials, which have the potential to improve the future success rate of adjuvant chemotherapy.

Goal of Therapy

The goal of adjuvant chemotherapy for breast cancer is to eradicate any micrometastases while their overall volume is low, thus eliminating the risk of systemic relapse.

Patient Selection

Several factors should be taken into consideration in deciding whether adjuvant chemotherapy is appropriate for an individual patient:

1. The absolute reduction in the risks of relapse and death for the individual. While systemic therapy is efficacious for most individuals with breast cancer, the absolute benefit gained from chemotherapy should be compared with the benefits possible from other treatment modalities.
2. The toxicity of the proposed treatment. The absolute benefit for the patient should be balanced against the risks and side effects associated with the proposed chemotherapy. The estimate of toxicity should take into consideration the patient's preexisting medical conditions and any other influencing factors that could impede the safe and timely delivery of therapy.
3. The patient's own beliefs and goals. For some women, the absolute risk reduction from systemic chemotherapy is not enough to change quality of life. Patients should be thoroughly counseled about the options available to them and the risks and benefits of each possible course of action.

Timing of Therapy in Relation to Surgery and Radiation Therapy

The optimal timing of adjuvant chemotherapy for breast cancer is still unknown. In most clinical trials, patients receive adjuvant chemotherapy starting less than 8 weeks after surgery. A retrospective review conducted at M. D. Anderson found no decrease in overall survival when adjuvant chemotherapy was delayed up to 18 weeks after surgery (Buzdar et al, 1982). In addition, no benefit has been found for chemotherapy given in the early postoperative period compared with chemotherapy initiated 4 to 5 weeks after surgery. At M. D. Anderson, we currently recommend that chemotherapy begin within 4 to 6 weeks after surgery.

Delay of adjuvant radiation therapy due to administration of adjuvant chemotherapy has not proven to decrease disease-free survival or overall survival, although in some studies, local control has been impaired. However, the opposite strategy—delay of adjuvant chemotherapy due to administration of adjuvant radiation therapy—may jeopardize the opportunity for cure. One study found that patients with stage I or II breast cancer who were randomly assigned to receive chemotherapy before or after radiation therapy were more likely to have distant recurrences if chemotherapy was delayed for radiation therapy (Recht et al, 1996). Given the possibility of systemic micrometastases at the time of diagnosis and the associated risk of distant treatment failure, most patients should receive chemotherapy before radiation therapy in the adjuvant setting.

Neoadjuvant Chemotherapy

The role of neoadjuvant (preoperative) chemotherapy in the treatment of operable breast cancer is currently under intensive investigation. Neoadjuvant chemotherapy has several theoretical benefits (Table 11–1). It may kill tumor cells before drug resistance develops. In addition, because this therapy is delivered before the tumor has been excised, neoadjuvant chemotherapy allows clinicians to evaluate the sensitivity of the tumor to a specific chemotherapeutic regimen. In theory, the effect of chemotherapy on the primary tumor is a reflection of the effect on occult micrometastases. Thus, neoadjuvant chemotherapy allows clinicians to limit the use of ineffective agents and optimize treatment choices. Another potential benefit of neoadjuvant chemotherapy is that it can downstage the primary tumor and thus improve the chances for breast conservation therapy and an improved cosmetic outcome.

Multiple trials have shown the ability of neoadjuvant chemotherapy to make breast-conserving surgery possible in patients with operable breast cancer who initially would have required a mastectomy. The National Surgical Adjuvant Breast and Bowel Project (NSABP) B-18 trial compared neoadjuvant doxorubicin and cyclophosphamide (AC) with adjuvant AC in the treatment of stage I and II breast cancer (Fisher et al, 1998). Patients were evaluated for surgical treatment plan prior to randomization. Among the patients randomly assigned to neoadjuvant chemotherapy, 69 (27%) of the 256 who originally planned to undergo mastectomy were

Table 11–1. Advantages and Disadvantages of Neoadjuvant Chemotherapy

Advantages	Disadvantages
• Less drug resistance	• Can induce drug resistance
• Permits in vivo determination of sensitivity to therapy	• Pathology findings more difficult to correlate with future prognosis (e.g., axillary lymph node number)
• Limits use of ineffective therapy	
• May enable breast conservation	• Reduced ability to evaluate biological appearance of primary tumor
• Improved cosmetic results	
• Intact tumor vasculature	

candidates for segmental mastectomy after neoadjuvant therapy. Overall, no advantage in disease-free or overall survival was seen for patients treated with neoadjuvant chemotherapy. Given the overall equivalent efficacy of neoadjuvant and adjuvant chemotherapy, physicians are encouraged to utilize a multidisciplinary approach in the selection of neoadjuvant therapy for early-stage breast cancer to aid in optimizing care for each individual patient.

Duration of Therapy

In the initial trials of adjuvant chemotherapy, patients received chemotherapy for 12 to 24 months. The overview of polychemotherapy for early breast cancer found that regimens lasting longer than 6 months conferred no benefit beyond that seen with regimens lasting 6 months or less (Early Breast Cancer Trialists' Collaborative Group, 1998). The overview also showed that regimens lasting less than 36 weeks were associated with decreased survival duration compared with regimens lasting 36 weeks or longer. The standard duration of adjuvant chemotherapy is now 3 to 8 months depending on the regimen used.

Evaluation before Therapy

Before adjuvant chemotherapy is initiated, careful disease staging is performed to rule out gross metastatic disease and to provide a baseline for future evaluations. Staging is usually performed before definitive surgical intervention so that unnecessary surgical procedures can be avoided in patients with more advanced disease. The specific tests performed are selected on the basis of the clinical or pathologic disease stage and information gathered from review of systems and physical examination (Table 11–2).

For patients with clinical stage I or II breast cancer, routine laboratory tests are performed to evaluate hematopoietic, renal, and liver function. Bilateral mammograms (with sonograms as indicated) and a chest radiograph are obtained. When patients present with focal symptoms to suggest bony metastases or an elevated alkaline phosphatase level, bone scans with plain-film radiographs of abnormal areas are ordered. Given the low likelihood of gross metastatic disease in patients with stage I or II disease, computerized tomography of the chest and abdomen is not routinely recommended. Additional tests are ordered as clinically indicated if the patient's history, physical examination, or initial staging raises suspicion of distant metastases.

For patients with clinical or pathologic stage III disease, the risk of metastatic disease is increased. Therefore, routine bone scans and imaging of the liver (with sonography, computed tomography, or magnetic resonance imaging) are indicated.

For all patients with operable breast cancer treated at M. D. Anderson, tissue samples are submitted for determination of estrogen receptor (ER)

Table 11–2. Staging Evaluation

Stage	Laboratory Evaluation	Radiographic Evaluation
I, IIA, IIB	CBC with platelet and differential BUN and creatinine AST, ALT, LDH, total bilirubin Alkaline phosphatase	Bilateral mammogram Breast sonogram* Chest radiograph
IIIA, IIIB	CBC with platelet and differential BUN and creatinine AST, ALT, LDH, total bilirubin Alkaline phosphatase	Bilateral mammogram Breast sonogram* Chest radiograph Bone scan** Liver imaging with sonography, computed tomography, or magnetic resonance imaging

*Breast sonography and sonography of the axillae should be ordered as clinically indicated.
**Abnormal areas on bone scans should be evaluated with plain radiographs.
ALT, alanine aminotransferase; AST, aspartate aminotransferase; BUN, blood urea nitrogen; CBC, complete blood count; LDH, lactate dehydrogenase.

and progesterone receptor (PR) status, HER-2/*neu* expression, S-phase fraction, and DNA index. The prognostic information gained from pathologic review helps guide future treatment recommendations.

Adjuvant Chemotherapy Regimens

In the United States, the chemotherapy regimens used most frequently in the adjuvant setting are 5-fluorouracil, doxorubicin (Adriamycin), and cyclophosphamide (FAC or CAF); AC; and cyclophosphamide, methotrexate, and 5-fluorouracil (CMF). At M. D. Anderson, most patients treated in the adjuvant setting are given a doxorubicin-containing regimen (FAC). The CMF regimen is reserved for patients with comorbid medical conditions that preclude administration of an anthracycline and some patients with stage I disease.

Doxorubicin-Containing Regimens

The anthracycline doxorubicin is one of the most active agents against breast cancer. Multiple trials have confirmed the efficacy of anthracycline-containing regimens in breast cancer. When doxorubicin is given as single-agent treatment for metastatic breast cancer, response rates are typically 40% to 65% and can be as high as 80%. Only a few studies have directly compared anthracycline-containing regimens with CMF. However, evidence from these few trials shows that anthracycline-containing regimens are superior to non-anthracycline-containing regimens in the adjuvant treatment of breast cancer. Initially, trials proved that doxorubicin-containing regimens such as FAC and CAF were superior to CMF and CMF-type regimens. The NSABP B-15 trial found that 4 cycles of AC (60/600 mg/m²) was equivalent to 6 cycles of CMF for patients with node-positive disease in terms of both relapse-free and overall survival (Fisher et al, 1990a). The NSABP has completed accrual of clinical trial B-23, which compares AC with or without tamoxifen with CMF with or without tamoxifen as adjuvant therapy for patients with node-negative, ER-negative tumors. The results of this trial are eagerly anticipated. In the early 1990s, the National Cancer Institute of Canada Clinical Trials Group conducted a trial that directly compared 5-fluorouracil, epirubicin, and cyclophosphamide with CMF in premenopausal women with high-risk, node-positive breast cancer. The epirubicin-containing regimen was found to be superior to CMF in terms of both relapse-free and overall survival (Levine et al, 1998). Another trial comparing CAF with CMF was an Intergroup trial that compared these regimens in patients with node-negative breast cancer. Researchers found that the anthracycline-containing regimen prolonged both disease-free and overall survival ($P = 0.03$) (Hutchins et al, 1998).

Some of the most convincing evidence supporting the use of doxorubicin in the adjuvant setting comes from the recent world overview data from the Early Breast Cancer Trialists' Collaborative Group. In 1998, as part of the overview meta-analysis, this group reviewed 11 trials that compared anthracycline-containing regimens with CMF. The anthracycline-containing regimens produced an additional 12% proportional reduction in the risk of recurrence compared with CMF. The absolute reduction in the risk of recurrence was 3.2%. Anthracycline-containing regimens also produced an 11% proportional reduction in the risk of death compared with CMF (absolute benefit, 2.7%) (Early Breast Cancer Trialists' Collaborative Group, 1998). As results from these trials mature, it is possible that an even greater overall benefit from anthracycline-containing regimens will be seen. Although 70% of the women in these studies were younger than 50 years of age, doxorubicin-containing regimens were found to be superior to CMF for women in all age groups.

For many years, FAC has been the standard adjuvant chemotherapy regimen given to most women with breast cancer at M. D. Anderson. This regimen is both effective and safe. The initial study of adjuvant FAC at M. D. Anderson found that the 10-year survival rate was 62% for patients with stage II breast cancer and 40% for patients with stage III breast cancer (Buzdar et al, 1989). Additional calculations suggested that adjuvant FAC was associated with a 55% reduction in the odds of recurrence for women younger than 50 years and a 37% reduction in the odds of recurrence for women 50 years of age and older.

At M. D. Anderson, the doxorubicin component of FAC is administered as a continuous infusion over 48 to 72 hours to minimize the risk of cardiac damage. The risk of cardiac damage increases as the cumulative dose of doxorubicin increases, but studies have shown that this risk is decreased when peak levels of doxorubicin are lower. Infusing doxorubicin over a prolonged period facilitates administration of a higher cumulative dose with a lower systemic peak drug level. Studies at M. D. Anderson in metastatic breast cancer show that continuous-infusion doxorubicin given over 48 to 96 hours decreases the risk of cardiotoxicity (Hortobagyi et al, 1989). The decrease in cardiac toxicity seen in patients with metastatic breast cancer can also be seen in patients receiving doxorubicin in the adjuvant setting. Continuous infusion of doxorubicin benefits patients who may have future relapses, for which the repeated use of doxorubicin can be very effective.

Additional incentive to use doxorubicin-based regimens in the adjuvant setting has come from recent investigations of chemotherapy for patients with tumors that overexpress HER-2/*neu* (for more information, see chapter 10). Several studies have suggested that overexpression of HER-2/*neu* predicts decreased benefit from or possible chemoresistance to CMF (Gusterson et al, 1992; Allred et al, 1992). Amplification of HER-2/*neu* has also been associated with heightened responsiveness to doxorubicin-containing therapy (Muss et al, 1994). Given the possible suboptimal outcome with CMF for patients whose tumors overexpress HER-2/*neu*, doxorubicin-containing therapy might be preferable in the adjuvant setting for this patient group. However, it should be recognized that the data showing a relationship between HER-2/*neu* overexpression and increased or decreased responsiveness to cytotoxic therapy are derived entirely from retrospective analyses. These results were obtained using different methods of HER-2/*neu* testing and are based on incomplete data sets.

Regimens Containing Doxorubicin and Paclitaxel

Recently, the remarkable responses seen with paclitaxel (Taxol) in patients with metastatic disease have sparked interest in use of this agent in the adjuvant setting. Paclitaxel is an antimicrotubular agent isolated from the stem bark of *Taxus brevifolia*, the Western (Pacific) yew tree. Unlike other antimicrotubular agents, paclitaxel acts by promoting the formation of unusually stable microtubules, inhibiting the normal dynamic reorganization of the microtubular network required for mitosis and cell proliferation.

In a phase II study conducted at M. D. Anderson, 25 patients with metastatic breast cancer in whom a doxorubicin-containing chemotherapy regimen had failed to produce an adequate response were treated with paclitaxel (250 mg/m^2 infused over 24 hours every 21 days). The objective response rate was 56% (complete response rate, 12%; partial response rate, 44%) (Holmes et al, 1991). This significant response rate for patients who had experienced disease progression after treatment with one of the most active agents against breast cancer was encouraging.

The efficacy of single-agent paclitaxel is similar to the efficacy of single-agent doxorubicin. Intergroup study E1193 compared doxorubicin versus paclitaxel versus the combination of doxorubicin and paclitaxel in patients with metastatic breast cancer. There were no significant differences in the overall response rates produced by doxorubicin or paclitaxel. The combination of the 2 agents produced a higher response rate but did not improve overall survival (Sledge et al, 1997).

In a recent study conducted at M. D. Anderson, paclitaxel was compared with FAC in the neoadjuvant setting, and the 2 regimens were found to produce equivalent clinical results. Patients received either paclitaxel 250 mg/m^2 as a continuous intravenous infusion over 24 hours or FAC (5-fluorouracil 500 mg/m^2 days 1 and 4; doxorubicin 50 mg/m^2 as a continuous infusion over 72 hours starting on day 1; cyclophosphamide 500 mg/m^2 on day 1). Each regimen was given every 3 weeks for 4 cycles before surgery. The clinical overall response rate was 79.3% for patients who received FAC and 80.2% for patients who received paclitaxel. Estimated 2-year relapse-free survival rates were similar for the 2 groups (Buzdar et al, 1999).

The sequential use of doxorubicin-based regimens and paclitaxel has been evaluated in the adjuvant setting in an effort to optimize cytotoxicity and the possibility of cure. Paclitaxel and doxorubicin have different mechanisms of action: paclitaxel inhibits normal microtubule function, and doxorubicin functions as both a topoisomerase inhibitor and an anti-metabolite. It is hypothesized that the individual cells of a tumor vary in their ability to resist drugs. If this is indeed the case, then the use of drugs with different mechanisms of action, such as paclitaxel and doxorubicin, may be a means of circumventing drug resistance and increasing tumor cell kill. In addition, using agents such as doxorubicin and paclitaxel that affect cells at different phases of the cell cycle can enhance cytotoxicity.

Early results of 2 studies suggest a benefit with the sequential use of doxorubicin and paclitaxel in the adjuvant setting. In a 1998 study, Henderson and colleagues randomly assigned patients with node-positive breast cancer to receive AC ($60/600$ mg/m^2 every 21 days) for 4 cycles or AC (same dosage) for 4 cycles followed by paclitaxel (175 mg/m^2 every 21 days) for 4 cycles. Initially there was a statistically significant reduction in the odds of both recurrence and death for the group that received paclitaxel (Henderson et al, 1998). This study is also significant for the finding that increasing doses of doxorubicin did not result in improved relapse-free or overall survival rates. Further follow-up continues to show significant reduction in the odds of recurrence; however, the survival advantage originally seen is less clear. At M. D. Anderson, paclitaxel (250 mg/m^2 over 24 hours every 21 days) for 4 cycles followed by FAC ($500/50/500$ mg/m^2 every 21 days) for 4 cycles was compared with 8 cycles of FAC in the neoadjuvant and adjuvant settings. At a median follow-up time of 36 months, the addition of paclitaxel reduced the risk of recurrence by 24%. At the time of this analysis, the data were not yet mature enough to permit determination of the impact on overall survival (Thomas et al, 2000). To date there is not yet conclusive evidence that the addition of paclitaxel to anthracycline-based chemotherapy significantly improves survival. As data from the M. D. Anderson and Cancer and Leukemia Group B trials mature and as additional trials complete accrual, the use of taxanes in the adjuvant setting will be further defined.

Treatment Guidelines by Disease Stage

Doxorubicin-containing regimens form the foundation of all chemotherapy regimens at M. D. Anderson. We recommend that patients participate in randomized clinical trials; however, for those patients unable to enroll in trials, the following guidelines are used. Again, treatment is often guided by multiple factors, and a multidisciplinary approach to treatment planning should be utilized whenever possible.

Noninvasive Breast Cancer

Adjuvant chemotherapy currently has no role in the treatment of patients with noninvasive breast cancer. The use of adjuvant tamoxifen in this group is discussed in chapter 1.

Stage I Breast Cancer

Most patients with stage I breast cancer have a small risk of local recurrence, metastasis, or death from their tumor. The overall risk of recurrence and death from breast cancer in this group is less than 25% at 10 years. The risk of recurrence and death increases with increasing tumor size; therefore, adjuvant chemotherapy may be appropriate for some patients with stage I disease. Tumor size, hormone receptor status, and other prognostic factors should guide treatment for each patient.

Tamoxifen is given to all patients with ER-positive tumors. The use of tamoxifen for patients with tumors that are ER negative and PR positive is often advised. Adjuvant therapy with tamoxifen is not indicated for patients with tumors that lack expression of both ER and PR.

Estrogen Receptor–Positive Disease. Currently, all premenopausal and postmenopausal women with ER-positive stage I disease are given tamoxifen for 5 years after definitive surgical treatment. In women with tumors smaller than 1 cm, adjuvant chemotherapy does not significantly improve outcomes and thus is not indicated. However, as the size of the primary tumor increases, the risk of recurrence also increases, and the potential benefits of adjuvant chemotherapy become more significant. At M. D. Anderson, most patients with ER-positive tumors between 1 and 2 cm are treated with 6 cycles of FAC ($500/50/500$ mg/m^2 every 21 days) followed by tamoxifen 20 mg per day for 5 years (Table 11–3). Under

Table 11–3. Adjuvant Chemotherapy Regimens Commonly Used at M. D. Anderson

FAC

   5-Fluorouracil 500 mg/m^2 IV days 1 and 4
   Doxorubicin 50 mg/m^2 as continuous IV infusion over 72 hours day 1
   Cyclophosphamide 500 mg/m^2 IV day 1

   Cycle is repeated every 21 days for 6 cycles.
   Chemotherapy is given if absolute neutrophil count greater than 1500 and
      platelet count greater than 100,000.

FAC-Paclitaxel

   Paclitaxel 225 mg/m^2 as continuous IV infusion over 24 hours on day 1
   Cycle is repeated every 21 days for 4 cycles.

   Followed by:
   5 Fluorouracil 500 mg/m^2 IV days 1 and 4
   Doxorubicin 50 mg/m^2 as continuous IV infusion over 72 hours day 1
   Cyclophosphamide 500 mg/m^2 IV day 1
   Cycle is repeated every 21 days for 4 cycles.

   Chemotherapy is given if absolute neutrophil count greater than 1500 and
      platelet count greater than 100,000.

special circumstances, such as comorbid medical conditions that preclude doxorubicin-containing therapy, CMF is used in place of FAC. The CMF regimen is also considered for patients with tumors between 1 and 2 cm with good prognostic indicators.

Estrogen Receptor–Negative Disease.   As is the case in patients with ER-positive stage I disease, the use of adjuvant chemotherapy in patients with ER-negative stage I disease depends on tumor size. No systemic adjuvant therapy is recommended for patients with invasive tumors 0.5 cm or smaller.

Patients with tumors between 0.6 and 1.0 cm generally have a good prognosis. However, some studies have reported decreased survival (72% at 5 years) for invasive tumors in this size range. Review of other prognostic factors in combination with open discussion with the patient should guide the use of adjuvant therapy in this population (Chen et al, 1998).

For patients with stage I tumors larger than 1.0 cm, adjuvant chemotherapy with FAC is recommended. The CMF regimen is sometimes considered for patients with tumors between 1 and 2 cm with good prognostic indicators. Currently, adjuvant chemoendocrine therapy (chemotherapy followed by tamoxifen) is not routinely given to patients with ER-negative, PR-negative disease.

Stage II Breast Cancer

The overall survival rate for patients with stage II breast cancer is greater than 70% at 5 years. However, patients with stage II disease have a significant risk of recurrence and death from breast cancer. For example, in 1 study, patients with T2N0M0 invasive ductal carcinoma were found to have a 33% chance of recurrence at 20 years for tumors 2.1 to 3.0 cm and a 44% chance of recurrence at 20 years for tumors 3.1 to 5.0 cm (Rosen et al, 1991).

Tamoxifen is given to all patients with ER-positive tumors. The use of tamoxifen for patients with tumors that are ER negative and PR positive is often advised. Adjuvant therapy with tamoxifen is not indicated for patients with tumors that lack expression of both ER and PR.

Node-Negative Disease.   At M. D. Anderson, patients with node-negative stage II breast cancer are usually treated with FAC (500/50/500 mg/m^2) every 21 days for 6 cycles. After chemotherapy, patients with ER-positive tumors receive tamoxifen 20 mg daily for 5 years.

Node-Positive Disease.   Given the initial encouraging results seen with the addition of paclitaxel to anthracycline-based therapy and given the possibility of enhanced cytotoxicity from treatment with non-cross-resistant drugs, patients with node-positive, ER-negative tumors are treated with a combination of paclitaxel and FAC (Table 11–3). Currently, administration of this combination to patients with node-positive, ER-positive disease is not recommended outside the context of a clinical trial. Patients with ER-positive tumors should be treated with FAC for 6 cycles followed by tamoxifen 20 mg daily for 5 years.

Locally Advanced Breast Cancer

Patients with locally advanced breast cancer (LABC) have advanced tumor size, extensive nodal involvement, or both. Patients with inflammatory carcinoma are also considered to be part of this group for the purposes of treatment planning. Patients with stage IV disease with metastases confined to the ipsilateral supraclavicular or infraclavicular fossa are sometimes included in this group as well. When treated with a combined-modality approach, these patients with stage IV disease can have 10-year disease-free survival rates exceeding 30%. Thus, these patients should be treated with curative intent.

Patients with LABC have a poor prognosis, with 5-year survival rates ranging from 30% to 60% depending on nodal status and other prognostic indicators. Given this poor prognosis, patients with LABC should be considered for participation in clinical trials. To ensure the optimal sequencing of treatment modalities and the optimal choice of regimen, the care of patients with LABC is best guided by a multidisciplinary team. Despite the intriguing data from trials evaluating high-dose chemotherapy with stem cell transplantation as treatment for LABC (and other stages of breast cancer), this approach is investigational and should be performed only in the context of a randomized clinical trial.

Tamoxifen is given to all patients with ER-positive tumors. The use of tamoxifen for patients with tumors that are ER negative and PR positive is often advised. Adjuvant therapy with tamoxifen is not indicated for patients with tumors that lack expression of both ER and PR.

Operable Locally Advanced Breast Cancer. Most patients with operable stage III disease are candidates for neoadjuvant chemotherapy (see the section Inoperable Locally Advanced Breast Cancer later in this chapter), which can shrink tumors, thus permitting less aggressive surgery and possibly decreasing morbidity. At M. D. Anderson, most patients with operable LABC are treated with neoadjuvant chemotherapy. However, surgical excision (modified radical mastectomy with axillary lymph node dissection) followed by adjuvant chemotherapy is also an established, effective treatment option for this group. In the adjuvant setting, the use of non-cross-resistant drugs to improve the opportunity for tumor cell kill is recommended. Paclitaxel (225 mg/m^2 over 24 hours every 21 days) for 4 cycles followed by FAC (500/50/500 mg/m^2 every 21 days) for 4 cycles is currently recommended. Patients with ER-positive tumors should receive tamoxifen 20 mg daily for 5 years after the completion of chemotherapy. The use of tamoxifen for patients with tumors that are ER-negative and PR-positive is often advised.

Conventional CMF is not recommended for patients with operable stage III disease because of the advantages seen with doxorubicin-containing regimens in terms of both response rates and survival. The combination of CMF plus doxorubicin may be appropriate, however. One study randomly assigned patients to receive adjuvant CAF for 6 months followed by 6 months of CMF plus vincristine and prednisone or 12 months of CMF plus vincristine and prednisone. Patients treated with the anthracycline-based regimen had a trend towards improved disease-free survival (Casper et al, 1987). Adding doxorubicin to CMF can improve response in some patients. Bonadonna and colleagues found that in the adjuvant setting, single-agent doxorubicin for 4 cycles followed by CMF for 8 cycles was superior to alternating use of the same drugs for patients with more than 3 lymph nodes involved by tumor (Bonadonna et al, 1995b). Because doxorubicin-containing and paclitaxel-containing regimens produce similar clinical responses in the neoadjuvant setting and because anthracycline-containing regimens are superior to CMF, the combination of FAC and paclitaxel is currently administered at M. D. Anderson.

Inoperable Locally Advanced Breast Cancer. The benefit of neoadjuvant therapy for patients with inoperable stage III disease is established. Previously, 4 cycles of FAC was the standard neoadjuvant treatment given to these patients at M. D. Anderson. However, recent studies show superior response rates with the combination of docetaxel (Taxotere) and an anthracycline in the metastatic setting. Because of this finding and the improved survival seen with anthracycline/taxane sequential therapy in the adjuvant setting, we have recently changed the standard of care at M. D. Anderson for treatment of patients with inoperable stage III disease with the goal of improving response rates and, hopefully, survival.

There is increasing evidence that docetaxel will benefit patients with inoperable LABC. At M. D. Anderson, these patients receive neoadjuvant doxorubicin and docetaxel (50/75 mg/m^2 every 21 days) for 4 cycles. Patients with objective response undergo surgical therapy (modified radical mastectomy or segmental mastectomy) as indicated. Adjuvant chemotherapy with CMF (600/40/600 mg/m^2 every 21 days) is administered for 4 cycles followed by 5 years of tamoxifen (20 mg per day) for patients with ER-positive tumors.

Patients who do not respond to neoadjuvant chemotherapy with docetaxel and doxorubicin are candidates for crossover to CMF or radiation therapy as guided by a multidisciplinary team. If patients are technically operable, surgery also can be considered at this time. Involvement of a multidisciplinary team is essential in guiding patient care for these poor-prognosis patients. After the completion of chemotherapy and local therapy, treatment with tamoxifen (20 mg per day) for 5 years is recommended for patients with ER-positive tumors.

Side Effects and Their Management

The FAC regimen and paclitaxel are associated with significant yet acceptable acute side effects (Table 11–4). In patients treated with these drugs, a medical history and physical examination should be performed before each chemotherapy cycle. In general, dose reduction by 25% is recommended in the case of nonhematologic grade 3 or 4 side effects. Dose reduction for reasons other than side effects has the potential to decrease the therapeutic benefit. Antiemetics and growth factors are given as indicated by the American Society of Clinical Oncology (ASCO) guidelines (Gralla et al, 1999; ASCO, 1996). Routine use of growth factors is not indicated for either regimen unless patients develop febrile neutropenia after receiving therapy.

The combination of docetaxel and doxorubicin used for patients with LABC is associated with a high incidence of febrile neutropenia. At M. D. Anderson, patients treated with this regimen receive prophylactic growth factors (granulocyte-macrophage colony-stimulating factor 250 mcg/m^2 subcutaneously daily for 10–14 days).

A long-term risk associated with adjuvant chemotherapy is premature ovarian failure in premenopausal women. The risk of premature ovarian failure is age related: most women younger than 30 will continue to menstruate during and after chemotherapy, but approximately 90% of women over the age of 40 who are treated with chemotherapy will have permanent ovarian failure.

Myelodysplastic syndrome and acute leukemia are also possible long-term consequences for patients who receive cyclophosphamide and other

Table 11–4. Common Acute Side Effects Associated with Adjuvant
              Chemotherapy

Regimen	Side Effects
FAC	Alopecia
	Nausea
	Vomiting
	Stomatitis
	Diarrhea
	Neutropenia and risk of neutropenic fever
Paclitaxel	Alopecia
	Peripheral sensory neuropathy
	Rash/nail changes
	Neutropenia and risk of neutropenic fever
	Nausea
	Constipation

alkylating agents or topoisomerase II inhibitors. The risk of myelodysplastic syndrome or leukemia increases with increasing numbers of alkylating agents and increasing doses of these agents. Longer duration of therapy and younger age have also been associated with increased risk. A review of patients treated with FAC at M. D. Anderson found that the 10-year estimated rate of developing leukemia was 1.5% for all patients and 0.5% for patients treated with chemotherapy without radiation therapy.

Surveillance After Chemotherapy

The risk of breast cancer recurrence is highest during the first 2 years after initial therapy but remains high for 5 years. Physical examination is recommended every 4 months for the first 2 years after treatment, every 6 months for the next 3 years, and then annually. Patients should have annual mammograms as part of their follow-up care. Patients who received systemic chemotherapy should have a yearly complete blood count with differential and platelet counts and review of alanine aminotransferase, alkaline phosphatase, and lactate dehydrogenase levels. These laboratory values will help to indicate any long-term sequelae from chemotherapy and possibly warn of recurrent disease. Breast cancer can recur 20 years or later after diagnosis. A high index of suspicion and continued follow-up by a physician from the treatment team are ideal.

CHEMOTHERAPY FOR METASTATIC BREAST CANCER

Despite the advances in adjuvant therapy for breast cancer, a significant number of patients with breast cancer have a relapse and die of their disease. It is estimated that 20% to 30% of patients with node-negative disease and 50% to 60% of patients with node-positive disease will eventually have a recurrence. The most common sites of recurrence include the liver, lungs, and bones. As with cancer in general, the clinical course for patients with metastatic breast cancer varies from patient to patient. As a group, patients with metastatic breast cancer have a median survival of 24 months. Patients with bone-only metastases tend to live longer than patients with visceral-organ involvement. With therapy, patients with visceral metastases have an average survival of 21 months, whereas patients with bone-only disease have longer average survival time—up to 60 months in some reviews.

Goals of Therapy

As a general rule, there is no cure for metastatic breast cancer. However, some studies have shown prolonged remissions in patients who receive systemic chemotherapy for metastatic breast cancer. A review of patients with metastatic breast cancer treated at M. D. Anderson shows that among individuals who have a complete remission after anthracycline-containing therapy, 17% (3% of the overall population) will remain free of disease for more than 5 years (Greenberg et al, 1996). Currently, the primary goals of chemotherapy for metastatic breast cancer should be palliation of symptoms attributable to cancer and prolongation of life. It is the physician's duty to balance the benefits of therapy with possible toxic effects and to fully discuss therapeutic options with patients.

Work-up before Therapy

In the majority of cases, metastatic breast cancer is detected because of symptoms or changes found during physical examination and routine radiographic surveillance. The work-up to document recurrence should include a complete blood count with differential and platelet counts; liver function tests (bilirubin, alkaline phosphatase, aspartate aminotransferase, alanine aminotransferase, lactate dehydrogenase); and chest radiography and bone scan, with plain films of abnormal or suspicious regions. Other tests should be conducted as guided by patient symptoms and findings on physical examination. Recurrence should be documented with tissue diagnosis. The hormone receptor status and HER-2/*neu* level should be determined if these are not already known.

Choosing between Chemotherapy and Hormonal Therapy

The decision whether to use chemotherapy or hormonal therapy for initial treatment of metastatic disease should be guided by several factors (Figure 11–1). Patients with symptomatic visceral disease or life-threatening disease should be considered for treatment with systemic chemotherapy regardless of hormone receptor status because systemic therapy offers faster palliation of symptoms for most patients.

Among women who do not have life-threatening or symptomatic visceral disease, those whose tumors are negative for ER and PR should be considered for systemic chemotherapy. Those whose tumors are positive for ER or PR should be treated with hormonal therapy. Multiple agents are active against hormone-responsive tumors. Hormonal therapy tends to be associated with fewer side effects and helps to maintain quality of life for many patients. If the tumor does not respond to hormonal therapy or becomes unresponsive to hormonal therapy, systemic chemotherapy should be initiated. The use of hormonal therapy in the treatment of metastatic breast cancer is discussed in chapter 13.

Duration of Chemotherapy

The optimal duration of chemotherapy for metastatic breast cancer is controversial. Several studies have compared continuous (maintenance) che-

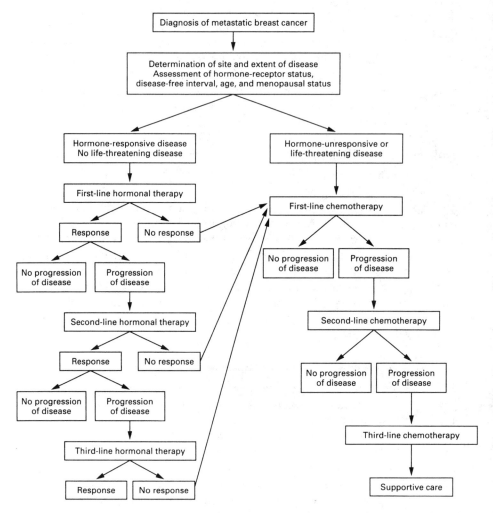

Figure 11–1. Treatment schema for patients with metastatic breast cancer. Reprinted with permission from *The New England Journal of Medicine* (1998;339:974–984). Copyright 1998, Massachusetts Medical Society. All rights reserved.

motherapy with intermittent therapy as treatment of metastatic breast cancer. Five studies found that continuous therapy was associated with a longer time to relapse (Falkson et al, 1998; Muss et al, 1991; Coates et al, 1987; Ejlertsen et al, 1993; Gregory et al, 1997). One study found that patients receiving continuous therapy experienced worse side effects (Muss et al, 1991). None of the individual studies comparing continuous and intermittent therapy showed prolongation of life with continuous therapy. However, a recent meta-analysis of these data showed a statistically significant improvement in survival for patients receiving chemotherapy for longer, as compared with shorter, durations (Stockler et al, 1997). Some regimens, such as anthracycline-containing treatments, have inherent dose-limiting toxic effects that prohibit prolonged continued use. Other agents—such as trastuzumab (Herceptin) and, possibly, low-dose taxanes given weekly—lend themselves to indefinite continued therapy. Many trials are constructed to treat patients until they have progression of disease or for 2 to 3 cycles after maximum benefit is seen. Currently there is no single right answer regarding treatment duration except that the right choice is the one that provides the most benefit for the patient. Open communication between the patient and clinician is essential to determine the correct length of treatment.

Selection of Agents

The patient's previous therapies, comorbid conditions, and HER-2/*neu* level should be taken into account in the design of treatment for metastatic breast cancer. Several factors predict improved response to chemotherapy in the metastatic setting (Table 11–5). Full-dose chemotherapy within the conventional range of doses is associated with higher response rates than is "low-dose chemotherapy." In the setting of metastatic disease, as in the adjuvant setting, high-dose chemotherapy with stem cell transplantation remains investigational and should be used only in the context of a randomized clinical trial. For most patients, an anthracycline-based regimen is the initial treatment of choice.

Doxorubicin-Containing Regimens

Patients who have metastatic breast cancer at initial diagnosis should be treated with a doxorubicin-containing regimen. Doxorubicin-containing regimens are also the initial treatment of choice for patients with meta-

Table 11–5. Predictors of Improved Response to Chemotherapy in the Metastatic Setting

Low tumor burden
Normal organ function
Good performance status
No recent weight loss
No prior chemotherapy or radiation therapy
Soft-tissue metastases
Premenopausal status
Prolonged disease-free interval after adjuvant chemotherapy
Prolonged disease-free interval after adjuvant chemotherapy with an
   anthracycline-based regimen

static breast cancer who previously received non-anthracycline-containing chemotherapy in the adjuvant setting. Patients who received doxorubicin in the adjuvant setting and had a prolonged disease-free interval before the appearance of metastatic disease occasionally benefit from repeat administration of this drug. However, given the increasing number of active agents available to treat metastatic breast cancer, repeat treatment with doxorubicin should be reserved for patients in whom other treatments have failed.

Several studies have confirmed the benefits of anthracyclines in the treatment of metastatic breast cancer. A 20-year analysis of published randomized trials of chemotherapy and hormonal therapy for metastatic breast cancer was presented at the 1998 annual meeting of ASCO (Fossati et al, 1998). Fossati and colleagues found that trials published between 1975 and 1994 showed benefit in terms of both response rates and survival for polychemotherapy regimens compared with single-agent therapies. In addition, polychemotherapy regimens containing doxorubicin were associated with improved response and a trend towards improved survival compared with other polychemotherapy regimens (Fossati et al, 1998). An analysis published in 1993 by A'Hern and colleagues compared doxorubicin-containing regimens (primarily CAF) with CMF or its variants. Again, doxorubicin-containing therapy was associated with better response rates, failure-free survival, and overall survival (A'Hern et al, 1993).

Single-agent doxorubicin as treatment for metastatic breast cancer produces overall response rates ranging from 40% to 65%. These results can be improved by combining doxorubicin with other active agents. An analysis was recently published of 18 successive trials at M. D. Anderson that investigated doxorubicin-based regimens in metastatic breast cancer. The analysis included 1581 patients. The overall response rate was 65%, and the complete response rate was 16.6%. The median overall survival time was 21.3 months (Rahman et al, 1999).

Until the recent widespread use of trastuzumab and chemotherapy in the metastatic setting, FAC (500/50/500 mg/m^2 every 21–28 days) was the standard initial regimen recommended to all women with metastatic breast cancer treated at M. D. Anderson. With this regimen, chemotherapy is given for 6 to 8 cycles (unless progression of disease is evident), and objective responses are seen in 50% to 80% of patients. However, at cumulative doses of 500 mg/m^2 or greater, the cardiotoxicity of doxorubicin becomes dose limiting. Current standard practice at M. D. Anderson is to administer doxorubicin as a continuous infusion over 72 hours through a central venous catheter. Administering doxorubicin by prolonged continuous infusion rather than as a bolus decreases the incidence of cardiotoxicity by more than 75% at cumulative doses of 450 mg/m^2 or greater compared with bolus-dosing schedules.

Multiple variations of FAC have been used in the metastatic setting. Efforts to improve response with dose intensification of FAC have failed to provide increases in overall response or survival but have significantly increased toxicity.

Paclitaxel

As previously stated, paclitaxel has significant antitumor activity against breast cancer. At M. D. Anderson, paclitaxel is used as a first-line therapy against metastatic breast cancer for patients previously treated with anthracyclines and patients in whom doxorubicin is contraindicated. In addition, paclitaxel (or docetaxel; see the next section) is used as second-line therapy for patients who have disease progression after treatment with FAC.

An initial phase II trial conducted at M. D. Anderson in the early 1990s evaluated paclitaxel 250 mg/m^2 administered as a continuous intravenous infusion over 24 hours every 21 days. Of the 25 patients evaluated, 23 (92%) had received prior therapy with anthracyclines, and 15 (60%) had visceral disease. The overall response rate was 56%, and 12% of the patients had a complete response. A significant number of patients became neutropenic; however, only 5% experienced neutropenic fever (Holmes et al, 1991). Other trials have confirmed the activity of paclitaxel in metastatic breast cancer.

The ideal dose and schedule of paclitaxel are not yet known. Paclitaxel was initially administered over a prolonged period in an effort to decrease the hypersensitivity reactions seen in phase I studies. Later studies revealed that premedication with dexamethasone permitted safe administration of paclitaxel over a shorter duration. Paclitaxel given as second-line (or later) therapy for metastatic breast cancer at doses ranging from 135 mg/m^2 to 250 mg/m^2 administered over 3 hours every 3 weeks results in response rates ranging from 21% to 60%.

As with the initial phase II trial conducted at M. D. Anderson, many trials suggested improved response rates with increased duration of infusion of paclitaxel. The NSABP B-26 trial compared paclitaxel 250 mg/m^2 given over 24 hours or 3 hours as first-line therapy for metastatic breast cancer and confirmed improved response rates for longer infusion of paclitaxel (51% vs 40%; $P = 0.02$) (Mamounas et al, 1998). Grade 4 neutropenia was more common among patients receiving the prolonged infusion of chemotherapy, but no other significant differences in toxicity were seen.

Continuous infusion of paclitaxel has practical disadvantages, including patient inconvenience. As in NSABP B-26, the main toxic effect seen with continuous-infusion (24-hour) paclitaxel is the high incidence of grade 3 or 4 neutropenia. To help improve the response rate with shorter infusion of paclitaxel and possibly decrease the risk of infection, the Cancer and Leukemia Group B compared 3 doses of paclitaxel—175, 210, and 250 mg/

m²—administered over 3 hours. No improvement in overall response rate or survival was seen with increasing dose; however, progression-free survival was prolonged with the highest dose (Winer et al, 1998). In a randomized phase II trial published in 1996 by Nabholtz and colleagues, the overall response rate among patients who received paclitaxel 175 mg/m² over 3 hours every 21 days as first-line therapy for metastatic breast cancer was 36%. In the same study, the overall response rate among patients with anthracycline-resistant breast cancer was 26% (Nabholtz et al, 1996). Sixty-four percent of women experienced grade 3 or 4 neutropenia; however, only 4% had neutropenic fever.

Response rates with continuous-infusion paclitaxel are superior to those with paclitaxel given over shorter periods. However, these differences do not translate into prolongation of survival, so many investigators have elected the convenience of shorter infusion schedules. Paclitaxel is phase specific, with ability to block dividing cells. Continuous-infusion schedules and schedules that involve more frequent drug dosing offer the greatest theoretical benefit in terms of cell kill. To improve efficacy and decrease toxicity in the metastatic setting, researchers developed treatment schedules in which lower doses of paclitaxel are given weekly. Studies have found decreased myelotoxicity with weekly doses of paclitaxel ranging from 80 to 100 mg/m² per week. With higher doses of paclitaxel (>100 mg/m²), increased neurotoxicity is seen, manifested primarily as glove-and-stocking peripheral sensory neuropathy. Response rates range from 40% to 60% for this weekly, lower-dose schedule (Seidman et al, 1999). Also encouraging is evidence that weekly, low-dose paclitaxel can provide further tumor regression for patients who experienced disease progression during or after every-3-week paclitaxel.

At M. D. Anderson, paclitaxel is given every 3 weeks as a continuous infusion of 225 mg/m² over 24 hours. Unpublished data show this regimen to be very effective, with a decreased incidence of febrile neutropenia compared with higher doses. Another alternative is weekly administration of paclitaxel at a dose of 80 to 90 mg/m². Both regimens are highly effective in the treatment of metastatic breast cancer.

Docetaxel

Docetaxel, like paclitaxel, is a taxane that can promote tubulin polymerization and inhibit depolymerization. Preclinical studies suggest that in addition to preventing cell division, docetaxel may induce apoptosis. Docetaxel has significant activity against breast cancer cells. A phase II study conducted at M. D. Anderson evaluated docetaxel 100 mg/m² administered over 1 hour every 21 days (Valero et al, 1995). Patients had either primary or secondary anthracycline resistance—that is, their disease either did not respond to initial anthracycline therapy or progressed after an initial response to an anthracycline. In this poor-prognosis population, 53% of patients treated with docetaxel had a partial response, and 35%

had stable disease. The median duration of response was 23.5 weeks, and the median time to progression was 4 months. The median overall survival was 9 months; however, for patients who responded to therapy, median survival improved to 13.5 months. The ability to achieve a high response rate in patients with anthracycline resistance is encouraging. The activity of docetaxel in this patient population has been confirmed by other studies. Other agents have significantly less effect on this same population. For example, paclitaxel is associated with overall response rates of only 6% to 48% in anthracycline-resistant patients. Docetaxel has also been proven effective for patients previously treated with paclitaxel, with response rates approaching 20%.

A review of single-agent phase III trials (Burris, 1999) confirmed the high activity of docetaxel in the treatment of metastatic breast cancer. Three different studies published in 1998 found overall response rates of 30% to 43% when docetaxel was used to treat patients whose disease progressed after anthracycline-containing therapy. In addition, each study compared docetaxel with combination chemotherapy regimens previously used in this patient population. In each study, docetaxel was found to be superior to the combination therapy. Of particular interest, the International 304 Study Group trial found that docetaxel produced a statistically significant improvement in overall survival compared with other salvage therapy.

In addition to its remarkable activity, a second benefit of docetaxel in heavily pretreated patients is that it is less likely than paclitaxel to cause neuropathy and myalgias. Docetaxel 100 mg/m^2 every 3 weeks induces levels of neutropenia similar to those seen with standard paclitaxel regimens given every 3 weeks. One unique side effect of docetaxel is the development of significant fluid retention in patients who receive cumulative doses greater than 300 mg/m^2 and are not treated with steroids. This fluid retention can lead to anasarca and pleural effusions in some patients. The addition of steroid premedication to docetaxel significantly reduces the magnitude of fluid retention. The optimal dose and schedule of steroid premedication is unknown; however, most regimens utilize dexamethasone before and after chemotherapy. At M. D. Anderson, patients receive dexamethasone orally (4 mg twice a day for 3 days) beginning the day prior to chemotherapy administration.

Several phase I and II studies have investigated weekly administration of docetaxel as a possible means of increasing efficacy and decreasing hematologic toxicity and sensory neurotoxicity, which is often dose limiting. One study presented at the ASCO meeting in 1999 found an overall response rate of 41% for patients with metastatic breast cancer who received docetaxel 40 mg/m^2 over 1 hour every week for 6 weeks followed by a 2-week break. Thirty-eight percent of patients in this study had previously been treated with anthracyclines. This treatment was well tolerated; no grade 3 or 4 toxic effects were reported (Burstein et al, 1999).

The current role of docetaxel in the treatment of metastatic breast cancer has yet to be defined. Docetaxel appears to be the most active agent against anthracycline-refractory breast cancer identified in the past 25 years. Multiple phase III studies of docetaxel are under way, and when these trials are completed, the use of docetaxel is expected to increase in both the adjuvant and metastatic settings. Currently, however, docetaxel has 2 recommended uses in the metastatic setting: treatment of metastatic breast cancer that has shown primary resistance to anthracycline-based therapy and treatment of metastatic breast cancer that has progressed within 12 months of treatment with an anthracycline. While the weekly dosing schedule appears to be effective and less toxic than the traditional every-3-weeks schedule, greater clinical experience exists with the traditional schedule. Discussion between physician and patient should help guide treatment choice.

Taxane-Doxorubicin Combinations

As with paclitaxel and doxorubicin, several studies suggest that docetaxel and doxorubicin have similar efficacy against breast cancer cells. Paclitaxel and docetaxel have both been combined with anthracyclines for treatment of metastatic breast cancer.

Paclitaxel-doxorubicin combinations have been tested in a variety of schedules and doses. Initial phase I and II studies revealed an unexpected pharmacokinetic interaction between the 2 drugs when paclitaxel was given before doxorubicin. Continuous infusion of paclitaxel 24 hours before continuous infusion of doxorubicin resulted in excessive accumulation and decreased clearance of the anthracycline. The resulting toxic effects were severe mucositis and bone marrow suppression (Holmes et al, 1999). Other investigators found that bolus doxorubicin followed by paclitaxel given over 3 hours is associated with decreased mucositis and bone marrow suppression. Unfortunately, this schedule was associated with significant cardiotoxicity and the development of irreversible congestive heart failure. Although the initial combinations of bolus doxorubicin and 3-hour paclitaxel had impressive activity, subsequent clinical results were more modest. However, recent randomized clinical trials showed this combination to be significantly superior to AC or FAC in terms of response rate, time to progression, and survival. Unfortunately, the paclitaxel-containing combination is associated with greater toxicity.

Docetaxel-doxorubicin combinations have been suggested to be superior to paclitaxel-doxorubicin combinations in the treatment of metastatic breast cancer. Phase II studies evaluating docetaxel-doxorubicin as first-line therapy for metastatic breast cancer are reviewed in a recent publication by Nabholtz (1999). Response rates range from 57% to 77%, and the combination has significant activity against visceral disease. Median survival has not been reached for these studies; however, at 2-year follow-up, survival rates ranged from 57% to 66%. Median time to progression is reported to be between 47 and 59 weeks.

In a phase III trial comparing AC (60/600 mg/m^2) with a docetaxel-doxorubicin combination (docetaxel 75 mg/m^2 plus doxorubicin 50 mg/m^2) as first-line treatment for metastatic breast cancer, the reported overall response rate for the docetaxel-doxorubicin combination was greater (60% vs 47% $P = 0.008$). The docetaxel-doxorubicin regimen was also associated with a higher complete remission rate. The main side effects seen with both regimens were neutropenia and febrile neutropenia; these were more common with the docetaxel-doxorubicin regimen. In contrast to what was seen with the paclitaxel-doxorubicin combination, the docetaxel-doxorubicin combination was not associated with increased cardiotoxicity. Another phase III trial is currently comparing a combination of doxorubicin, docetaxel, and cyclophosphamide versus FAC. As results of these studies mature, combinations of doxorubicin and taxanes are expected to be highly utilized in the metastatic, adjuvant, and neoadjuvant settings. For now, the use of doxorubicin-docetaxel combinations is a reasonable alternative to AC or FAC.

Trastuzumab

Trastuzumab is the first humanized monoclonal antibody approved in the United States for the treatment of metastatic breast cancer. Trastuzumab targets the protein product of the proto-oncogene HER-2/*neu*. A trial evaluating the benefit of trastuzumab as monotherapy for metastatic breast cancer was presented at the ASCO meeting in 1998 (Cobleigh et al, 1998). This single-arm trial enrolled 222 women, more than 60% of whom had received more than 2 prior therapies for metastatic disease. A total of 213 patients received trastuzumab. At 11 months, the overall response rate was found to be 15% by an independent response evaluation committee. The median response duration was 8.4 months, and the estimated median survival duration was 13 months. Treatment was well tolerated, with only 2 patients discontinuing therapy because of side effects. Fever and chills during the first infusion were the most prominent side effects. However, 9 patients (5%) had reduction of greater than 10% in left ventricular ejection fraction, and in 6 of these patients, the compromised cardiac function was symptomatic. These results showed that trastuzumab has impressive efficacy in a heavily pretreated group of patients.

Preclinical investigation has shown cytotoxic synergy between chemotherapy and monoclonal antibodies to HER-2/*neu*. Trastuzumab has been combined with several agents in the treatment of metastatic breast cancer. For example, the combination of trastuzumab and single-agent cisplatin is more active than cisplatin alone. Trastuzumab also enhances the efficacy of paclitaxel and doxorubicin against HER-2/*neu*–overexpressing breast cancer cells. A randomized trial comparing trastuzumab plus standard chemotherapy with standard chemotherapy alone as front-line treatment for metastatic breast cancer was presented at the ASCO meeting in 1998 (Slamon et al, 1998). A total of 469 patients whose tumors overexpressed HER-2/*neu* were enrolled. Patients without previous anthracycline exposure were given AC and randomly assigned to receive treatment with or without trastuzumab. Patients with previous anthracycline exposure were given paclitaxel with or without trastuzumab. With a median follow-up of 10.5 months, investigators found an overall benefit of chemotherapy plus trastuzumab versus chemotherapy alone. In both the AC and paclitaxel groups, the median time to progression was 8.6 months for patients who received chemotherapy plus trastuzumab versus 5.5 months for patients who received chemotherapy alone. Treatment with the trastuzumab/chemotherapy combination also produced higher response rates (62% vs 6.2%) (Slamon et al, 1998). An updated analysis at a median follow-up of 25 months revealed that patients who received trastuzumab had better overall survival than patients who received chemotherapy alone (25.4 months vs 20.9 months) (Norton et al, 1999).

Of concern was the grade 3 or 4 cardiac toxicity seen with the combination of trastuzumab and chemotherapy. Congestive heart failure occurred more often in patients receiving doxorubicin and trastuzumab (18%) than in those receiving paclitaxel and trastuzumab (2%). The combination of anthracycline and trastuzumab caused greater cardiac toxicity than was seen in the phase II trial evaluating trastuzumab as monotherapy. This increase in toxicity implicates an interaction of the 2 drugs.

Given the benefit seen with single-agent trastuzumab and the combination of trastuzumab and paclitaxel, trastuzumab should be considered for treatment of patients whose tumors overexpress HER-2/*neu*. However, because of the potential for cardiac damage, trastuzumab should not be given with anthracyclines outside the context of a clinical trial. Patients with newly diagnosed metastatic breast cancer with significant amplification of HER-2/*neu* may receive either an anthracycline-based regimen (based on the benefit of anthracyclines as treatment for tumors overexpressing HER-2/*neu*) without trastuzumab or a combination of paclitaxel and trastuzumab. At M. D. Anderson, doxorubicin-based regimens are generally utilized first. This allows for later use of trastuzumab in combination with other chemotherapies. Continuation of trastuzumab after progression of disease with the combination of paclitaxel and trastuzumab should be considered and is currently under evaluation. Trastuzumab enhances the effects of many agents in vitro and could possibly be of benefit in vivo.

Capecitabine

Capecitabine (Xeloda) is a commercially available prodrug of 5-fluorouracil approved by the Food and Drug Administration for treatment of metastatic breast cancer resistant to anthracyclines and taxanes. Capecitabine is activated by a cascade of enzymes that increases release of 5-fluorouracil in tumor cells. In a phase II trial of capecitabine for treatment of metastatic breast cancer, the overall response rate was 20%, and the median survival duration was 12.8 months (Blum et al, 1998).

Capecitabine is an oral medication with relatively few side effects. The recommended dose is 2500 mg/m^2 in 2 divided doses daily for 14 days, with a 7-day drug-free interval before the next course is started. With this schedule and dose, the most frequently experienced side effects include hand and foot syndrome, diarrhea, stomatitis, and fatigue. Nausea and vomiting have been reported but are less severe than with other chemotherapies commonly given for breast cancer. Capecitabine is recommended for patients in whom therapy with anthracycline- and taxane-based regimens fails. Current studies are evaluating the role of capecitabine as front-line therapy for the treatment of metastatic breast cancer in women over the age of 55.

Other Active Agents

In the metastatic setting, continued use of chemotherapy is controversial beyond the administration of 3 different regimens. Studies evaluating quality of life have found that improvement in a patient's sense of well-being is closely correlated with the response achieved with chemotherapy. With each additional regimen given, the likelihood of response to additional therapy decreases. When a patient's performance status falls to 3 or less on the Eastern Cooperative Oncology Group scale, a move to supportive care should be discussed. As with all therapy, the potential risks and benefits of any proposed treatment should be discussed thoroughly with the patient. In patients with metastatic breast cancer in whom standard regimens have failed, vinorelbine (Navelbine) or gemcitabine (Gemzar) may be useful.

Vinorelbine is a semisynthetic vinca alkaloid that produces overall response rates of 41% to 50% when it is used as a single agent as first-line therapy for metastatic breast cancer. When used as second-line therapy for breast cancer previously treated with taxanes or anthracyclines, vinorelbine produces overall response rates of 20% to 30%. Phase II trials showed that vinorelbine 30 mg/m^2 given intravenously over 20 minutes on days 1 and 8 every 3 weeks resulted in an overall response rate of 47% in previously untreated patients (Terenziani et al, 1996). The primary side effects seen with this regimen include neutropenia (dose-limiting), pain with infusion, flulike symptoms, and gastrointestinal symptoms (e.g., nausea and constipation). Longer infusion schedules (96-hour infusion) do not result in increased efficacy or decreased toxicity. Vinorelbine is currently being evaluated in combination with other agents in clinical trials. Vinorelbine is appropriate as third-line (or later) therapy for patients with metastatic breast cancer.

Gemcitabine is a nucleoside analogue active against breast cancer cells. The unique ability of gemcitabine to escape DNA repair enzymes may enhance its activity in cancer cells. Gemcitabine has been tested in multiple phase II trials. One study evaluated a dose of 800 mg/m^2 administered over 30 minutes once a week for 3 weeks (Carmichael et al, 1995). The patients then had a 1-week rest without chemotherapy before the cycle was restarted. In 40 patients who were previously untreated or had received only 1 prior treatment for breast cancer, the overall response rate was 25%. For patients who responded to gemcitabine, the median survival duration was 18.6 months. For all patients, however, median survival was 11.5 months. Grade 3 or 4 toxic effects seen in this study included neutropenia (30% of patients) and nausea and vomiting (25% of patients). In general, gemcitabine is well tolerated; few patients treated with this agent have alopecia or infections. The unique mechanism of action of gemcitabine has prompted investigation of this agent in polychemotherapy trials. At present, gemcitabine is appropriate as palliative treatment for patients with metastatic breast cancer in whom standard regimens have failed.

FUTURE DIRECTIONS

Systemic chemotherapy improves both the disease-free and overall survival of patients with operable breast cancer. Efforts to develop more effective adjuvant cytotoxic regimens are ongoing. Taxanes are being investigated in a variety of schedules and doses, and biologic agents, such as trastuzumab, are also being evaluated. Systemic chemotherapy also produces improvements in survival and quality of life in patients with metastatic breast cancer. As our understanding of the mechanisms of cell growth and death increases, new therapies will be developed to attack tumor-specific targets. Many new agents are in clinical development, including angiogenesis inhibitors, matrix metalloprotease inhibitors, intracellular signaling inhibitors, novel molecules that inhibit growth factors, vaccines, and new biologic agents. In addition, the role of other approaches utilizing chemotherapy (such as high-dose chemotherapy with stem cell transplantation) will continue to be defined. Despite our advances, the prognosis for many women with breast cancer is still grim. Only with continued investigation of new ideas and approaches will outcomes improve.

KEY PRACTICE POINTS

- A recent meta-analysis has confirmed the role of systemic chemotherapy in the treatment of most subsets of women with operable breast cancer.

- Anthracycline-containing regimens are superior to non-anthracycline-containing regimens.

- The addition of paclitaxel to FAC improves overall survival in node-positive patients. Paclitaxel should be considered for the treatment of patients at high risk for recurrence. To ensure that each patient's care is optimal, a multidisciplinary approach should be utilized in the development of treatment plans.

- Neoadjuvant chemotherapy can improve cosmetic results and can make breast conservation feasible in patients who initially would have required mastectomy. Neoadjuvant therapy is used routinely for patients with LABC. Neoadjuvant chemotherapy should be thoroughly discussed with the patient and multidisciplinary team before this therapy is administered.

- Patients should be encouraged to participate in clinical trials to help improve treatment of breast cancer for all women.

- The use of high-dose chemotherapy and stem cell transplantation is investigational at this time and should be used only in the context of a clinical trial.

- Systemic chemotherapy can improve the survival of patients with metastatic breast cancer.

- Systemic chemotherapy produces durable remissions in a small percentage of patients with metastatic breast cancer.

- Patients with hormone-sensitive tumors and non-life-threatening metastatic disease should be evaluated for hormonal therapy before systemic chemotherapy is initiated.

- Antitumor activity generally correlates with improved quality of life for patients with metastatic breast cancer.

- Amplification of HER-2/*neu* is associated with increased aggressiveness of breast cancers. Trastuzumab should be utilized for patients with metastatic breast cancer whose tumors overexpress HER-2/*neu.*

SUGGESTED READINGS

A'Hern RP, Smith IE, Ebbs SR. Chemotherapy and survival in advanced breast cancer: the inclusion of doxorubicin in Cooper type regimens. *Br J Cancer* 1993;67:801–805.

Allred DC, Clark GM, Tandon AK, et al. HER-2/neu in node-negative breast cancer: prognostic significance of overexpression influenced by the presence of in situ carcinoma. *J Clin Oncol* 1992;10:599–605.

American Society of Clinical Oncology. Update of recommendations for the use of hematopoietic colony stimulating factors: evidence-based clinical practice guidelines. *J Clin Oncol* 1996;14:1957–1960.

Blum JL, Buzdar AU, LoRusso PM, et al. A multicenter phase II trial of Xeloda (capecitabine) in paclitaxel-refractory metastatic breast cancer (MBC). *Proc Am Soc Clin Oncol* 1998; 17:125A. Abstract 476.

Bonadonna G, Brusamolino E, Valagussa P, et al. Combination chemotherapy as an adjuvant treatment in operable breast cancer. *N Engl J Med* 1976;294:405–410.

Bonadonna G, Valagussa P, Moliterni A, Zambetti M, Brambilla C. Adjuvant cyclophosphamide, methotrexate, and fluorouracil in node-positive breast cancer: the results of 20 years of follow-up. *N Engl J Med* 1995a;332:901–906.

Bonadonna G, Zambetti M, Valagussa P. Sequential or alternating doxorubicin and CMF regimens in breast cancer with more than three positive nodes. Ten-year results. *JAMA* 1995b;273:542–547.

Burris HA III. Single-agent docetaxel (Taxotere) in randomized phase III trials. *Semin Oncol* 1999;26(suppl 9):1–6.

Burstein HJ, Younger J, Bunnell CA, et al. Weekly docetaxel (Taxotere) for metastatic breast cancer: a phase II trial. *Proceedings of the American Society of Clinical Oncology* 1999;18:127A. Abstract 484.

Buzdar AU, Kau SW, Smith TL, Hortobagyi GN. Ten-year results of FAC adjuvant chemotherapy trial in breast cancer. *Am J Clin Oncol* 1989;12:123–128.

Buzdar AU, Singletary SE, Theriault RL, et al. Prospective evaluation of paclitaxel versus combination chemotherapy with fluorouracil, doxorubicin, cyclophosphamide as neoadjuvant therapy in patients with operable breast cancer. *J Clin Oncol* 1999;17:3412–3417.

Buzdar AU, Smith TL, Powell KC, Blumenschein GR, Gehan EA. Effect of timing of initiation of adjuvant chemotherapy on disease-free survival in breast cancer. *Breast Cancer Res Treat* 1982;2:163–169.

Carmichael J, Possinger K, Phillip P, et al. Advanced breast cancer: a phase II trial with gemcitabine. *J Clin Oncol* 1995;13:2731–2736.

Casper ES, Guidera CA, Bosl GJ, et al. Combined modality treatment of locally advanced breast cancer: adjuvant combination chemotherapy with and without doxorubicin. *Breast Cancer Res Treat* 1987;9:39–44.

Chen YY, Schnitt SJ. Prognostic factors for patients with breast cancers 1 cm and smaller. *Breast Cancer Res Treat* 1998;51:209–225.

Coates A, Gebski V, Bishop JF, et al. Improving the quality of life during chemotherapy for advanced breast cancer. A comparison of intermittent and continuous treatment strategies. *N Engl J Med* 1987;317:1490–1495.

Cobleigh MA, Vogel CL, Tripathy D, et al. Efficacy and safety of Herceptin (humanized anti-HER2 antibody) as a single agent in 222 women with HER2 overexpression who relapsed following chemotherapy for metastatic breast cancer. *Proceedings of the American Society of Clinical Oncology* 1998;17:97A. Abstract 376.

Early Breast Cancer Trialists' Collaborative Group. Polychemotherapy for early breast cancer: an overview of the randomised trials. *Lancet* 1998;352:930–942.

Ejlertsen B, Pfeiffer P, Pedersen D, et al. Decreased efficacy of cyclophosphamide, epirubicin and 5-fluorouracil in metastatic breast cancer when reducing treatment duration from 18 to 6 months. *Eur J Cancer* 1993;29A:527–531.

Falkson G, Gelman RS, Pandya KJ, et al. Eastern Cooperative Oncology Group randomized trials of observation versus maintenance therapy for patients with metastatic breast cancer in complete remission following induction treatment. *J Clin Oncol* 1998;16:1669–1676.

Fisher B, Brown AM, Dimitrov NV, et al. Two months of doxorubicin-cyclophosphamide with and without interval reinduction therapy compared with 6 months of cyclophosphamide, methotrexate, and fluorouracil in positive-node breast cancer patients with tamoxifen-nonresponsive tumors: results from the National Surgical Adjuvant Breast and Bowel Project B-15. *J Clin Oncol* 1990a;8:1483–1496.

Fisher B, Bryant J, Wolmark N, et al. Effect of preoperative chemotherapy on the outcome of women with operable breast cancer. *J Clin Oncol* 1998;16:2672–2685.

Fisher B, Dignam J, Wolmark N, et al. Tamoxifen and chemotherapy for lymph node-negative, estrogen receptor-positive breast cancer. *J Natl Cancer Inst* 1997;89:1673–1682.

Fisher B, Redmond C, Legault-Poisson S, et al. Postoperative chemotherapy and tamoxifen compared with tamoxifen alone in the treatment of positive-node breast cancer patients aged 50 years and older with tumors responsive to tamoxifen: results from the National Surgical Adjuvant Breast and Bowel Project B-16. *J Clin Oncol* 1990b;8:1005–1018.

Fisher B, Slack N, Katrych D, Wolmark N. Ten year follow-up results of patients with carcinoma of the breast in a co-operative clinical trial evaluating surgical adjuvant chemotherapy. *Surg Gynecol Obstet* 1975;140:528–534.

Fossati R, Confalonieri C, Torri V, et al. Cytotoxic and hormonal treatment for metastatic breast cancer: a systematic review of published randomized trials involving 31,510 women. *J Clin Oncol* 1998;16:3439–3460.

Gralla RJ, Osoba D, Kris MG, Kirkbride P, et al. Recommendations for the use of antiemetics: evidence-based clinical practice guidelines. *J Clin Oncol* 1999; 17:2971–2994.

Greenberg PA, Hortobagyi GN, Smith TL, Ziegler LD, Frye DK, Buzdar AU. Long-term follow-up of patients with complete remission following combination chemotherapy for metastatic breast cancer. *J Clin Oncol* 1996;14:2197–2205.

Gregory RK, Powles TJ, Chang JC, Ashley S. A randomised trial of six versus twelve courses of chemotherapy in metastatic carcinoma of the breast. *Eur J Cancer* 1997;33:2194–2197.

Gusterson BA, Gelber RD, Goldhirsch A, et al. Prognostic importance of c-erbB-2 expression in breast cancer. International (Ludwig) Breast Cancer Study Group. *J Clin Oncol* 1992;10:1049–1056.

Henderson IC, Berry D, Demetri G, et al. Improved disease-free (DFS) and overall survival (OS) from the addition of sequential paclitaxel (T) but not from the escalation of doxorubicin (A) dose level in the adjuvant chemotherapy of patients (PTS) with node-positive primary breast cancer (BC). *Proceedings of the American Society of Clinical Oncology* 1998;17:101A. Abstract 390.

Holmes FA, Valero V, Walters RS, et al. Paclitaxel by 24-hour infusion with doxorubicin by 48-hour infusion as initial therapy for metastatic breast cancer: phase I results. *Ann Oncol* 1999;10:403–411.

Holmes FA, Walters RS, Theriault RL, et al. Phase II trial of taxol, an active drug in the treatment of metastatic breast cancer. *J Natl Cancer Inst* 1991;83:1797–1805.

Hortobagyi GN, Frye D, Buzdar AU, et al. Decreased cardiac toxicity of doxorubicin administered by continuous intravenous infusion in combination chemotherapy for metastatic breast carcinoma. *Cancer* 1989;63:37–45.

Hutchins L, Green S, Ravdin P, et al. CMF versus CAF with and without tamoxifen in high-risk node-negative breast cancer patients and a natural history follow-up study in low-risk node-negative patients: first results of intergroup trial INT 0102. *Proceedings of the American Society of Clinical Oncology* 1998;17. Abstract 1.

Kroman N, Jensen MB, Wohlfahrt J, Mouridsen HT, Andersen PK, Melbye M. Factors influencing the effect of age on prognosis in breast cancer: population based study. *BMJ* 2000;320:474–478.

Levine MN, Bramwell VH, Pritchard KI, et al. Randomized trial of intensive cyclophosphamide, epirubicin, and fluorouracil chemotherapy compared with cyclophosphamide, methotrexate, and fluorouracil in premenopausal women with node-positive breast cancer. National Cancer Institute of Canada Clinical Trials Group. *J Clin Oncol* 1998;16:2651–2658.

Mamounas E, Brown A, Smith R, et al. Effect of taxol duration of infusion in advanced breast cancer (ABC): results from NSABP B-26 trial comparing 3- to 24-h infusion of high-dose taxol. *Proceedings of the American Society of Clinical Oncology* 1998;17:101A. Abstract 389.

Muss HB, Case LD, Richards F III, et al. Interrupted versus continuous chemotherapy in patients with metastatic breast cancer. The Piedmont Oncology Association. *N Engl J Med* 1991;325:1342–1348.

Muss HB, Thor AD, Berry DA, et al. c-erbB-2 expression and response to adjuvant therapy in women with node-positive early breast cancer. *N Engl J Med* 1994;330:1260–1266.

Nabholtz JM. Docetaxel (Taxotere) plus doxorubicin-based combinations: the evidence of activity in breast cancer. *Semin Oncol* 1999;26(suppl 9):7–13.

Nabholtz JM, Gelmon K, Bontenbal M, et al. Multicenter, randomized comparative study of two doses of paclitaxel in patients with metastatic breast cancer. *J Clin Oncol* 1996;14:1858–1867.

Norton L, Slamon D, Leyland-Jones B, et al. Overall survival (OS) advantage to simultaneous chemotherapy (CRx) plus the humanized anti-HER2 monoclonal antibody Herceptin (H) in HER2 overexpressing (HER2 +) metastatic breast cancer (MBC). *Proceedings of the American Society of Clinical Oncology* 1999;18:127A. Abstract 483.

Rahman ZU, Frye DK, Smith TL, et al. Results and long term follow-up for 1581 patients with metastatic breast carcinoma treated with standard dose doxorubicin-containing chemotherapy: a reference. *Cancer* 1999;85:104–111.

Recht A, Come SE, Henderson IC, et al. The sequencing of chemotherapy and radiation therapy after conservative surgery for early-stage breast cancer. *N Engl J Med* 1996;334:1356–1361.

Rosen PP, Groshen S, Kinne DW. Prognosis in T2N0M0 stage I breast carcinoma: a 20-year follow-up study. *J Clin Oncol* 1991;9:1650–1661.

Seidman AD. Single-agent paclitaxel in the treatment of breast cancer: phase I and II development. *Semin Oncol* 1999;26(suppl 8):14–20.

Slamon DJ, Clark GM, Wong SG, Levin J, Ullrich A, McGuire WL. Human breast cancer: correlation of relapse and survival with amplification of the HER-2/ neu oncogene. *Science* 1987;235:177–182.

Slamon D, Leyland-Jones B, Shak S, et al. Addition of Herceptin (humanized anti-HER2 antibody) to first line chemotherapy for HER2 overexpressing metastatic breast cancer (HER2 + /MBC) markedly increases anticancer activity: a randomized, multinational controlled phase III trial. *Proceedings of the American Society of Clinical Oncology* 1998;17:98A. Abstract 377.

Sledge G, Neuberg D, Ingle J, Martino S, Wood W. Phase III trial of doxorubicin (A) vs. paclitaxel (T) vs. doxorubicin + paclitaxel (A + T) as first-line therapy for metastatic breast cancer (MBC): an intergroup trial. *Proceedings of the American Society of Clinical Oncology* 1997;16:1A. Abstract 2.

Stockler M, Wilcken N, Coates A. Chemotherapy for metastatic breast cancer— when is enough enough? *Eur J Cancer* 1997;33:2147–2148.

Terenziani M, Demicheli R, Brambilla C, et al. Vinorelbine: an active, non cross-resistant drug in advanced breast cancer. Results from a phase II study. *Breast Cancer Res Treat* 1996;39:285–291.

Thomas E, Buzdar A, Theriault R, et al. Role of paclitaxel in adjuvant therapy of operable breast cancer: preliminary results of prospective randomized clinical trial. *Proceedings of the American Society of Clinical Oncology* 2000;19. Abstract 285.

Valero V, Holmes FA, Walters RS, et al. Phase II trial of docetaxel: a new, highly effective antineoplastic agent in the management of patients with anthracycline-resistant metastatic breast cancer. *J Clin Oncol* 1995;13:2886–2894.

Winer E, Berry D, Duggan D, et al. Failure of higher dose paclitaxel to improve outcome in patients with metastatic breast cancer—results from CALGB 9342. *Proceedings of the American Society of Clinical Oncology* 1998;17:101A. Abstract 388.

Zambetti M, Bonadonna G, Valagussa P, et al. Adjuvant CMF for node-negative and estrogen receptor-negative breast cancer patients. *J Natl Cancer Inst Monogr* 1992;(11):77–83.

12 HIGH-DOSE CHEMOTHERAPY AS TREATMENT FOR HIGH-RISK PRIMARY AND METASTATIC BREAST CANCER

Naoto T. Ueno and Richard E. Champlin

CHAPTER OVERVIEW

Recent data from randomized trials of high-dose chemotherapy as treatment for high-risk primary and metastatic breast cancer provide important information about the risks and benefits of this treatment approach. Further research through well-designed, hypothesis-oriented clinical trials is needed to establish the role of high-dose chemotherapy in a multimodality treatment approach. M. D. Anderson Cancer Center continues to conduct such research.

INTRODUCTION

Many patients with high-risk primary breast cancer experience recurrence and micrometastatic disease even after receiving conventional combined-modality therapy (i.e., chemotherapy, surgery, and radiation therapy). Because metastatic breast cancer is generally considered incurable by conventional therapy, the treatment focus for this patient group is generally palliative care.

In preclinical and clinical studies of breast cancer, dose escalation of alkylating agents, such as cyclophosphamide, carboplatin, cisplatin, etoposide, carmustine, and thiotepa, has resulted in increased tumor response rates. High-dose chemotherapy (HDCT) with non-cross-resistant alkylating agents supported by autologous hematopoietic stem cell transplantation (AHST) has been explored for almost 2 decades as treatment for breast cancer. Initial data from early phase I and II studies suggested that HDCT plus AHST might be superior to standard-dose chemotherapy (SDCT) as both adjuvant therapy for primary breast cancer and therapy for metastatic disease. However, recent randomized trials have yielded conflicting results. Interpretation of published reports was further complicated by the revelation that some of the data from a study of adjuvant HDCT conducted in South Africa and reported by Bezwoda (1999) were falsified. Furthermore, oversimplified interpretations of existing data by the lay media, including some editorials, that suggested that HDCT was ineffective against breast cancer have slowed accrual to clinical trials designed to address the major issues regarding this approach. As of June 2000, the results of 6 randomized trials of HDCT for high-risk primary breast cancer and 4 randomized trials of HDCT for metastatic breast cancer have been reported, and the consensus is that further research is needed in this field.

This chapter will review the treatment processes involved in HDCT, the major issues surrounding HDCT, and results of randomized clinical trials of HDCT, including studies conducted at M. D. Anderson Cancer Center.

HIGH-DOSE CHEMOTHERAPY PLUS AUTOLOGOUS HEMATOPOIETIC STEM CELL TRANSPLANTATION

High-dose chemotherapy plus AHST is a multimodality process that also involves SDCT and other therapies. This section describes how the components of this process are integrated in breast cancer treatment at M. D. Anderson through the collaborative efforts of several disciplines. The process is also outlined in Table 12–1.

Table 12–1. Outline of High-Dose Chemotherapy Approach to Treatment of Breast Cancer

Process	Timeline
1. Patient assessment (consultation with Department of Blood and Marrow Transplantation)	Consultation: 1 day Restaging: 3–5 days
2. Induction therapy (standard-dose chemotherapy)	Time varies. Goal is to achieve maximum cytoreduction of metastatic breast cancer.
3. Stem cell collection after mobilization with cytokine alone or chemotherapy plus cytokine	6 days–4 weeks
4. Preparative therapy (high-dose chemotherapy, radiation therapy, or both)	3–5 days
5. Stem cell infusion (reinfusion or transplantation of collected stem cells)	1 day
6. Supportive therapy (administration of colony-stimulating factors)	10 days–3 weeks
7. Recovery	4–6 weeks
8. Assessment of treatment response and follow-up	• Every 3–4 months for first 2 years • Then every 6 months for 2–5 years • Every year thereafter for life

Patient Assessment

In a consultation conducted by a clinical staff member of the Department of Blood and Marrow Transplantation, a patient's eligibility for an HDCT clinical trial is assessed. The patient is made aware of the risks and benefits of HDCT plus AHST, and then clinical tests are performed on potential candidates to evaluate the status of vital organs such as the lungs, heart, kidneys, and liver. The tumor is restaged by radiographic and biochemical studies to determine the extent of disease. At the same time, medical and financial authorizations are obtained from the patient's third-party medical insurance carrier. Written informed consent is obtained before the patient enters the study.

Induction Therapy

The response to HDCT depends on the amount of tumor burden and the sensitivity of the tumor to chemotherapy. The longest survival durations have been observed in patients who had minimal or no tumor burden after SDCT. Therefore, induction SDCT is given prior to HDCT to maximally reduce the tumor burden.

Stem Cell Collection

Before HDCT is performed, hematopoietic stem cells are collected and cryopreserved for use in the AHST. Without AHST after HDCT, patients will experience prolonged periods of neutropenia, anemia, and thrombocytopenia, which result in infection, bleeding, and fatigue.

After cytoreduction (induction therapy), patients are given chemotherapy plus cytokine therapy or cytokine therapy alone to mobilize circulating peripheral blood stem cells (PBSCs). The chemotherapy mobilization regimen used at M. D. Anderson consists of cyclophosphamide, etoposide, and cisplatin (CVP). Other myelosuppressive chemotherapy agents, such as high doses of cyclophosphamide, ifosfamide, or paclitaxel, can also be used. The cytokines used are granulocyte colony-stimulating factor (G-CSF) or granulocyte-macrophage colony-stimulating factor (GM-CSF).

The hematopoietic stem cell source can be PBSCs or bone marrow cells. Peripheral blood stem cells are collected by leukapheresis, which is performed daily until an adequate volume of PBSCs is collected. Bone marrow cells are collected from the posterior superior iliac crests by multiple aspirations while the patient is under anesthesia. If an adequate volume of PBSCs is not mobilized, bone marrow cells are harvested and used along with the PBSCs.

In initial trials of HDCT, bone marrow cells alone were used as the hematopoietic stem cell source. However, it has been shown that hematopoietic recovery occurs significantly faster when cytokine-mobilized PBSCs are used. The shorter duration of neutropenia experienced with PBSCs reduces the period of risk for infection and allows for earlier hospital discharge. In all current ongoing trials at M. D. Anderson, PBSCs alone are used as the hematopoietic stem cell source.

Preparative Therapy

Preparative therapy involves the administration of intensive-dose radiation therapy or chemotherapy. For HDCT to be successful, the breast cancer must exhibit a dose-dependent response to chemotherapy or radiation therapy so that, in general, 1 course of treatment will eradicate the malignant cells. Bone marrow suppression is the dose-limiting toxicity of most chemotherapy agents and of radiation therapy as well. The dose of chemotherapy or radiation can be substantially elevated for maximum therapeutic effect if treatment is followed by transplantation of normal hematopoietic stem cells (PBSCs or bone marrow), which rescues patients from prolonged myelosuppression.

In breast cancer, most patients are treated with preparative regimens that utilize high doses of alkylating agents. Alkylating agents have moderate activity against breast cancer at standard doses, and preclinical experiments have suggested a steep dose-response correlation as well as lack of cross-resistance between these agents. Other investigators have incorporated drugs with higher activity against breast cancer (e.g., paclitaxel, epirubicin, and doxorubicin) into their regimens; however, the dose of these agents cannot be markedly escalated because they can cause nonhematologic side effects (e.g., cardiac or neurological toxicity). Some studies have evaluated the administration of multiple cycles of submyeloablative doses of chemotherapy with PBSC support, but no substantial improvement in event-free survival has been demonstrated.

The most common preparative regimens used as treatment for patients with breast cancer are cyclophosphamide, thiotepa, and carboplatin (CTCb) and cyclophosphamide, carmustine, and cisplatin (CBP). Phase II trials have shown that HDCT can convert partial responses (PRs) to SDCT into complete responses (CRs) in 20% to 40% of patients (CR conversion rate). At M. D. Anderson, our preparative HDCT regimen consists of cyclophosphamide, carmustine, and thiotepa (CBT), which has a CR conversion rate of 31%.

Close monitoring and meticulous supportive care are required to protect patients from the potential toxic effects of preparative regimens.

Stem Cell Infusion

After the administration of the preparative regimen, the collected PBSCs or bone marrow cells are infused intravenously. The stem cells circulate transiently and home to the bone marrow to restore hematopoiesis. Peripheral blood counts are profoundly suppressed owing to the effects of the preparative regimens but generally recover within 10 days to 2 weeks after a PBSC transplant or 2 to 3 weeks after a bone marrow transplant.

Supportive Therapy

Just after reinfusion of collected stem cells, the patient's blood counts will be low, and patients will be at risk for infections. Patients are isolated in private rooms and advised to limit visitations and to avoid eating raw fruits and vegetables. Patients receive prophylactic treatment to prevent bacterial, fungal, and parasitic infections. Either G-CSF or GM-CSF is given to shorten recovery of neutrophil counts. Use of these cytokines is generally continued until the absolute neutrophil count is greater than $1 \times 10^6/L$ for 3 consecutive days. If the patient's thrombocyte count decreases to less than $20 \times 10^6/L$, platelets are given to eliminate the risk of bleeding complications.

Recovery

The patient recovers strength and nutritional status over several weeks. After 4 to 6 weeks, the patient's general condition usually returns to their normal physical status.

Assessment of Treatment Response and Follow-up

After full recovery of bone marrow cells or PBSCs, response to treatment is assessed by radiographic and biochemical studies every 3 to 4 months for the first 2 years after the transplantation, every 6 months for 2 more years, and then once a year.

Progress in the Use of High-Dose Chemotherapy in Breast Cancer

Advances in supportive care and the technology of AHST have reduced the morbidity and largely eliminated the mortality associated with HDCT and have made this approach safer, more effective, and less expensive than it was 5 to 10 years ago, when most of the randomized trials of HDCT were designed and initiated. Progress with regard to the major issues surrounding HDCT is discussed here.

Morbidity and Mortality

In trials conducted in the 1980s, the mortality rate associated with HDCT plus AHST was as high as 23%. The major complications were infections occurring during prolonged periods of neutropenia (immunosuppression) and regimen-related toxic effects. With the use of cytokines for stem cell support, prophylactic antibiotics, and PBSCs as the stem cell transplant source, the rate of infections has been markedly reduced. Regimen-related toxic effects also appear to be reduced when hematopoietic recovery is accomplished rapidly. The transplant-related mortality rate is generally lowest at large centers experienced in delivering HDCT plus AHST. Data from the American Blood and Marrow Transplantation Registry show that 5% of patients with metastatic breast cancer die within 100 days of AHST, whereas only 2% to 3% of patients with high-risk primary breast cancer who undergo HDCT die in this time frame. In the past 3 years at M. D. Anderson, there have been no deaths among patients with high-risk primary breast cancer who received a transplant, and the mortality rate among patients with metastatic disease who received a transplant was only 2%. In terms of quality of life, patients who undergo HDCT usually do not receive any further treatment after transplantation for metastatic breast cancer; therefore, they may have a better quality of life compared with patients who undergo SDCT and must continue chemotherapy every 3 to 4 weeks for life.

Cost

Several factors have contributed to a dramatic reduction in the cost of HDCT. They are: shorter duration of neutropenia, which decreases morbidity and mortality; the use of prophylactic antibiotics; the early recognition of regimen-related toxic effects; and a shorter hospital stay. As well, the cost of transplantation for breast cancer is now less than $75,000, which is about equal to the total cost of SDCT for metastatic breast cancer.

Contamination of the Stem Cell Graft

The presence of large numbers of malignant cells in the PBSC or bone marrow autograft increases the patient's risk for systemic relapse. Thus, a variety of techniques have been proposed to "purge" the autograft of malignant cells. The 2 most common methods of purging are negative selection, in which malignant cells are targeted and depleted, and positive selection, in which healthy stem cells are separated from mature hematopoietic stem cells and tumor cells in the unsolicited fraction and the mature cells and tumor cells are discarded. Attempts have been made to deplete the malignant-cell content of the autograft by physical means, with drug treatment (4-hydroperoxycyclophosphamide), and with monoclonal antibody–based approaches. Although several purging methods have been shown to reduce the number of breast cancer cells in the PBSC or bone marrow autograft, no controlled studies have been performed to determine whether patients who receive the purged grafts have improved progression-free survival (PFS). A major problem is that recurrence might be caused by the cancer cells contaminating the autograft and cancer cells surviving HDCT. Effective purging will be essential in clinical settings to ensure that the preparative regimen successfully eliminates systemic disease.

UPDATE OF RANDOMIZED TRIALS OF HIGH-DOSE
CHEMOTHERAPY IN THE PUBLIC DOMAIN

This section describes the results of randomized trials in the public domain of HDCT in patients with metastatic and high-risk primary breast cancer.

Metastatic Breast Cancer

Standard-dose chemotherapy may produce a CR rate of 10% to 25% and an overall response rate of 45% to 70% in patients with chemotherapy-naïve metastatic breast cancer. The duration of response typically ranges from 12 to 18 months, and fewer than 5% of patients remain disease-free at 5 years after treatment. The most effective HDCT regimens used in patients with chemotherapy-responsive metastatic breast cancer significantly increase the overall CR rate to more than 50%, and approximately 15% to 20% of patients survive disease-free for more than 5 years. A substantial number of patients remain disease-free for more than 10 years after HDCT plus AHST. Favorable prognostic factors in these patients include an initial good response to SDCT, minimal tumor burden, minimal number of disease sites, absence of liver involvement, good performance status, and no history of adjuvant chemotherapy or radiation therapy. Long-term survivors tend to be younger, to have a lower tumor burden, and to have a better performance status.

Although the data from phase II studies appear encouraging, patient selection bias should be considered. To qualify for HDCT plus AHST, patients usually need to have good performance status, no major organ dysfunction, and no active infection and to be of physiological age younger than 60 years. These criteria should facilitate the selection of patients who have a relatively good prognosis and are likely to respond to either SDCT or HDCT. Some authors argue that the apparent favorable results of HDCT can be attributed entirely to the selection of patients with a relatively favorable prognosis. Greenberg et al (1996) published a report about long-term follow-up in patients with metastatic breast cancer who had a CR with doxorubicin-containing SDCT. Of the patients who had a CR, 19% remained progression-free for more than 5 years. Lead-time bias should be taken into account when considering these results. Most patients typically receive SDCT for only a few months before receiving HDCT, and most HDCT trials report overall survival (OS) and PFS from the time of stem cell infusion rather than from the initiation of SDCT. In this chapter, OS and PFS durations are measured from the day of stem cell infusion.

Most of the data about HDCT have been derived from phase I and II trials that confirm the feasibility of this treatment approach and the high tumor response rate and CR conversion rate. It is difficult to compare the results of single-arm HDCT trials with SDCT trials because of the different eligibility criteria, patient selection requirements, and time points for the measurement of OS and PFS rates and durations. Therefore, prospective randomized trials are needed to determine whether HDCT improves OS and PFS rates and durations compared with SDCT.

Four randomized clinical trials comparing HDCT with SDCT for metastatic breast cancer have been reported (Table 12–2). The largest is the PBT-1 trial reported by Stadtmauer et al (2000). Of 553 patients enrolled, 199 (36%) received SDCT with 5-fluorouracil, doxorubicin, and cyclophosphamide (FAC) or cyclophosphamide, methotrexate, and 5-fluorouracil (CMF). If a CR or PR was achieved, patients were randomly assigned to HDCT with CTCb or to SDCT with CMF as maintenance therapy for 2 years or until disease progression. With a median follow-up of 37 months, there was no difference between the 2 groups in median OS or PFS duration. It was not possible to identify patient or disease characteristics that favored either treatment arm. This study had several limitations. There was a high drop-out rate (33%) that could have obscured the final results. Only 45 patients were randomly assigned to maintenance CMF or CTCb after having a CR to SDCT; thus, there was inadequate power to detect a clinically significant difference in this important subgroup. Furthermore, among patients who had a PR to SDCT, there was only an 8% CR conversion rate by HDCT, which was not different from that of continued SDCT. This is the lowest CR conversion rate reported in any HDCT study.

Peters et al (1996) reported a trial of 96 patients with metastatic breast cancer who received SDCT with doxorubicin, 5-fluorouracil, and methotrexate (AFM) and, if a CR was reached, were then randomly assigned to immediate HDCT with CBP or delayed HDCT with CBP (delayed until relapse or progression). Patients who had immediate consolidation with high-dose CBP had longer duration of PFS compared with patients in whom high-dose CBP was delayed until relapse or progression (22.2 months vs 3.8 months; $P = .008$). However, OS duration was better among patients in whom high-dose CBP was delayed (38.4 months vs 20.4 months; $P = .04$). This is an interesting observation, and it suggests that delaying HDCT consolidation could provide the benefit of chemoresistance. A major criticism of this study was that the AFM regimen was given for only 2 to 4 cycles before randomization. There was an unusually short remission duration in the delayed CBP group, which was possibly due to an inadequate duration of standard-dose AFM administration.

Bezwoda et al (1995) randomly assigned 90 patients with untreated metastatic breast cancer to either 6 to 8 cycles of SDCT with cyclophosphamide, vincristine, and mitoxantrone (CNVc) or to 2 cycles of HDCT with cyclophosphamide, etoposide, and mitoxantrone (CNVp) plus AHST. Overall response rates were 53% with CNVc and 95% with CNVp, and CR rates were 4% and 51%, respectively. There were statistically significant improvements in the median PFS duration (18.6 months vs 7.9

months; $P < .01$) and median OS duration (21.0 months vs 10.5 months; $P < .01$), with both favoring HDCT with CNVp. The unconventional treatment regimens used in this trial were significantly different from regimens used in Europe and the United States. The CR rate of 4% and the response duration of 40 weeks achieved with SDCT were much lower than what had been reported in the literature. Bezwoda and colleagues, in their initial report of SDCT with CNVc, reported an overall response rate of 81% and a CR rate of 23%. Furthermore, all patients whose tumors responded were given tamoxifen at the end of chemotherapy, and more patients who underwent HDCT with CNVp received tamoxifen. Because of the misconduct reported in the more recent Bezwoda trial of HDCT for high-risk primary breast cancer (Bezwoda, 1999), data from the 1995 trial should not be considered reliable until their validity is confirmed. However, the concept of up-front HDCT in chemotherapy-naïve patients with metastatic breast cancer warrants investigation.

In the PEGASE 04 study conducted by Lotz et al (1999), 61 patients with metastatic breast cancer responding to SDCT were randomly assigned to either SDCT or HDCT with cyclophosphamide, mitoxantrone, and melphalan (CAN). The median OS duration of patients in the HDCT arm was double that of patients in the SDCT arm (36.1 months vs 15.7 months; $P = .08$). However, because of the small sample size, the difference was not statistically significant. At 5 years, there was still no difference in OS or PFS durations between these patient groups.

The PBT-1 and PEGASE 04 studies raise interest about the overall quality of life of patients during these treatments because patients who undergo HDCT do not receive any further chemotherapy, whereas patients who undergo SDCT continue receiving treatment.

The existing data are inconclusive with regard to the potential benefit of HDCT for patients with metastatic breast cancer. In each HDCT trial, the drug regimen and dose-intensification schedule was different, and each trial addressed different questions. It is clear, however, from available information from recent randomized studies, that HDCT has only a modest beneficial effect, if any, with a maximum improvement in OS of approximately 15%. The shorter treatment duration required with HDCT compared with SDCT to achieve a similar OS and PFS can be considered a desirable treatment parameter. Studies with larger numbers of patients are needed to provide the power required to detect such a difference. In addition, the subgroups of patients likely to benefit from HDCT need to be identified. The current data suggest that future studies should focus on patients with low tumor burden and chemotherapy-responsive disease. We continue to support ongoing randomized trials in Europe and the United States and await their final results. In addition to treatment efficacy, quality of life and cost-effectiveness are important issues to address in HDCT trials, particularly in the PBT-1 trial.

Table 12–2. Recent Trials of High-Dose Chemotherapy in Metastatic Breast Cancer

Study	No. of patients / Median follow-up / Trial design	Outcome	Highlights
Stadtmauer PBT-1 USA	• 553 patients • 3.1 years • 199 patients treated with SDCT with FAC or CMF; if CR or PR was achieved, patients were randomly assigned to SDCT with CMF maintenance therapy or HDCT with CTCb	No difference in OS or PFS duration • OS: 26 months (CMF maintenance) vs 24 months (CTCb) ($P = .23$) • PFS: 9 months (CMF maintenance) vs 9.6 months (CTCb) ($P = .31$)	• Very high dropout rate; only 33% of patients randomized • Very low CR conversion rate after HDCT (8%) • Similar PFS and OS achievable with a shorter treatment duration (HDCT arm)
Peters Duke USA	• 96 patients • 7 years • 2 to 4 cycles of SDCT with AFM; if CR was achieved, patients were randomly assigned to immediate HDCT with CBP or delayed HDCT with CBP	Statistical difference in OS and PFS duration • OS: 38.4 months (delayed arm) vs 20.4 months (immediate arm) ($P = .04$) • PFS: 22.2 months (immediate arm) vs 3.8 months (delayed arm) ($P = .008$)	• Small sample size • Possibly inadequate duration of initial SDCT (AFM) to achieve a CR; may have resulted in improved OS in delayed HDCT group • Issues associated with immediate vs delayed transplant

Bezwoda South Africa	• 90 patients • 5 years • SDCT with CNVc x 6 to 8 vs HDCT with CNVp x 2	Statistical difference in OS and PFS duration • OS: 21.0 months (HDCT with CNVp) vs 10.5 months (SDCT with CNVc) ($P < .01$) • PFS: 18.6 months (HDCT with CNVp) vs 7.9 months (SCDT with CNVc) ($P < .01$)	Falsification of data related to HDCT in primary breast cancer; these data should be discredited until external review is completed.
Lotz PEGASE 04 France	• 61 patients • 5 years • SDCT; if response was achieved, patients were randomly assigned to SDCT with CAN or HDCT with CAN	No difference in OS or PFS duration at 5 years • Median OS: 36.1 months (HDCT) vs 15.7 months (SDCT) ($P = .08$) • Median PFS: 26.9 (HDCT) vs 15.7 months (SDCT) ($P = .04$)	• Small sample size • There was a trend of doubling the OS and PFS by HDCT.

AFM, doxorubicin, 5-fluorouracil, and methotrexate; CAN, cyclophosphamide, mitoxantrone, and melphalan; CBP, cyclophosphamide, carmustine, and cisplatin; CMF, cyclophosphamide, methotrexate, and 5-fluorouracil; CNVc, cyclophosphamide, vincristine, and mitoxantrone; CNVp, cyclophosphamide, etoposide, and mitoxantrone; CR, complete response; CTCb, cyclophosphamide, thiotepa, and carboplatin; FAC, 5-fluorouracil, doxorubicin, and cyclophosphamide; HDCT, high-dose chemotherapy; OS, overall survival; PFS, progression-free survival; PR, partial response; SDCT, standard-dose chemotherapy.

High-Risk Primary Breast Cancer

High-risk primary breast cancer is generally defined as stage II or III disease with 10 or more positive axillary nodes and stage IIIB disease with inflammatory breast cancer. Five-year PFS rates after adjuvant SDCT are 25% to 50% in patients with 10 or more positive axillary nodes and 30% to 35% in patients with inflammatory breast cancer. High-dose chemotherapy is considered most likely curative if administered at a time of minimal tumor burden and before the tumor becomes drug resistant; therefore, it has been suggested that HDCT be administered after completion of adjuvant SDCT. In phase II studies, approximately 70% of patients with high-risk features survive disease-free for 5 years after HDCT. Although these data compare favorably with most studies of SDCT, in which the 5-year PFS rate is typically less than 50%, the results are confounded by patient selection bias and stage migration (rigorous staging of candidates for transplantation, eliminating those with occult stage IV disease). Six randomized studies of HDCT for high-risk primary breast cancer have been reported in the public domain (see Table 12–3). As shown in the discussion that follows, the results of these studies are mixed.

In 2 small studies, 1 by Rodenhuis et al (1998) and 1 by Hortobagyi et al (2000), which evaluated 81 and 78 patients, respectively, no benefit was found with HDCT, but the statistical power was designed to detect more than a 30% difference in OS and DFS rates. The Rodenhuis study involved patients with positive bone scans and bone marrow disease, which included patients with metastatic disease. Of these patients, 15% did not follow the protocol guidelines. Complete restaging was not done to rule out patients with metastatic disease prior to HDCT, which may have resulted in some patients with metastatic disease being treated with HDCT. The study by Hortobagyi et al evaluated patients with stage II or III breast cancer involving 10 or more lymph nodes after initial surgery or 4 or more lymph nodes after neoadjuvant chemotherapy. Patients received 8 cycles of SDCT with FAC and were then randomly assigned to 2 cycles of HDCT with CVP or observation. The 3-year PFS rates were 48% and 62%, respectively (P = .35). The OS rates were 58% and 78%, respectively (P = .23). In this study, a fairly significant number of patients (20.5%) did not follow the original treatment plan. Furthermore, CVP is not a true myeloablative regimen and can be given without AHST. Therefore, CVP alone may not be an effective myeloablative HDCT regimen.

Preliminary results of 3 other randomized trials comparing HDCT with SDCT in patients with high-risk primary breast cancer were reported at the American Society of Clinical Oncology meeting in 1999. Bezwoda (1999) reported superior PFS and OS rates with HDCT; however, an audit of this study revealed that some of the data were falsified, so the study must be totally disregarded. Bergh (1999) randomly assigned patients with multiple metastatic lymph nodes to individually adjusted, intensive-dose SDCT with 9 cycles of 5-fluorouracil, epirubicin, and cyclophospha-mide (FEC) or to SDCT with 3 cycles of FEC plus HDCT with CTCb. There was no difference between the 2 groups with regard to OS or PFS rates at 2 years, but the median follow-up was only 1.7 years. Furthermore, there were more patients with secondary myelodysplastic syndrome or acute myelogenous leukemia in the SDCT-alone arm. It should be noted that the cumulative dose intensity in the SDCT-alone arm was greater than that of the SDCT plus HDCT arm. Thus, this study compared 2 methods of ad-ministering intensive-dose chemotherapy.

In the largest study of its kind to date, Peters and colleagues (1999) treated 874 patients with high-risk primary breast cancer and 10 or more positive axillary lymph nodes with 4 cycles of standard-dose FAC and then randomly assigned them to HDCT with CBP plus AHST or intermediate-dose CBP plus G-CSF support. There were no differences in OS or PFS rates with a median follow-up of 3.5 years. However, the high-dose CBP arm did show a 34% decrease in relapse compared with the intermediate-dose CBP arm, which was offset by a higher rate of treatment-related mortality (8%) in the high-dose CBP arm. It is possible that the differences in relapse rates will translate into PFS and OS differ-ences with continued follow-up. The statistical power is designed to detect a 14% difference at 5 years. Long-term follow-up is needed in order to draw definitive conclusions. The unusually high mortality rate of 8% in the high-dose CBP arm may be related to the regimen used; as indicated in recent studies, the mortality rate in patients with high-risk primary breast cancer is less than 3%.

In another study by Rodenhuis and colleagues (2000), 885 patients with 4 or more positive axillary lymph nodes were randomly assigned to re-ceive SDCT with FEC alone or SDCT with FEC followed by HDCT with CTCb plus AHST. Only 289 patients were included in the analysis of the OS and PFS benefit of these regimens. There was a statistically significance difference in OS and PFS at 3 years median follow-up: the PFS rates were 62% in the standard-dose FEC-alone group and 77% in the group that received standard-dose FEC and high-dose CTCb plus AHST; the OS rates were 79% and 89%, respectively. The transplant-related mortality rate was 1%. This difference was statistically significant and favored transplanta-tion; however, longer follow-up is needed.

UPDATE OF HIGH-DOSE CHEMOTHERAPY TRIALS AT M. D. ANDERSON

In this section, we will discuss ongoing clinical trials of HDCT for both metastatic and high-risk primary breast cancer being conducted at M. D. Anderson.

Table 12–3.   Recent Trials of High-Dose Chemotherapy in High-Risk Primary Breast Cancer

Study	No. of Patients Median follow-up Trial design	Outcome	Highlights
Rodenhuis The Netherlands	• 81 patients • 4.5 years • 4 cycles of SDCT with FEC, then randomly assigned to HDCT with CTCb or observation	No OS or PFS difference	• Small sample size limited to detecting only 35% difference • 15% of patients were off study plan • Patients with positive bone scan and bone marrow disease were included.
Hortobagyi M. D. Anderson USA	• 78 patients • 4 years • 8 cycles of SDCT with FAC, then randomly assigned to HDCT with 2 cycles of CVP or observation	No OS or PFS difference	• Small sample size • Large number of patients did not follow the intended treatment plan. • CVP is not a myeloablative regimen.
Bezwoda South Africa	Data were falsified.		The study is discredited because the data were falsified.
Bergh Scandinavian Breast Cancer Study Group 9401 Scandinavia	• 525 patients • 1.7 years • Individually adjusted, intensive-dose SDCT with FEC (9 cycles) or SDCT with FEC (3 cycles) plus HDCT with CTCb	No OS or PFS difference	• SDCT arm can be considered intensive arm. • Short follow-up • Higher incidence of secondary leukemia in SDCT arm

| Peters CALGB 9082 USA | • 874 patients
• 3.5 years
• SDCT (FAC × 4), then randomly assigned to HDCT with CBP plus AHST or intermediate-dose CBP plus G-CSF | No difference in OS or PFS at 5 years; however, there was a 34% decrease in relapse rate in the HDCT arm. | • Less recurrence with HDCT compared with intermediate dose
• Inadequate duration of follow-up
• High transplant-related mortality rate (8%) in the HDCT arm |
| Rodenhuis The Netherlands | • 885 patients (first 289 patients analyzed)
• 3 years
• Randomly assigned to 4 cycles of SDCT with FEC alone or 4 cycles of SDCT with FEC plus HDCT with CTCb | Statistically significant difference in OS and PFS at 3 years
• OS rate at 3 years: 79% (SDCT) vs 89% (SDCT plus HDCT) (P = NA)
• PFS rate at 3 years: 62% (SDCT) vs 77% (SDCT plus HDCT) (P = NA) | • Less recurrence and improved survival in HDCT arm compared with SDCT arm
• Inadequate duration of follow-up
• Further analysis required with total patients |

CBP, cyclophosphamide, carmustine, and thiotepa; CTCb, cyclophosphamide, thiotepa, and carboplatin; CVP, cyclophosphamide, etoposide, and cisplatin; FAC, 5-fluorouracil, doxorubicin, and cyclophosphamide; FEC, 5-fluorouracil, epirubicin, and cyclophosphamide; HDCT, high-dose chemotherapy; NA, not available; OS, overall survival; PFS, progression-free survival; SDCT, standard-dose chemotherapy.

Metastatic Breast Cancer

At M. D. Anderson, 232 patients have undergone HDCT as treatment for metastatic breast cancer. With a median duration of follow-up of 2.3 years, the 5-year OS rate of these patients is 30%, and the PFS rate is 22%. Preliminary analysis has shown that achieving a CR after HDCT is an important prognostic factor for long-term OS and PFS durations. Therefore, at M. D. Anderson, our objective with HDCT for metastatic breast cancer is to induce a CR and to maintain this CR by immunomodulation or post-transplant biological therapy to eradicate minimal residual disease.

Allogeneic Transplantation

Patients with metastatic breast cancer may have multiple immune defects, so host immunosurveillance may not be effective in controlling the disease. Preclinical data suggest that immune defense cells (e.g., cytotoxic T lymphocytes and natural killer cells) can lyse breast cancer cells in vitro. Allogeneic transplantation has been shown to be effective in leukemia and lymphoma by inducing a graft-versus-tumor effect. Since 1995, we have explored the immunological effects of allogeneic hematopoietic transplantation in metastatic breast cancer. It is well established that in hematological malignancies, the success of allogeneic transplantation is dependent not only on the effect of the HDCT but also on the immunological antitumor effect of immunocompetent donor cells on residual malignant disease.

We have demonstrated that allogeneic transplantation is feasible in breast cancer and that a graft-versus-tumor effect can be achieved. Initially, this trial focused on patients with advanced disease and extensive bone marrow and liver involvement. Twenty-one patients, median age 42 years (range, 25–59 years), have been treated. Except for one patient who also had a myelodysplastic syndrome, metastatic breast cancer was the only malignancy for all patients. Thirteen patients had bone marrow involvement, and 9 had liver involvement. The median number of metastatic sites was 2 (range, 1–5 sites). One patient had a CR to SDCT, 4 had a PR, 14 had stable disease, and 4 had progressive disease. The patients then underwent allogeneic transplantation. In all cases, the stem cell donor was an HLA-identical sibling. The preparative regimen was high-dose CBT. For graft-versus-host-disease (GVHD) prophylaxis, 2 patients received cyclosporine and steroids, and 19 received tacrolimus and methotrexate. The median duration of follow-up was 445 days (range, 53–1396 days), and the median PFS duration was 227 days (range, 37–1127 days). Nine patients experienced acute GVHD, and 10 experienced chronic GVHD. Four patients had residual disease after HDCT, but the tumor regressed after immunosuppressive therapy was ceased. These data suggest that allogeneic transplantation may be a useful immunotherapy for treatment of metastatic breast cancer.

We currently use melphalan and fludarabine, a less toxic, nonmyeloablative preparative regimen, to reduce the risk of treatment-related mortality. We are investigating this approach in patients who have less-extensive metastatic disease and are responding well to induction SDCT. In these patients, we can incorporate allogeneic transplantation into the multimodality treatment approach (see Table 12–4, protocol DM 97–268).

For patients who do not have an HLA-identical donor, we are exploring the autologous transplantation of interleukin (IL)-2–activated PBSCs (see Table 12–4, protocol DM 97–323). In this strategy, the PBSCs are collected and stimulated with G-CSF and IL-2 to mobilize natural killer cells, T cells, and dendritic cells. These cells are further stimulated with IL-2 ex vivo and again by systemically administered IL-2 and GM-CSF after transplantation to eradicate breast cancer cells in the PBSC graft and to enhance the antitumor effect of the graft. Sixteen patients have undergone this treatment so far with no major side effects.

Treatment of HER-2/neu–Overexpressing Tumors

HER-2/neu overexpression may be predictive of response to SDCT or poor prognosis. In a large randomized study conducted by the Cancer and Leukemia Group B, patients with breast cancer overexpressing HER-2/neu benefited from escalated doses of doxorubicin-based chemotherapy, whereas patients whose tumors did not overexpress HER-2/neu did not. Our preliminary analysis also shows that HER-2/neu overexpression is predictive of shorter duration of PFS and OS for patients with metastatic breast cancer who undergo HDCT. Clinical trials have been proposed that will determine whether HDCT combined with anti-HER-2/neu antibody (trastuzumab) may be effective in this patient group.

Weekly administration of trastuzumab and paclitaxel has resulted in high response rates and minimal toxicity in patients with metastatic breast cancer. Therefore, we recently opened a study of patients with HER-2/neu–overexpressing metastatic breast cancer whose tumors show sensitivity to SDCT (see Table 12–4, protocol ID 99–004). Our goal is to reduce the volume of breast cancer by HDCT and then eradicate minimal residual disease by weekly administration of trastuzumab and paclitaxel.

Treatment of Bone-Only Metastasis

In some patients, breast cancer metastasizes to the bone only. We have used the radioisotope holmium as a preparative therapy for this subset of patients (see Table 12–4, protocol DM 96–103). Holmium-DOTMP is a phosphonate chelate that can localize to active areas of bone turnover. Therefore, high-dose beta radiation can be delivered directly to bone metastases and to the adjacent bone marrow without major visceral toxicity. The treatment is intended for patients in whom conventional chemother-

Table 12–4. Trials of High-Dose Chemotherapy for Metastatic Breast Cancer at M. D. Anderson

Protocol Number and Eligibility Criteria	Treatment Plan	Highlights
DM 97–268 • Tumor responding to SDCT • Related HLA-matched donor (6 out of 6 or 5 out of 6 match) • Unrelated HLA-matched donor (6 of 6) for patients who have recurrent disease after autologous transplantation	• Allogeneic transplantation • Immunomodulation by withdrawing immunosuppressants or donor lymphocyte infusion if residual disease detected at 100 days after allogeneic transplantation	• Allogeneic stem cells or lymphocytes may enhance graft-vs-tumor effect, which may eradicate breast cancer. • Melphalan and fludarabine will be used to reduce toxicity.
DM 97–323 • Tumor responding to SDCT • No HLA-matched sibling and low HER-2/neu overexpression	• Stimulation of stem cells with G-CSF and IL-2 • HDCT with CBT • Posttransplantation stimulation with IL-2 and GM-CSF	• To enhance autologous graft-vs-tumor effect by IL-2 • Treatment of stem cells with IL-2 will eradicate contaminated breast cancer cells in the stem cell product
ID 99–004 • Tumor responding to SDCT • HER-2/neu–overexpressing tumor	• HDCT with CBT • Weekly trastuzumab and paclitaxel after HDCT	HDCT will reduce tumor volume to minimal residual disease status, which may allow maximum response to trastuzumab and paclitaxel.
DM 96–103 • Bone-only disease • Failure of first-line treatment	High-dose holmium with AHST	Bone-seeking radioisotope is expected to deliver high-dose radiation to bone without major toxicity.

AHST, autologous hematopoietic stem cell transplantation; CBT, cyclophosphamide, carmustine, and thiotepa; G-CSF, granulocyte colony-stimulating factor; GM-CSF, granulocyte-macrophage colony-stimulating factor; HDCT, high-dose chemotherapy; HLA, human leukocyte antigen; IL, interleukin; SDCT, standard-dose chemotherapy.

apy and hormonal therapy (in cases of estrogen receptor–positive tumor) fail to produce adequate response.

High-Risk Primary Breast Cancer

At M. D. Anderson, our goal in the treatment of high-risk primary breast cancer is to deliver the safest yet most effective preparative regimen. We have a strong interest in the role of HDCT as part of a multimodality approach for treating locally advanced breast cancer. Locally advanced breast cancer is commonly treated with neoadjuvant chemotherapy with the goals of reducing the tumor burden, which allows for less invasive surgery, and determining chemotherapy responsiveness. In our investigations, we have focused on patients whose tumors respond poorly to neoadjuvant chemotherapy. These patients can be categorized as those whose tumors can be removed surgically when neoadjuvant chemotherapy fails to produce a response and patients whose tumors cannot be removed surgically. Patients who are operable undergo surgical resection and then HDCT with a combination of CVP and CBP followed by irradiation as consolidation therapy. Patients who are not eligible for surgery undergo up-front HDCT, with the goal of rendering the tumor resectable, and then radiation therapy for consolidation.

We initially hypothesized that patients without overt metastases could possibly be rescued by HDCT using non-cross-resistant alkylating agents. So far, we have treated 16 patients (median age 46 years; range, 36–58 years) in a study of HDCT for patients with chemoresistant primary breast cancer (see Table 12–5, DM 95–046). Of these patients, 5 had stage II primary breast cancer, 5 had stage IIIA primary breast cancer, and 6 had stage IIIB primary breast cancer. All patients had poor response (minor response, stable disease, or progressive disease) to neoadjuvant chemotherapy (FAC or FAC plus a taxane). After a median follow-up of 381 days (range, 165–682 days) from the day of transplantation, 14 patients remained disease-free. The PFS rate at 1 year was 80%. The median PFS duration was 381 days (range, 165–682 days) from the day of transplantation and 655 days (range, 296–905 days) from the day of initiation of neoadjuvant chemotherapy. One patient died of multi-organ failure at 344 days without disease. Compared with our historical experience with patients with locally advanced breast cancer refractory to neoadjuvant chemotherapy, the PFS and OS rates of patients who underwent HDCT were substantially improved.

Patients who have involvement of 10 or more lymph nodes after initial primary surgery for primary breast cancer or those with involvement of 4 or more lymph nodes after neoadjuvant chemotherapy and primary surgery continue to have a 50% to 70% risk of recurrent disease even after treatment with a combination of surgery, chemotherapy, and radiation therapy. The use of a doxorubicin-containing regimen such as FAC, FAC plus paclitaxel, or doxorubicin plus cyclophosphamide as neoadjuvant chemotherapy continues to improve patients' long-term survival dura-

Table 12–5. Trials of High-Dose Chemotherapy for High-Risk Primary Breast Cancer at M. D. Anderson

Protocol Number and Eligibility Criteria	Treatment Plan	Highlights
DM 95–046 Neoadjuvant chemotherapy–refractory primary breast cancer	• Resectable breast cancer: Surgical resection, then chemomobilization (CVP/G-CSF) and HDCT with CBT plus AHST • Unresectable breast cancer: Chemomobilization (CVP/G-CSF) then HDCT with CBT plus AHST; patients who are eligible will proceed with surgical resection • All patients will proceed with radiation therapy	Preliminary data suggest that HDCT has been significantly active among patients who are considered chemoresistant.
DM 95–047 ≥ 10 positive axillary nodes after primary surgery or ≥ 4 positive axillary nodes after neoadjuvant chemotherapy and primary surgery	HDCT with CBT plus AHST after completion of adjuvant chemotherapy for 4–8 cycles	• Patients are randomly assigned to receive either moderate HDCT with CVP plus G-CSF or G-CSF alone to collect PBSC. • Double intensity may reduce the recurrence rate more than single intensity.
DM 97–135 > 4 positive axillary nodes after primary surgery	Patients randomly assigned to intensive-dose, sequential SDCT plus G-CSF or SDCT with AC (4 cycles) and HDCT with CTCb for consolidation	Two different types of dose intensification are compared among patients at moderately high risk for recurrence.
ID 00–226 Newly diagnosed, inoperable breast cancer	Randomization between up-front HDCT (CVP-CBT) vs (AT × 4 cycles)	Comparison to determine regimen that will achieve a high pathological CR rate and increase operability of the tumor.

AC, doxorubicin and cyclophosphamide; AHST, autologous hematopoietic stem cell transplantation; AT, adriamycin and taxotere; CBT, cyclophosphamide, carmustine, and thiotepa; CR, complete response; CTCb, cyclophosphamide, thiotepa, and carboplatin; CVP, cyclophosphamide, etoposide, and cisplatin; G-CSF, granulocyte colony-stimulating factor; HDCT, high-dose chemotherapy; SDCT, standard-dose chemotherapy.

tion. However, disease relapse is still a major problem. We are currently comparing the effect of double-regimen HDCT with that of single-regimen HDCT to see which produces the longest duration of PFS. In the double-regimen approach, patients receive CVP with G-CSF to mobilize the PBSC. After PBSC collection, patients receive high-dose CBT and AHST. In the single-regimen approach, the PBSCs are mobilized with G-CSF alone, and then patients receive high-dose CBT and AHST (see Table 12–5, protocol 95–047).

Patients with high-risk primary breast cancer with involvement of more than 4 lymph nodes after combined-modality therapy are also at high risk (30%–50%) for recurrence. We are participating in the Southwest Oncology Group 9623 study in which patients with this status are randomly assigned to intensive-dose, sequential SDCT (doxorubicin $\rightarrow$ paclitaxel $\rightarrow$ cyclophosphamide) plus G-CSF or 4 cycles of SDCT with doxorubicin plus cyclophosphamide consolidated with high-dose CTCb (see Table 12–5, protocol DM 97–135).

Pathological CR achieved with standard-dose neoadjuvant chemotherapy has been shown to be predictive of long-term survival in patients with locally advanced breast cancer. Therefore, we initiated a randomized clinical trial to compare the rates of pathological CR achieved with high-dose CVP and CBT plus AHST with that achieved with standard-dose doxorubicin and docetaxel in patients with inoperable primary breast cancer (see Table 12–5, protocol ID 00–226). The study will also show which group of patients will become eligible for surgery after treatment. Secondary goals of this study are to compare the symptoms and the quality of life of women receiving an HDCT regimen versus a SDCT regimen. We expect that a high pathological CR rate achieved by HDCT may translate into longer disease-free survival.

CONCLUSIONS

A major question with regard to HDCT as treatment for high-risk primary and metastatic breast cancer remains whether it provides a benefit in terms of OS or PFS rates and durations. Another key question is whether prognostic factors such as response to SDCT (reduction in tumor burden) prior to transplantation can identify patient groups that can benefit from HDCT. In recent clinical trials, high CR rates have been reported with HDCT in metastatic breast cancer. As well, improvements in transplantation technology have resulted in lower morbidity and mortality and reduced costs associated with HDCT plus AHST. Continuation of randomized clinical trials is warranted to determine the role of HDCT in the treatment of high-risk primary and metastatic breast cancer. Results of maturing and ongoing clinical trials at established research centers will help to resolve the major issues in the field.

KEY PRACTICE POINTS

- High-dose chemotherapy reduces tumor volume and produces a high CR rate. Immunotherapy, chemotherapy, and the use of novel biological agents are now incorporated after AHST in new trials to maintain this CR.

- The morbidity, mortality, and costs associated with HDCT have been substantially reduced by improved transplantation technology.

- High-dose chemotherapy should be administered through well-designed clinical trials.

- Current data from randomized trials in both high-risk primary breast cancer and metastatic breast cancer continue to support the need for research in this field.

SUGGESTED READINGS

Antman K, Rowlings PA, Vaughan WP, Pelz CJ, Fay JW, Fields KK. High-dose chemotherapy with autologous hematopoietic stem-cell support for breast cancer in North America. *J Clin Oncol* 1997;15:1870–1879.

Bergh J. Results from a randomized adjuvant breast cancer study with high dose chemotherapy with CTCb supported by autologous bone marrow stem cells versus dose escalated and tailored FEC therapy. *Proceedings of the American Society of Clinical Oncology* 1999;18:Abstract 3.

Bezwoda WR. Randomized, controlled trial of high dose chemotherapy (HD-CNVp) versus standard dose (CAF) chemotherapy for high risk, surgically-treated, primary breast cancer. *Proceedings of the American Society of Clinical Oncology* 1999;18:Abstract 4.

Bezwoda WR, Seymour L, Dansey RD. High-dose chemotherapy with hematopoietic rescue as primary treatment for metastatic breast cancer: a randomized trial. *J Clin Oncol* 1995;13:2483–2489.

Eibl B, Schwaighofer H, Nachbaur D, et al. Evidence for a graft-versus-tumor effect in a patient treated with marrow ablative chemotherapy and allogeneic bone marrow transplantation for breast cancer. *Blood* 1996;88:1501–1508.

Greenberg PA, Hortobagyi GN, Smith TL, et al. Long-term follow-up of patients with complete remission following combination chemotherapy for metastatic breast cancer. *J Clin Oncol* 1996;14:2197–2205.

Hortobagyi GN. Evolving concepts in high-dose chemotherapy for breast cancer. ASCO Educational Book for Fall 1999.

Hortobagyi GN, Buzdar AU, Theriault RL, et al. Randomized trial of high-dose chemotherapy and blood cell autografts for high-risk primary breast carcinoma. *J Natl Cancer Inst* 2000;92:225–233.

Lotz JP, Curé H, Janvier M, et al. High-dose chemotherapy (HD-CT) with hematopoietic stem cell transplantation (HSCT) for metastatic breast cancer: results of the French Protocol Pegase 04. *Proceedings of the American Society of Clinical Oncology* 1999;18:Abstract 161.

Peters WP. High-dose chemotherapy and stem-cell support for primary and metastatic breast cancer. ASCO Educational Book for Fall 1999.

Peters WP, Jones RB, Vredenburgh J, et al. A large, prospective, randomized trial of high-dose combination alkylating agents (CPB) with autologous cellular support (ABMS) as consolidation for patients with metastatic breast cancer achieving complete remission after intensive doxorubicin-based induction therapy (AFM). *Proceedings of the American Society of Clinical Oncology* 1996; Abstract 149.

Peters WP, Rosner G, Vredenburgh J, et al. A prospective, randomized comparison of two doses of combination alkylating agents (AA) as consolidation after CAF in high-risk primary breast cancer involving ten or more axillary lymph nodes (LN): preliminary results of CALGB 9082/SWOG 9114/NCIC MA-13. *Proceedings of the American Society of Clinical Oncology* 1999;18:Abstract 2.

Rahman ZU, Frye DK, Buzdar AU, et al. Impact of selection process on response rate and long-term survival of potential high-dose chemotherapy candidates treated with standard-dose doxorubicin-containing chemotherapy in patients with metastatic breast cancer. *J Clin Oncol* 1997;15:3171–3177.

Rizzieri DA, Vredenburgh JJ, Jones R, et al. Prognostic and predictive factors for patients with metastatic breast cancer undergoing aggressive induction therapy followed by high-dose chemotherapy with autologous stem-cell support. *J Clin Oncol* 1999;17:3064–3074.

Rodenhuis S, Botenbal M, Beex LVAM, et al. Randomized phase III study of high-dose chemotherapy with cyclophosphamide, thiotepa and carboplatin in operable breast cancer with 4 or more axillary lymph nodes. *Proceedings of the American Society of Clinical Oncology* 2000;19:Abstract 286.

Rodenhuis S, Richel DJ, van der Wall E, et al. Randomized trial of high-dose chemotherapy and hemopoietic progenitor-cell support in operable breast cancer with extensive axillary lymph-node involvement. *Lancet* 1998;352:515–521.

Stadtmauer EA, O'Neill A, Goldstein LJ, et al. Conventional-dose chemotherapy compared with high-dose chemotherapy plus autologous hematopoietic stem-cell transplantation for metastatic breast cancer. *N Engl J Med* 2000;342:1069–1076.

Ueno NT, Rondon G, Mirza NQ, et al. Allogeneic peripheral blood progenitor cell transplantation for poor-risk patients with metastatic breast cancer. *J Clin Oncol* 1998;16:986–993.

Weiss RB, Rifkin RM, Stewart FM, et al. High-dose chemotherapy for high-risk primary breast cancer: an on-site review of the Bezwoda study. *Lancet* 2000; 355:999–1003.

13   ENDOCRINE THERAPY FOR BREAST CANCER

Aman U. Buzdar

CHAPTER OVERVIEW

Endocrine therapy can result in palliation of disease in 50% to 60% of patients with hormone receptor–positive breast cancer. The choice of agents for endocrine therapy depends on the menopausal status of the patient. In premenopausal women, luteinizing hormone-releasing hormone agonists or tamoxifen can be used as initial therapy. In postmenopausal women, aromatase inhibitors or tamoxifen can be used as initial therapy. The use of anastrozole, an aromatase inhibitor, as initial therapy in postmenopausal women with estrogen receptor–positive tumors results in increased response rates, longer control of disease, and fewer side effects. Patients who respond to initial therapy have a higher probability of response to secondary and tertiary endocrine therapies. There is a partial lack of cross-resistance between steroidal and nonsteroidal aromatase inhibitors; thus, these agents may provide palliation of disease if used sequentially in patients with hormone receptor–positive tumors. Endocrine therapy alone or with chemotherapy can significantly reduce the risk of recurrence and has a favorable impact on survival. A number of new endocrine agents are in clinical development, and preliminary data from these studies are encouraging. The role of these agents in the treatment of breast cancer will be evaluated in ongoing trials.

INTRODUCTION

Manipulation of the endocrine system as a treatment for metastatic breast cancer was first introduced in 1896, when Beatson demonstrated objective regression of the disease following oophorectomy. A number of endocrine therapies are now used as palliative treatment for patients with hormone-sensitive metastatic disease and as adjuvant treatment of early breast cancer. Endocrine therapies are directed at either reducing the synthesis of estrogen or blocking estrogen receptors in hormone-dependent tumors.

HORMONE RECEPTOR STATUS AS AN INDICATOR OF RESPONSE TO ENDOCRINE THERAPY

The presence of estrogen receptors (ERs) or progesterone receptors (PRs) on tumors is predictive of a higher likelihood of response to endocrine therapy. As shown in Table 13–1, more than 50% of patients whose tumors

Table 13–1. Hormone Receptor Status and Probability of Response to Endocrine Therapy

Estrogen Receptor	Progesterone Receptor	Probability of Clinical Benefit
Positive	Positive	High, 50% to 70%
Positive	Negative	Intermediate, 33%
Negative	Positive	Intermediate, 33%
Negative	Negative	Low, less than 10%

are both ER and PR positive experience clinical benefit from endocrine therapy, compared with fewer than 10% of patients with tumors that are both ER and PR negative. Patients with hormone receptor–positive tumors also live 2 to 3 times longer after development of metastases than do patients with ER-negative tumors. These receptors can now be measured on archival tissue. The assays have become much simpler, and immunohistochemical analysis can be performed to determine whether patients have ER- or PR-positive tumors and thus whether they are appropriate candidates for endocrine therapy. For patients whose tumor tissue cannot be easily accessed for evaluation of receptor status, the clinical criteria used to determine eligibility for endocrine therapy are longer disease-free interval, no vital-organ involvement, no major dysfunction of the organs involved by the disease, minimal or moderate visceral involvement, and metastasis limited to the soft tissue or bone (Table 13–2).

Types of Endocrine Therapy

The primary source of estrogen in premenopausal women is the ovaries. After menopause, estrogen is produced in peripheral tissues such as fat, muscle, liver, and the breast tumor tissues through the aromatization of androgens produced by the adrenals. The amount of estrogen produced by this pathway is considerably less than that produced by the ovaries prior to menopause, but it is still sufficient to support the growth of estrogen-dependent tumors in postmenopausal women. Approximately 100 ng of estrone is produced daily by aromatization of androstenedione, which results in a plasma estradiol level of 10 to 20 pg/mL. Several types of endocrine therapy are available for use in managing metastatic breast cancer, including ovarian ablation, hormonal agonists, synthetic agents, and nonselective aromatase inhibitors (Table 13–3). The treatment schema utilized at M. D. Anderson Cancer Center in applying endocrine therapies is illustrated in Figure 13–1.

Ovarian Ablation

Ovarian function can be ablated by surgery, irradiation, or pharmacologic intervention. All treatment modalities result in a similar response rate;

Table 13–2. Clinical Criteria Used to Determine Eligibility for Endocrine Therapy

Positive ER or PR status
Disease-free interval of more than 2 years
Disease limited to soft tissue or bone or low-volume visceral disease
Previous response to endocrine therapy
Candidate for additional endocrine therapies

however, surgical ablation is the fastest means of deterring estrogen production. Ovarian ablation can be performed laparoscopically. One of the disadvantages of surgical ablation is that it is irreversible. Radiation-induced ablation is a rather slow process. Because it is difficult to isolate the ovaries from the nearby small and large intestine, the radiation therapy may cause gastrointestinal disturbances. Radiation therapy may also affect the bone marrow to a limited extent.

Luteinizing Hormone-Releasing Hormone Agonists

Luteinizing hormone-releasing hormone (LHRH) agonists, also known as gonadotropin-releasing hormone agonists, suppress ovarian function to a degree similar to surgical ablation. Luteinizing hormone-releasing hormone agonists reduce the release of estrogen by providing a constant high level of pituitary-releasing hormone receptors and shutting down gonadotropin production. Several different forms of LHRH agonists are available for clinical use, but only goserelin acetate is approved for treatment of metastatic breast cancer, and it is only approved for use in premenopausal women. There are limited data to support that LHRH agonists have activity in postmenopausal women. Luteinizing hormone-releasing hormone agonists may have a direct antitumor effect because some tumors have LHRH receptors.

Table 13–3. Types of Endocrine Therapy for Breast Cancer

Type of Therapy	Example(s)
Ovarian ablation	Surgery, irradiation, pharmacologic intervention
LHRH agonists	Goserelin acetate
Progestins	Megestrol acetate Medroxyprogesterone acetate
Androgens	
Nonselective aromatase inhibitors	Testolactone Aminoglutethimide
Selective aromatase inhibitors	Formestane Anastrozole Letrozole Exemestane Fadrozole
Selective estrogen receptor modulators	Tamoxifen Toremifene Raloxifene Arzoxifene hydrochloride
Estrogen receptor downregulators	Faslodex

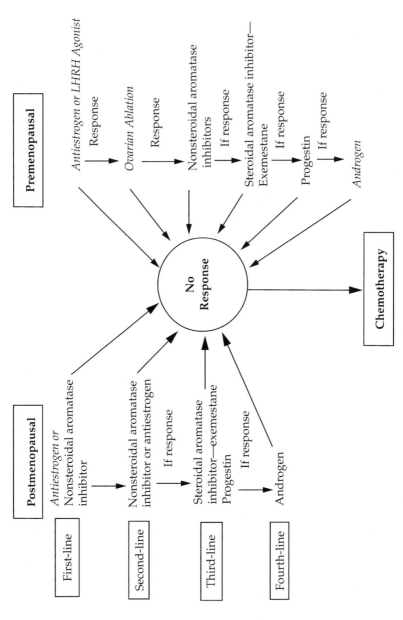

Figure 13–1. Schema of endocrine therapies used as treatment for patients with metastatic breast cancer.

Administration of LHRH agonists may cause an initial rise in gonadotropin levels, which may be associated with tumor flare. Chronic administration of LHRH agonists is associated with serum estrogen and progesterone levels comparable with levels in women who have undergone oophorectomy. Luteinizing hormone-releasing hormone agonists are now available in a slow-release form that can be injected at 1- to 3-month intervals. The objective response rates with LHRH agonists are similar to those with ablative surgery.

Progestins

Progestins are synthetic derivatives of progesterone that have a progesterone-agonist effect. Progestins such as megestrol acetate and medroxyprogesterone acetate are effective in treating metastatic disease; however, their exact mechanism of action is unknown. They have antiestrogenic properties and may result in interruption of the pituitary-ovarian axis. It has also been suggested that increased levels of progestin may mimic pregnancy. In vitro, progestins have direct cytotoxic effects. Progestins have been extensively evaluated and utilized as a second-line therapy but are associated with a number of side effects, including dyspnea, vaginal bleeding, nausea, fluid retention, hot flashes, skin rash, and thromboembolic complications. Megestrol acetate is the only progestin indicated and approved by the U.S. Food and Drug Administration (FDA) for treatment of advanced breast cancer. Progestins were once used as second-line therapy for palliative treatment for metastatic disease. With the introduction of aromatase inhibitors, however, progestins have moved down in the sequential order of therapy for this disease (Figure 13–1).

Androgens

Androgens have been evaluated and are still utilized as a fourth-line therapy in patients with metastatic breast cancer.

Aromatase Inhibitors

In postmenopausal women, estrogen is produced by an aromatization reaction, and only low levels of the hormone are produced. A wide range of aromatase inhibitors have been evaluated as treatments for metastatic breast cancer. The objective in developing aromatase inhibitors was to produce drugs that had a specific activity and a good safety profile. These compounds can be broadly categorized as nonselective and selective aromatase inhibitors. Nonselective inhibition of steroid hormone production results in significant side effects, and in a number of situations—for example, when the patient is under acute stress—replacement therapy is required. On the other hand, selective inhibition of aromatase enzymes alters only the estrogen level and does not affect steroid hormone levels (Figure 13–2).

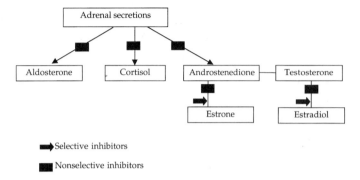

Figure 13–2. Site of action of selective and nonselective aromatase inhibitors.

There are 2 general types of aromatase inhibitors. Suicidal inhibitors (type 1) are steroidal compounds, and competitive inhibitors (type 2) are generally nonsteroidal agents. Both types mimic normal substrates (androgen), competing with the substrate in binding to the normal site on the enzyme.

After initial binding, the next step differs for suicidal and competitive inhibitors. Once the suicidal inhibitor is bound to the active site, the enzyme initiates its typical sequence of hydroxylations, but hydroxylation produces an unbreakable covalent bond between the inhibitor and the enzyme. Enzyme activity is thus permanently blocked even if all the unattached inhibitor is removed. Enzyme activity can only be restored by new enzyme synthesis. Competitive inhibitors reversibly bind to the active enzyme site, and either no enzyme activity is triggered or it causes no effect. The inhibitor remains and can dissociate from the binding site, allowing renewed competition between inhibitor and substrate for binding to the active enzyme site. As a result, the effectiveness of competitive inhibitors depends on the relative concentration and affinity of the inhibitor and the substrate. Continued activity requires the constant presence of the inhibitor.

To compete for binding to the active site, both suicidal and competitive inhibitors must necessarily share important structural features with the natural substrate. Suicidal inhibitors and androgens share a structural feature that allows them to interact with catalytic residues of the enzyme. This renders the suicidal inhibitor inherently selective. Competitive inhibitors interact with heme iron, a common feature of all cytochrome p450 enzymes. Some may also bind to highly conserved oxygen-binding sites in addition to the substrate-binding site. Thus, unless the specificity of a competitive inhibitor is reinforced through other structural features, this inhibitor may block the activity of a wide variety of p450 enzymes, such as aminoglutethimide.

Aromatase inhibitors are used only in women with no ovarian function. In women with intact ovarian function, aromatase inhibition may increase estrogen production by increasing gonadotropin-releasing hormone levels; the follicle-stimulating hormone level; aromatase production; the luteinizing hormone level; and ovarian steroid synthesis, particularly synthesis of androstenedione, the substrate for aromatase.

Nonselective Aromatase Inhibitors

Testolactone was the first aromatase inhibitor investigated as a treatment for advanced breast cancer. This drug was initially considered an androgen, although it lacked virilizing properties. Its potential was not fully recognized until the introduction of aminoglutethimide.

Aminoglutethimide blocks cholesterol side-chain cleavage, inhibiting steroid synthesis and leading to significant reduction in glucocorticoids and thus requiring steroid supplementation. The initial half-life of aminoglutethimide is 12.3 ± 2.6 hours; however, this drug induces the enzyme that catalyzes its own elimination, so with prolonged use, the half-life decreases to 7.3 ± 2.14 hours. Aminoglutethimide has been prospectively compared with hypophysectomy and adrenalectomy in metastatic disease, and its antitumor activity was similar to that of ablative surgical procedures. Aminoglutethimide has also been compared with tamoxifen as a first-line therapy. In 3 of the 4 studies, there was no notable difference in response rates or median survival rates between the 2 agents. In the other study, there was some suggestion that patients treated with aminoglutethimide had higher response rates than patients treated with tamoxifen, but there were no differences in survival rates. In other studies, no overall difference in response rate was noted. Aminoglutethimide was also compared with progestin, and these results suggested that the antitumor activity of aminoglutethimide is similar to that of progestins. Aminoglutethimide-associated adverse effects include lethargy, central nervous system toxicities, and skin rash. These adverse effects are observed in 20% to 40% of patients.

Selective Aromatase Inhibitors

The selective aromatase inhibitors include formestane, anastrozole, letrozole, exemestane, and fadrozole.

Formestane (4-hydroxyandrostenedione). Formestane was the first selective suicidal aromatase inhibitor to be discovered. Its half-life when administered orally is 2 to 3 hours. In clinical studies, formestane has been shown to have no effect on serum levels of androstenedione, testosterone, dihydrotestosterone, aldosterone, cortisol, or 17-hydroxyprogesterone. Formestane has weak androgenic properties as reflected by a 15% fall in the serum level of the sex-hormone-binding globulin following oral administration. The fact that this effect is not induced following intramuscular injection probably reflects that hepatic exposure to formestane is reduced by this route. The safety profile of formestane is superior to that of aminoglutethimide. The major drawback of formestane is that it needs to be administered by injection. A small number of patients experience local reaction at the injection site. Although formestane is not available in the United States, it has been shown to have significant antitumor activity and has been extensively evaluated and utilized in European countries.

Anastrozole.   Anastrozole is a selective, competitive inhibitor of aromatase that has no activity against desmolase or other enzymes involved in steroid biosynthesis. Oral absorption of this drug is rapid, and peak concentration is reached within 2 hours. The average plasma half-life is approximately 50 hours in postmenopausal women. Studies have shown that administration of up to 10 mg for 14 days does not alter basal cortisol or aldosterone levels or response to adrenocorticotropic hormone stimulation. Two large randomized trials compared the efficacy of anastrozole at doses of 1 and 10 mg/day, respectively, with megestrol acetate at 40 mg 4 times a day. Initial results at a median follow-up of 6 months showed no differences in time to disease progression or survival duration, but anastrozole was associated with fewer side effects than megestrol acetate. However, with additional follow-up (31 months), there was significant improvement in survival duration for patients treated with 1 mg of anastrozole compared with progestin.

Anastrozole was recently evaluated as first-line therapy for metastatic disease in postmenopausal women in 2 double-blind, placebo-controlled trials. The control in both studies was tamoxifen. In both studies, the antitumor activity of anastrozole was similar to that of tamoxifen, and in patients with ER-positive tumors, anastrozole was superior to tamoxifen. A higher fraction of patients with ER-positive tumors had clinical benefit (complete response, partial response, or stable disease for more than 24 weeks) with anastrozole. Anastrozole also produced a longer time to treatment failure in this subset of patients. The safety profile of anastrozole was more favorable than that of tamoxifen. Anastrozole produced fewer episodes of thromboembolism and vaginal bleeding. The FDA recently approved anastrozole as initial therapy for postmenopausal women with hormonally responsive disease.

Letrozole.   Letrozole is a selective competitive inhibitor of the aromatase enzyme system. Letrozole does not cause any clinically relevant changes in plasma levels of cortisol, aldosterone, 17-hydroxyprogesterone, androstenedione, testosterone, or gonadotropins in healthy, postmenopausal women treated with doses ranging from 0.1 to 5 mg/day. Letrozole markedly suppresses the plasma level of estradiol, estrone, and estrone sulfate within 2 weeks of initiation of treatment at a dose of 1 mg/day. In a European study, the safety and efficacy of letrozole and aminoglutethimide were compared in postmenopausal women. Time to progression, time to treatment failure, and overall survival duration were superior in the letrozole-treated patients compared with the aminoglutethimide group. In another European study, letrozole was compared with progestin. In this study, patients treated with letrozole had significantly higher objective response rates compared with patients treated with progestin (following progression on tamoxifen). Indirect comparison of these data with data documenting the use of anastrozole in a similar patient population suggests that letrozole and anastrozole produce similar overall clinical benefits; if anything, the trend favors anastrozole. Prospective, randomized studies are needed to compare the safety and antitumor activity of these newer aromatase inhibitors. Anastrozole and letrozole have become the agents of choice for treatment of metastatic breast cancer in postmenopausal women following tamoxifen therapy.

Letrozole was recently evaluated as first-line therapy for metastatic disease in postmenopausal women in a large, double-blind controlled trial. Patients in the control group received tamoxifen. The fraction of patients with clinical benefit was higher in the letrozole group. Letrozole was also associated with longer time to treatment failure. The FDA recently approved letrozole as initial therapy for postmenopausal women with hormonally responsive disease.

Exemestane.   Exemestane is a selective suicidal aromatase inhibitor. It is a derivative of steroidal androgen. Because of the androgen-like structure of steroidal compounds, the potential exists for androgenic side effects following treatment. In early clinical trials, some patients treated with high doses of exemestane (up to 200 mg/day) had androgenic symptoms that included alopecia, hoarseness, and a decrease in the level of plasma sex-hormone-binding globulin (a sensitive endocrine androgenic side effect). Exemestane also effectively suppresses the estradiol level similarly to anastrozole and letrozole. In 2 prospective trials, exemestane was evaluated as a third-line therapy in women treated with aminoglutethimide, formestane, or both; 20% of the patients in both trials had major responses. In 2 other studies, exemestane was evaluated as a second-line therapy following the use of competitive aromatase inhibitors. A fraction of patients had objective responses, and a sizable fraction of patients had stable disease. These data imply a partial lack of cross-resistance between steroidal and nonsteroidal aromatase inhibitors.

In a large phase III study, exemestane was evaluated in postmenopausal women following tamoxifen therapy. The study design was similar to the design of studies of anastrozole or letrozole as second-line therapies. The control in this study was megestrol acetate. The study demonstrated that the activity of exemestane was similar to that of anastrozole and letrozole. The limited cross-resistance between exemestane and these 2 nonsteroidal aromatase inhibitors suggests that this drug is appropriate for use as a third-line therapy for patients who experience disease progression while on one of the nonsteroidal aromatase inhibitors.

Fadrozole. Fadrozole is a competitive aromatase inhibitor that is more selective than aminoglutethimide but less selective than letrozole. Fadrozole has little or no effect on the desmolase enzyme; however, it does partially inhibit the 11-hydroxylase and 18-hydroxylase enzymes. The half-life of fadrozole is 10.5 hours, and maximal effects are seen with 2 to 4 mg/day. In 2 double-blind, prospective studies, megestrol acetate and fadrozole were compared in postmenopausal patients with metastatic breast cancer following tamoxifen therapy. No significant differences were detected between the treatment groups with respect to time to progression, duration of response, objective response rate, survival duration, or safety. Patients treated with fadrozole had a lower incidence of weight gain and thromboembolic complications. This drug is currently available for clinical use in Japan.

Antiestrogens

Antiestrogens, also referred to as selective estrogen receptor modulators (SERMs), are generally the preferred first-line endocrine therapy for breast cancer. These drugs block the action of estrogenic compounds such as 17-β-estradiol and estrone, which bind to and activate the ER, and they have a variable effect on different organs and tissues.

Tamoxifen

The antiestrogen tamoxifen has been available for treatment of breast cancer for 30 years. It is an established and effective palliative treatment for metastatic disease and is used as adjuvant therapy for patients with primary breast cancer. Tamoxifen was compared with diethylstilbestrol in a study of women with metastatic breast cancer, and the drugs were shown to have comparable antitumor activity. Tamoxifen is readily absorbed and reaches peak plasma concentration approximately 5 hours after a single oral dose. The terminal half-life of tamoxifen is about 5 to 7 days. Tamoxifen is extensively metabolized by demethylation and to a small degree by subsequent deamination and by hydroxylation. It is metabolized to N-desmethyltamoxifen and 4-hydroxytamoxifen. The major metabolite, N-desmethyltamoxifen, is a weak antiestrogen with an affinity for ER that is similar to that of tamoxifen, whereas 4-hydroxytamoxifen is believed to provide the major antiestrogenic activity. Tamoxifen is approved by the FDA as a first-line therapy for metastatic breast cancer in both pre- and postmenopausal women as well as in men and also as an adjuvant therapy in patients with node-positive or node-negative hormone receptor–positive tumors. Recently, tamoxifen was also approved for use in reducing the risk of breast cancer in women who are at increased risk for this disease and in patients who have ductal carcinoma in situ only. In premenopausal women, response rates to tamoxifen vary from 15% to 53%, and higher response rates were observed in patients with hormone receptor–positive disease. The response and survival durations associated with tamoxifen were comparable with those associated with ovarian ablation or ovarian irradiation.

Patients with tumors that overexpress HER-2/*neu* have a poor prognosis, and limited data suggest that these patients may be less likely to gain clinical benefit from endocrine therapy. Prospective studies are needed to definitively establish the value of endocrine therapy alone or in combination with trastuzumab (Herceptin) in this subset of patients.

Toremifene

Toremifene is a triphenylethylene analogue of tamoxifen. It is rapidly absorbed when given orally, and its peak plasma half-life is reached within 3 hours of administration. Linear pharmacokinetics have been reported after single-dose administration for which the plasma half-life is 4 hours and the elimination half-life is about 5 days. The major metabolites of toremifene are N-demethyltoremifene and deaminohydroxytoremifene. Toremifene is approved by the FDA as first-line therapy for metastatic breast cancer in patients with ER-positive tumors or tumors of unknown ER status. In a controlled clinical trial, the safety and efficacy of toremifene were shown to be similar to those of tamoxifen. In experimental endometrial cancer models, the activity of toremifene has been shown to be similar to that of tamoxifen, indicating that toremifene may increase the risk of endometrial cancer similarly to tamoxifen. A couple of small studies have evaluated the antitumor effect of toremifene against tamoxifen-resistant cancers, and a very small number of patients showed clinical benefit with the use of toremifene. As more mature clinical data are derived from ongoing trials of adjuvant therapies, the superiority, if any, of toremifene over tamoxifen may be established.

ADJUVANT ENDOCRINE THERAPY

The use of endocrine therapy at M. D. Anderson in the treatment of early breast cancer is outlined in Table 13–4. Patients at low risk include women with ER-positive tumors 1 cm or smaller and negative nodes. The addition of chemotherapy to the treatment regimen is discussed with each woman

Table 13–4. Recommended Adjuvant Endocrine Therapy in Patients with Hormone Receptor–Positive Tumors

Risk of Recurrence	Treatment
Low	Tamoxifen (and possibly chemotherapy)
Intermediate	Chemotherapy followed by tamoxifen
High	Chemotherapy followed by tamoxifen

in this subset of patients; however, further therapeutic gains with the addition of chemotherapy are marginal because of the side effects associated with chemotherapy.

Ovarian Ablation

The use of ovarian ablation as an adjuvant treatment has been shown to significantly improve disease-free and overall survival rates. Recently, the results of a meta-analysis conducted by the Early Breast Cancer Trialists' Collaborative Group revealed that adjuvant ovarian ablation resulted in an 18% proportional reduction in the risk of death in women younger than 50 years of age who had early breast cancer.

Tamoxifen

In the overview data from 55 randomized trials of adjuvant tamoxifen versus no tamoxifen reported by the Early Breast Cancer Trialists' Collaborative Group, 8000 of the 37,000 women had ER-low or ER-negative tumors, and the others had ER-positive tumors or unknown ER status. The duration of tamoxifen treatment varied from 1 to 5 years. The reduction in risk of recurrence based on ER status is shown in Table 13–5. Tamoxifen given for 5 years to patients with ER-unknown or ER-positive tumors significantly reduced the risk of recurrence and had a favorable impact on survival. The reductions in the annual rate of recurrence were 18%, 25%, and 42% with 1, 2, and 5 years of tamoxifen therapy, respectively. The corresponding reductions in mortality rates were 10%, 15%, and 22%, respectively. From these data, it could be concluded that 5 years of tamoxifen treatment provides greater benefit than 1 or 2 years. Two studies have prospectively evaluated longer durations of tamoxifen use (beyond 5 years) and have shown no further improvement in disease-free or overall survival. In studies of tamoxifen plus chemotherapy versus chemotherapy alone, the overview data illustrate that risk of recurrence was reduced by

Table 13–5. Reduction in Recurrence and Mortality Rates with Adjuvant Tamoxifen Therapy by Estrogen Receptor Status

Estrogen Receptor Status	Proportional Reduction in Breast Cancer Recurrence Rates at 10 Years (%)	Proportional Reductions in Breast Cancer Mortality Rates at 10 Years (%)
All women	42	22
ER poor	6	3
ER unknown	37	21
ER positive and ER unknown	47	26
ER positive	50	28

Source: Tamoxifen for early breast cancer: an overview of the randomised trials. Early Breast Cancer Trialists' Collaborative Group. *Lancet* 1998;351:1451–1467.

28% and risk of death was decreased by 20% with tamoxifen plus chemotherapy. Preliminary results of National Surgical Adjuvant Breast and Bowel Project (NSABP) study B-20 also support the use of endocrine therapy plus chemotherapy for patients with ER-positive tumors.

In a large NSABP study (B-24), 1804 patients with ductal carcinoma in situ were randomly assigned to treatment with local therapy or local therapy plus tamoxifen for 5 years. After a median follow-up of 74 months, the incidence of invasive and noninvasive breast cancer was significantly reduced in the tamoxifen group compared with the control group ($P = .0009$). These data are summarized in Table 13–6.

Luteinizing Hormone-Releasing Hormone Agonists

Luteinizing hormone-releasing hormone agonists have been evaluated alone and in combination with tamoxifen as adjuvant therapy in randomized trials. In these trials, patients in the control arm were treated with cyclophosphamide, methotrexate, and 5-fluorouracil (CMF), and LHRH agonists were administered for 2 to 3 years. At a median follow-up time of 4 to 5 years, the results of these studies demonstrate that ovarian suppression by LHRH agonists results in benefit similar to that produced by CMF in premenopausal women with ER-positive disease.

ENDOCRINE THERAPY FOR BREAST CANCER PREVENTION

Data from earlier trials of tamoxifen as adjuvant therapy for breast cancer suggested that tamoxifen may reduce the risk of breast cancer development in the contralateral breast. Overview data from randomized trials of adjuvant tamoxifen versus no tamoxifen provided further, stronger evidence that this drug may be able to prevent the development of new breast

Table 13–6. Tamoxifen for Ductal Carcinoma in Situ: Results of the National Surgical Adjuvant Breast and Bowel Project B-24 Trial

| | No. of Invasive and Noninvasive Breast Cancer Cases | | | |
| | Tamoxifen | Placebo | | |
Patient Group	($n = 899$)	($n = 899$)	Rate Ratio	P Value
All breast cancer	84	130	0.63	0.0009
Ipsilateral breast cancer	63	87	0.70	0.04
Contralateral breast cancer	18	36	0.48	0.01

Source: Fisher B, Dignam J, Wolmark N, et al. Tamoxifen in treatment of intraductal breast cancer: National Surgical Adjuvant Breast and Bowel Project B-24 randomised controlled trial. *Lancet* 1999;353:1993–2000.

cancer in the contralateral breast. On the basis of these findings, the role of tamoxifen in breast cancer prevention was evaluated.

Tamoxifen

The NSABP P-1 trial was the first trial to specifically examine whether a therapeutic agent could also lower the risk for development of breast cancer in a high-risk population. This study included 13,388 healthy women aged 35 years or older whose risk of developing breast cancer was similar to that of a woman 60 years of age or older. Participants in this trial were randomly assigned to tamoxifen or placebo for 5 years. At 53-month follow-up, there was an approximate 50% reduction in the risk of breast cancer development in the tamoxifen-treated group. The data from this study demonstrated a 49% reduction in the risk of invasive breast cancer and a 50% reduction in the risk of noninvasive breast cancer. There was also a 45% reduction in the incidence of hip fractures, but there was no impact on the incidence of ischemic heart disease. There was an increased risk of thromboembolic complications and endometrial cancer in women over age 50 years.

Raloxifene

Raloxifene is a nonsteroidal SERM developed for use in preventing postmenopausal osteoporosis. In a recent clinical trial, raloxifene was found to have a beneficial effect in reducing the risk of breast cancer. In this study, at a median follow-up of 40 months, raloxifene reduced the risk of second primary breast cancer by 76%. However, the study sample was small, and breast cancer prevention was a secondary end point. Currently, the NSABP P-2 study is comparing the safety and efficacy of raloxifene and tamoxifen in postmenopausal women who are at high risk for the development of breast cancer. Until data from this trial become available, it would be inappropriate to use raloxifene outside the context of a clinical trial.

Arzoxifene Hydrochloride

Arzoxifene hydrochloride (LY353381) is a SERM 3 or a benzothiophene SERM that is structurally related to raloxifene. Arzoxifene hydrochloride has significantly superior antitumor activity in experimental systems and is currently being evaluated in phase II studies. Initial phase II data are encouraging and have indicated that this drug has antitumor activity similar to that of tamoxifen. Prospective randomized trials to compare the efficacy of arzoxifene hydrochloride and tamoxifen are planned, and M. D. Anderson will be a study site.

Faslodex

Faslodex (ICI 182,780) is an ER downregulator with an affinity for receptors that is similar to that of estradiol and 50 times greater than that of

KEY PRACTICE POINTS

- Patients with hormone receptor–positive tumors are candidates for endocrine therapy.
- In metastatic disease, selective utilization of endocrine therapy agents can have palliative benefits.
- In the adjuvant setting, endocrine therapy reduces the risk of recurrence and improves survival, even after chemotherapy.

tamoxifen. This drug has significant antitumor activity in tamoxifen-resistant experimental systems, and in a limited phase II study, it had substantial antitumor activity in patients who were treated with tamoxifen. The duration of disease control observed when this agent was used as a second-line therapy was substantially longer than that observed with other agents. Faslodex is currently being tested in phase III trials, and data from these studies should become available in the very near future.

Suggested Readings

Buzdar AU, Hortobagyi GN. Recent advances in adjuvant therapy in breast cancer. *Semin Oncol* 1999;26:21–27.
Buzdar AU, Hortobagyi GN. Update on endocrine therapy for breast cancer. *Clin Cancer Res* 1998;4:527–534.

14 GYNECOLOGIC PROBLEMS IN PATIENTS WITH BREAST CANCER

Pedro T. Ramirez and Ralph S. Freedman

CHAPTER OVERVIEW

Many patients with breast cancer experience gynecologic problems during or after breast cancer treatment. Some of these problems are caused by chemotherapy or hormonal therapy; others are caused by low estrogen levels; and still others are unrelated to breast cancer or its treatment. Women who receive myelosuppressive chemotherapy are more likely to suffer vulvar and vaginal infections, as the chemotherapy can affect ovarian function and thus alter the vaginal ecosystem. Dyspareunia in patients with breast cancer may be due to loss of secretion of the secondary sexual glands, spasm of muscles around the vagina, or aggravation of psychosexual problems that existed before the breast cancer diagnosis. Patients taking tamoxifen are at increased risk for endometrial carcinoma and require careful monitoring. Low estrogen levels can exacerbate urinary incontinence. The evaluation of abnormal vaginal bleeding, uterine or vaginal prolapse, and uterine or ovarian enlargement in breast cancer patients is similar to the evaluation of these problems in patients without breast cancer. Vaginal sonography and hysteroscopy are useful diagnostic tools in patients with vaginal bleeding or other pelvic symptoms. More and more women are asking gynecologists about prophylactic oophorectomy. This surgery may be appropriate in women with a genetic predisposition to ovarian cancer.

Introduction

Many patients with breast cancer experience gynecologic problems during or after breast cancer treatment. Some of these problems result from the effects of cytotoxic or hormonal therapies; other problems are unrelated to breast cancer treatment but may require special management in the patient with breast cancer or the breast cancer survivor. It is hoped that this chapter will increase awareness of special gynecologic problems affecting patients with breast cancer among the physicians who are involved in the care of these patients.

In this chapter, we will discuss the diagnosis and management of clinical problems that are frequently seen among breast cancer patients referred to the Gynecologic Oncology Center at M. D. Anderson Cancer Center. Several of these problems, including infections of the vulva and vagina, vaginal bleeding, and dyspareunia, are often related to estrogen deprivation or the myelosuppressive effects of chemotherapy. We will also discuss tamoxifen-related gynecologic problems; genital prolapse; urinary incontinence; uterine and ovarian enlargement; and prophylactic oophorectomy. The use of vaginal sonography and hysteroscopy as aids for assessing gynecologic problems in patients with breast cancer will also be discussed.

Vulvovaginitis

Among patients who are undergoing active treatment for breast cancer, infections of the genital tract are a frequent reason for referral to the Gynecologic Oncology Center. Vulvovaginitis may occur in women treated with standard or high-dose chemotherapy. Vulvovaginitis can occur during or after chemotherapy and may result from an alteration in the vaginal ecosystem due to loss of normal ovarian function. Loss of ovarian function is usually associated with an increase in the vaginal pH due to a decrease in the vaginal epithelial glycogen content. Normal vaginal pH ranges from 3.8 to 4.2. Myelosuppressive chemotherapy can cause higher pH and neutropenia, which may facilitate the pathogenic behavior of bacteria, fungi, and protozoans coincidentally present in the vagina.

Vaginal infections are usually accompanied by a discharge that is troublesome to the patient. The patient will describe the discharge as being offensive and associated with "itching" or a "burning" sensation at the introitus or urethra. The discharge resulting from vaginal infections is different from the discharge that many women experience normally, which is white but sometimes leaves a brownish stain on underclothing. More than 1 type of vaginal infection can be present at the same time, and therefore careful work-up is essential.

Bacterial Vaginosis

Bacterial vaginosis is the most frequent type of vaginal infection, accounting for approximately 50% of all cases of vaginitis. Bacterial vaginosis was previously also known as *Corynebacterium vaginalis* infection and subsequently as *Gardnerella vaginalis* infection after H. L. Gardner, the clinician who first described it. The pathologic state is believed to involve multiple bacteria, and the incubation period is usually 5 to 10 days.

The following bacteria are commonly found in the vagina (approximate frequencies of specific infections are shown in parentheses): gram-positive rods such as *Diphtheriods* (40%); gram-positive cocci such as *Staphylococcus epidermidis* (55%), *S. aureus* (5%), β-hemolytic streptococci (20%), and group D streptococci (55%); gram-negative organisms such as *Escherichia coli* (30%) and *Klebsiella* (10%); and anaerobics such as *Bacteroides* (40%), *Clostridium* (20%), *Peptococcus* (65%), and *Peptostreptococcus* (35%).

Women with bacterial vaginosis usually complain of a fishy malodorous discharge. The odor becomes more pronounced after intercourse and during the menstrual cycle because aromatic amines are produced in the setting of an alkalotic environment. The discharge is usually dark gray, with low viscosity and homogeneous consistency, and it is primarily localized and adherent to the vaginal walls. Pruritus is not a common complaint. Three criteria aid in the diagnosis of bacterial vaginosis. First, the pH of the vaginal discharge is usually greater than 4.5. Second, when the discharge is mixed with potassium hydroxide, there is an amine-like odor. Third, "clue cells" are usually present. These are vaginal epithelial cells covered with clusters of coccobacilli, which give the cells a granular appearance.

Treatment options are shown in Table 14–1. Treatment of sex partners remains controversial. Most studies demonstrate no benefit from treating the partner after the first episode. However, in patients with recurrent infections, treatment of the partner may be indicated.

Vulvovaginal Candidiasis

Up to 30% of healthy women may harbor candidal organisms, but these women usually do not have symptoms. In contrast, patients with a history of diabetes or immunosuppression (e.g., because of HIV infection, malignancy, or chemotherapy) are at much higher risk for developing vulvovaginal candidiasis. Up to 70% of patients who receive antibiotics for prolonged periods are affected by this infection. Lactobacilli have been shown to regulate the growth of candidal organisms in the vagina. When the concentration of lactobacilli declines, the growth of candidal colonies increases. Vulvovaginal candidiasis is often recurrent.

Table 14–1. Treatment of Common Genital Tract Infections

Disease	Medication	How Supplied	Dosage
Bacterial vaginosis	Metronidazole	Topical–0.75%	b.i.d. x 5 days
		Oral–500 mg	b.i.d. x 7 days
		–250 mg	t.i.d. x 7 days
		–2 g	Single dose
	Clindamycin	Topical–2%	Apply q.i.d. x 7 days
		Oral–300 mg	b.i.d. x 7 days
	Amoxicillin/ clavulanic acid	Oral–500 mg	q.i.d. x 7 days
Vulvovaginal candidiasis	Fluconazole	Oral–150 mg	Single dose
	Clotrimazole	Tablet–100 mg	Apply vaginally x 7 days
		Tablet–500 mg	Apply vaginally x 1 day
	Miconazole	Suppository–200 mg	Apply vaginally x 3 days
	Nystatin	Tablet–100,000 U	Apply vaginally q.h.s. x 14 days
	Terconazole	Cream (0.8%)	Apply vaginally q.h.s. x 3 days
		Suppository–80 mg	Apply vaginally q.h.s. x 3 days
Trichomonas vaginitis	Metronidazole	Oral–2 g	Single dose
		–500 mg	b.i.d. x 7 days

It is important to note that vulvovaginal candidiasis is not associated with sexually transmitted diseases and is not itself considered a sexually transmitted disease. Patients with this infection report an odorless discharge, and many complain of a burning sensation of the vulva. The symptoms may be worsened by intercourse. In the vagina, the discharge usually appears whitish and floccular in consistency, is very viscous, and adheres to the vaginal walls. Slight bleeding may occur when the discharge is removed. The vulva often becomes red and moist, with an inflammatory reaction that extends to the labial-crural folds, and cheese-like deposits are often present in the vagina.

The diagnosis of vulvovaginal candidiasis is made by inspection and may be confirmed using a potassium hydroxide slide preparation (vaginal discharge diluted with saline and 10% potassium hydroxide). In 70% of affected individuals, hyphae or budding yeast cells are seen when the slide is examined under a microscope. Diagnosis by the above criteria is sufficient to initiate treatment; cultures are occasionally needed for confirmatory diagnosis.

Treatment options are shown in Table 14–1. Treatment of sex partners is unnecessary except in the case of uncircumcised partners, who may harbor the infection under the prepuce, and in cases of persistent or recurrent disease.

Trichomonas Vaginitis

Trichomonas vaginitis is the most prevalent nonviral sexually transmitted disease in women. The disease is caused by a flagellated protozoan, *Trichomonas vaginalis,* and primarily affects women during the reproductive years. The incubation period is usually 4 to 28 days. *Trichomonas vaginalis* has been isolated in 30% to 40% of male partners of infected women. Trichomonas infections are often recurrent.

The main symptom of trichomonas infection is usually profuse vaginal discharge. The discharge may be gray, yellow, or green, and it has been described as having a "frothy" appearance. The discharge has a foul odor and may also cause dysuria. Punctate reddened areas may be present on the vaginal and cervical mucosa. The classically described sign of "strawberry cervix and upper vagina" is seen in only about 25% of cases. Observation of flagellated mobile organisms on a wet mount provides a more conclusive diagnosis. The sensitivity of this test is approximately 80% to 90%. Patients who are asymptomatic but have *Trichomonas vaginalis* identified during a routine Papanicolaou examination should be treated because 30% of such patients will become symptomatic within 3 months if no treatment is given.

Treatment options are shown in Table 14–1. The woman's sex partner is usually treated because the risk of reinfection is 2.5-fold greater when the partner is not treated.

Viral Infections

Viral infections caused by human papillomavirus (HPV), herpes simplex virus, and herpes zoster ("shingles") are occasionally found in breast cancer patients.

Human Papillomavirus Infection

Condylomata acuminata of the vulva, vagina, and perianal area are usually associated with forms of HPV that have low oncogenic potential. In the case of such lesions, specific HPV typing is not usually performed. A simple biopsy of one of the lesions will confirm the diagnosis of condylomata and differentiate the lesions from vulvar or vaginal in situ lesions or invasive carcinoma. Biopsy is necessary because early invasive squamous carcinoma of the vulva may appear similar to condyloma. Condylomata acuminata can be treated in a variety of ways, including simple excision, laser ablation, and topical administration of 5-fluorouracil 1 to 2 days per week. Treatment with 5-fluorouracil may be required for 1 to 2 months. Recently, 5% imiquimod in a cream base has been used. The cream is applied 3 times weekly before bedtime, and the area is washed off the next day with mild soap and water. The surrounding normal skin should be protected when therapeutic creams are applied because they can be very irritating. We have also had success with the use of recombinant interferon-alpha made up in a cream base by the M. D. Anderson pharmacy.

For specific diagnosis of oncogenic forms of HPV—including HPV 16 and 18, which account for approximately 75% of the infections with oncogenic types of HPV—polymerase chain reaction methodology is required. However, polymerase chain reaction is used primarily in epidemiologic studies, and standardization of these assays is required. Certain HPV infections of the "high risk" or oncogenic type may be associated with or may predispose to cervical, vaginal, or vulval neoplasms. Furthermore, there is presently no effective treatment that will eliminate HPV, and HPV typing does not preclude the need for regular cytology screening on an annual basis or more frequently if indicated by an atypical Papanicolaou test. Vaccines that target early or late envelope proteins are currently at different stages of development.

Herpes Simplex Virus Infection

Herpes simplex virus infection is highly contagious; 75% of sex partners will be affected. The incubation period ranges from 3 to 7 days.

Herpes simplex virus infection typically presents as multiple small vesicles followed by 1 or more painful, shallow ulcers. These ulcers can occur on any part of the vulva and can be extremely painful when they occur on the labia minora or close to the urethra. Symptoms, including the vesicular phase, may persist for 10 to 14 days. The patient will often report a prior history of herpetic lesions that begin as a vesicular rash. Herpetic lesions may also be associated with tender inguinal lymphadenopathy. The lesions last for a few days, during which time they remain infectious. Viral cultures can be done to confirm the diagnosis, but it takes 2 to 4 days to get the results, and it is usually not practical to delay treatment until the results are received. Acyclovir administered in a cream base or orally may alleviate the pain and accelerate healing of the ulcers (Table 14–2). Topical treatment with solutions that contain aluminum acetate and acetic acid is soothing.

Herpes Zoster Infection

Herpes zoster infection (shingles) of the vulva is exceedingly rare. The presentation and management of this vulvar infection are the same as the presentation and management of infections at other sites. Patients with herpes zoster infection who are receiving chemotherapy, particularly high-dose chemotherapy, should be treated with the same antiviral agents that are used to treat herpes simplex virus. In certain instances intravenous treatment may be required. These patients should also usually receive antiviral agents as prophylaxis during and immediately after the administration of high-dose chemotherapy. Treatment should include the following regimen: valacyclovin (Valtrex) 1000 mg three times a day for 10 days.

VAGINAL BLEEDING

In the premenopausal female, vaginal bleeding is considered abnormal when menstrual cycles become heavier or more prolonged than is typical for the patient or when vaginal bleeding occurs between cycles or after a physical examination or coitus. As menopause approaches, menstrual cycles may become irregular, resulting in periods of amenorrhea followed by episodes of prolonged and usually painless vaginal bleeding.

Abnormal vaginal bleeding can be a sign of endometrial pathology and therefore must be evaluated carefully. Abnormal vaginal bleeding is cause for concern in patients who have been diagnosed with breast cancer because these patients are at increased risk for the development of endo-

Table 14–2. Treatment of Herpes Simplex Virus Infection of the Vulva

Indication	Acyclovir (Zovirax) Dosage
Initial episode	400 mg p.o. t.i.d. × 7–10 days
Recurrent episode	200 mg p.o. 5 × day × 5 days
	400 mg p.o. t.i.d. × 5 days
Herpes prophylaxis	400 mg p.o. b.i.d.

metrial cancer. In addition, prolonged use of certain anticancer drugs, such as tamoxifen, may be associated with a higher risk of developing endometrial cancer (see the section Tamoxifen Use and Endometrial Abnormalities later in this chapter). Tamoxifen can also be associated with the development of benign endocervical or endometrial polyps or endometrial hyperplasia, and both of these conditions can present with vaginal bleeding.

It is important to consider endometrial malignancy in any postmenopausal woman who presents with any vaginal bleeding and any premenopausal woman who presents with abnormal vaginal bleeding. Approximately 5% of all cancers of the endometrium occur in premenopausal women.

In a patient who presents with vaginal bleeding, obtaining a careful history of the bleeding is essential. The history may reveal other common sites of bleeding, such as the urinary tract and the lower intestinal tract. Patients sometimes have difficulty identifying the site of origin of the bleeding. Similar bleeding episodes may have occurred previously. The patient may have a history of endometrial or endocervical polyps or fibroids or recent use of hormonal agents; any of these factors could contribute to vaginal bleeding. Patients who develop oligomenorrhea (infrequent menstruation) within a year preceding menopause may develop episodes of uterine bleeding due to changes in their estrogen levels.

The initial clinical evaluation of abnormal bleeding should include a pregnancy test, if appropriate; a coagulation profile; and determination of the following laboratory values: fasting serum prolactin level, thyroid-stimulating hormone level, and follicle-stimulating hormone level. The luteinizing hormone level is rarely useful because it varies considerably during the day.

An examination of the abdomen and pelvis is always necessary to determine the site and cause of the bleeding. Clinical findings might include a friable cervix with nabothian follicles, suggesting chronic cervicitis; polyps extruding from the cervix, particularly in a patient undergoing treatment with tamoxifen; or an enlarged and irregularly shaped uterus, suggesting a diagnosis of leiomyomata. The majority of endometrial polyps are benign; however, histopathologic evaluation of polyps, including their base, is necessary to rule out endometrial malignancy. An estrogen-producing tumor of the ovary may be the cause of bleeding, although this situation is rare.

A complete gynecologic examination should include examination of cytologic material from the ectocervix and endocervix and, if there is a suspicion of malignancy, a tissue sample from the cervix, endocervix, or endometrial cavity. In the patient who has had previous vaginal deliveries, endometrial tissue samples can be obtained using methods that are easily performed in the outpatient setting. In patients who are nulliparous, however, dilatation of the cervix while the patient is under some form of anesthesia may be required. In our practice, we have found the pipelle instrument to be useful for outpatient procedures that do not require anesthesia (Figure 14–1). The larger suction curette permits access to a larger amount of tissue for diagnosis.

If the information from the cytologic examination and outpatient endometrial biopsy fails to explain the cause of the bleeding or if the bleeding continues, an examination under anesthesia involving hysteroscopy and diagnostic dilation and curettage may be necessary. This examination is often preceded by vaginal sonography, which provides useful information on the thickness of the endometrial stripe and the presence and anatomic location of polyps. It may also reveal an early carcinoma of the endometrium or endocervix. Vaginal sonography is also useful for evaluating the size and morphologic features of the ovaries.

A case from our own experience illustrates the importance of careful evaluation of vaginal bleeding. A patient who started having vaginal bleeding while undergoing chemotherapy for breast cancer was evaluated in the Gynecologic Oncology Center. Because of stenosis of the cervix, an endometrial biopsy could not be performed in the clinic. The cervix was dilated and a hysteroscopy was performed under general anesthesia. Hysteroscopy revealed an irregularity of the surface of the endocervix and endometrium. Samples were obtained by curettage from the endocervix and endometrium and revealed the presence of metastatic breast cancer, which was otherwise unsuspected (Figure 14–2). In this case, because of lack of mobility of the uterus and concerns about periuterine invasion, a

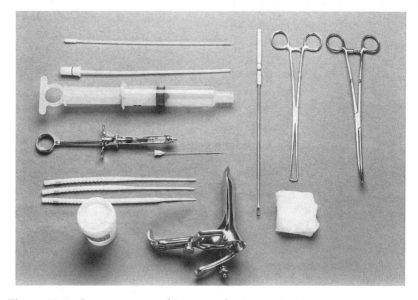

Figure 14–1. Instruments used in gynecologic examinations.

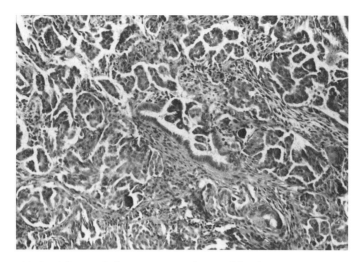

Figure 14–2. Metastatic breast cancer detected by hysteroscopy in a patient who presented with vaginal bleeding while undergoing chemotherapy for breast cancer.

combination of external and intracavitary radiation therapy was used instead of hysterectomy to control the bleeding.

Depending on the results of diagnostic studies, the patient may require a hysterectomy. Before hysterectomy, hysteroscopy may be performed to confirm the findings on vaginal sonography and determine whether any previous attempt at polyp removal has been successful. The findings on hysteroscopy may encourage a nonhysterectomy approach.

Whether a bilateral salpingo-oophorectomy is performed in addition to hysterectomy depends on several factors, including the age of the patient, her preferences, and whether her family history indicates an elevated risk of ovarian cancer. If endometrial cancer is detected or if active endometriosis contributes to symptoms, a bilateral salpingo-oophorectomy must be performed. However, because patients who have undergone oophorectomy may experience severe estrogen-deprivation symptoms, the indications for oophorectomy should be clear and carefully explained to the patient. The issue of estrogen deprivation is especially important for women who have been diagnosed with breast cancer because estrogen replacement therapy is not considered an option for the majority of these patients—especially for those who have estrogen receptor–positive tumors (see chapter 17).

DYSPAREUNIA

In patients with breast cancer, sexual dysfunction is a relatively frequent complaint both during and after treatment. Anxiety about the illness, concerns about disfigurement related to mastectomy, and loss of physiological hormone support, in particular endogenous estrogen, as a result of chemotherapy can all contribute to a lack of interest in sexual activity.

Dyspareunia in the patient with breast cancer may be due to loss of secretion from the secondary sexual glands, such as Bartholin's glands, Skene's glands, and the endocervical glands, or to spasm of the muscles around the vagina, particularly the levator ani muscles. Muscle spasms may result from painful coitus associated with vaginal dryness. Sudden onset of dyspareunia indicates the possibility of a vulvar or vaginal infection (see the section Vulvovaginitis earlier in this chapter).

Another possible cause of dyspareunia in the breast cancer patient is preexisting psychosexual problems, which may be aggravated by the cancer situation. If sexual activity has been interrupted by extended or intensive treatment for breast cancer, the patient and partner may express concerns as to whether resuming coitus can be harmful.

In the Gynecologic Oncology Center, our main objective in the evaluation of breast cancer patients presenting with dyspareunia is to determine whether mechanical barriers or disease states exist that might interfere with sexual activity. These might include scarring or atrophy of the vaginal mucosa, acute infections, and other inflammatory conditions, such as endometriosis or chronic pelvic inflammatory disease. Endometriosis is sometimes symptomatic even in the absence of normal ovarian function. It is also important to determine whether the problem may have preceded the diagnosis of breast cancer. The patient who has obvious atrophy of the vulva and vagina needs to be reassured and given guidance about using sterile lubricants, using dilators, and changing coital postures as appropriate to her individual situation. It is preferable to have the sex partner participate in discussions about these issues. If the problem is not resolved by more straightforward measures, then referral to a sex therapist can be suggested (see chapter 18).

UTERINE OR VAGINAL PROLAPSE

Except for a rare congenital form of the condition, genital prolapse occurs most commonly after multiple vaginal births, and it is more common in women of higher parity. We have also seen genital prolapse in women who have undergone hemipelvectomy or partial sacrectomy. As is the case with any other hernia, uterine prolapse is initiated by loss of supporting fascial structures above the pelvic diaphragm, including condensations or thickening of the fascia that comprise the uterosacral and pubocervical ligaments. In patients who have not had a hysterectomy, uterine prolapse can be associated with prolapse of the anterior or posterior vaginal wall. Vaginal prolapse, however, can occur in the absence of uterine descent.

Early symptoms may include lower-back pain, frequent need to urinate, and, sometimes, constipation associated with a large rectocele. As with other hernias, uterine prolapse is aggravated by conditions that increase intra-abdominal pressure, such as chronic pulmonary disease (frequently seen in smokers or patients with a history of chronic obstructive airway disease) and obesity.

In most patients with uterine prolapse, the degree of prolapse is not severe enough to compromise bladder or bowel function. Even in more severe cases, the use of a pessary may be sufficient to deal with the problem while therapy for breast cancer is ongoing. Vaginal pessaries come in different shapes and sizes. The most common types include Hodge's pessary and the ring, cube, cup, and stem pessaries. In our experience, a cube pessary is efficient and relatively easy for the patient to use with appropriate instruction. When prolapse contributes to difficulty in emptying the bladder or rectum, a surgical approach may be needed. The goal of the surgical approach is to correct the fascial defect, restore anal sphincter function, and remove redundant vaginal mucosa. If an enterocele is detected at surgery, the peritoneal sac must be entered, and the defect must be closed. Patients in whom the uterus prolapses partially or completely outside of the introitus, either spontaneously or with minimal increases in intra-abdominal pressure, usually require a suspensory operation that attaches the vaginal vault to the sacrospinous ligaments after removal of the uterus.

Most patients do not experience incapacitating symptoms from vaginal prolapse. Even patients who have the worst degree of prolapse may benefit from the use of a vaginal pessary until a better opportunity is presented for surgery, i.e., the treatment of breast cancer has been completed with an adequate follow-up period. Nonsurgical or conservative measures should be utilized if the patient has other significant medical problems that would increase the risk of the operation or if the patient has progressive cancer or a significant risk of progression. In some patients, the use of pessaries may have to be definitive.

URINARY INCONTINENCE

Urinary incontinence is reported in 10% to 25% of women younger than the age of 65 and in more than 50% of patients who are bedridden. Urinary incontinence may be exacerbated when estrogen levels are low. Breast cancer patients with urinary incontinence may not initially report the problem voluntarily because issues related to the cancer assume a higher priority for them. Because urinary incontinence may sometimes be related to a significant underlying pelvic pathology, it is important for the physician to inquire about this condition.

Multiple factors may contribute to incontinence, including older age; multiple vaginal births; smoking; neurologic, gastrointestinal, and pulmonary disease; genetic factors; and certain drugs—for example, anti-hypertensives, dopaminergic agonists, cholinergic agonists, neuroleptics, adrenergic β-agonists, and xanthines.

The 3 major types of incontinence are stress urinary incontinence, urge incontinence, and overflow incontinence.

Stress Urinary Incontinence

True stress incontinence occurs when increased intra-abdominal pressure is transmitted equally to the bladder and the functional part of the urethra. Stress incontinence is caused by loss of anatomic support of the urethra, bladder, and urethrovesical junction, which allows the urethra to be displaced below the pelvic floor. When intra-abdominal pressure in addition to intravesical pressure exceeds the urethral closing pressure, involuntary loss of urine will occur. The most common causes of stress incontinence are traumatic vaginal birth, multiple pregnancies, and, in aging women, tissue atrophy secondary to decrease in periurethral vascularity and atrophy of the mucous membrane of the urethra.

Urge Incontinence

Urge incontinence, also known as detrusor instability, is characterized by involuntary loss of urine associated with an abrupt and strong desire to void. Urge incontinence is usually a chronic condition. It is caused by sudden, spontaneous contraction of the detrusor muscle of the bladder, which is thought to be triggered by uninhibited stimulation of detrusor muscle receptors. Urine leakage may occur when the patient is in any position and is more frequent with changes in position. Also, patients with urge incontinence may report an inability to stop their urine stream during voiding.

Urge incontinence can be differentiated from stress incontinence on the basis of symptoms. Whereas stress incontinence usually disappears at night, urge incontinence is often associated with nocturia.

Sudden onset of urge incontinence in a patient diagnosed with breast cancer should raise suspicion of a bladder infection or a pelvic mass (associated with enlargement of the uterus or ovaries) pressing on the bladder. A pelvic examination should reveal any such pelvic mass.

Overflow Incontinence

Overflow incontinence occurs when the bladder becomes overdistended because it cannot empty properly. Overflow incontinence is usually caused by interference with normal neurologic control of the bladder. Patients will report that they void small quantities of urine and afterwards still feel that their bladder is full.

Although overflow incontinence can be caused by medical conditions such as multiple sclerosis, diabetic neuropathy, and trauma, in the patient with breast cancer it is important to rule out metastatic lesions in the lumbar sacral area of the spine. Patients with such lesions will often report loss of bowel continence and neuropathy—typically a loss of S1 sensation on the soles of the feet. Cystoscopic and neurologic assessment will establish the diagnosis. Appropriate radiologic studies, including bone scans and magnetic resonance imaging studies of the lumbar sacral spine, are necessary to identify metastatic sites that could be causing neurogenic bladder.

Diagnosis and Management

Because each type of incontinence presents with characteristic symptoms and findings, the history is the most important factor in the diagnostic work-up. The work-up should also include a culture of the urine, which may reveal a bladder infection, and a pelvic examination, which will often provide some information on the type of incontinence and may also reveal a causative factor, such as a pelvic mass. If physical examination does not reveal a causative factor, a short course of a detrusor inhibitor such as oxybutynin chloride extended-release can be offered. Patients who complain of stress incontinence should generally be referred to a urogynecologist, a physician who specializes in the evaluation and management of urogenital-tract problems in women.

It is not uncommon for a woman to have coexisting stress incontinence and urge incontinence; thus, proper evaluation is essential for successful management of incontinence.

TAMOXIFEN USE AND ENDOMETRIAL ABNORMALITIES

Approximately 80,000 women in the United States are receiving tamoxifen therapy annually as part of their treatment for breast cancer. Currently, adjuvant treatment with tamoxifen is being recommended for 5 years.

Tamoxifen is an antiestrogen, but it also acts as a partial estrogen agonist on the endometrium. Administration of unopposed estrogen can lead to endometrial proliferation and occasionally to carcinoma. Tamoxifen use has been associated with certain histopathologic changes in the endometrium, including increased endometrial thickness, increased uterine volume, proliferative changes, simple and complex atypical endometrial hyperplasia, endometrial polyps, and, rarely, endometrial carcinoma. In the National Surgical Adjuvant Breast and Bowel Project P-1 trial, which included patients at increased risk for the development of breast cancer and which examined the value of tamoxifen in preventing second breast cancers, patients were randomly assigned to receive either tamoxifen 20 mg daily or placebo. The cumulative rate for endometrial cancer was 13.0 cases per 1000 women in the tamoxifen-treatment group compared with 5.4 cases per 1000 women in the placebo control group. The increased risk in tamoxifen-treated women appeared at 1 year and increased progressively beyond 5 years. The relative risk of developing endometrial cancer after tamoxifen treatment increases with higher cumulative doses of tamoxifen and longer duration of exposure.

It is hoped that the introduction of other selective estrogen receptor modulators, such as raloxifene, into hormonal therapeutics for breast cancer may eliminate or reduce the problems of treatment-associated endometrioid polyps or even endometrial cancer. However, such changes in practice will have to await the conclusion of the National Surgical Adjuvant Breast and Bowel Project's ongoing P-2 trial, which compares tamoxifen with raloxifene.

In women treated for breast cancer, the benefits of tamoxifen in reducing the risk of breast cancer recurrence far outweigh the small risk of endometrial cancer. However, because of the risk of endometrial cancer, women taking tamoxifen must have frequent and thorough examinations. Table 14–3 shows the American College of Obstetrics and Gynecology guidelines for care of patients undergoing treatment with tamoxifen (ACOG, 1996).

Sonography has proven to be useful in evaluating the endometrium in patients taking tamoxifen. Typical sonographic appearances of the endometrium in patients taking tamoxifen include thick, homogeneous hyper-

Table 14–3. American College of Obstetrics and Gynecology Recommendations for Women Taking Tamoxifen (1996)

- Women with breast cancer should have annual gynecologic examinations, including Pap tests and bimanual and rectovaginal examinations.
- Any abnormal bleeding, including bloody discharge, spotting, or any other gynecologic symptoms, should be evaluated thoroughly. Any bleeding or spotting should be investigated by biopsy.
- Practitioners should be alert to the increased incidence of endometrial malignancy. Screening procedures or diagnostic tests should be performed at the discretion of the individual gynecologist.
- Women without breast cancer who are being treated with tamoxifen within a chemopreventive trial should be monitored closely for the development of endometrial hyperplasia or cancer.
- If atypical hyperplasia develops, use of tamoxifen should be discontinued, and dilation and curettage or other appropriate gynecologic management should be instituted within an appropriate interval.
- If tamoxifen therapy must be continued, hysterectomy should be considered in women with atypical endometrial hyperplasia.
- Tamoxifen use may be reinstituted following hysterectomy for endometrial carcinoma in consultation with the physician responsible for the woman's breast care.

Reprinted with permission from ACOG committee opinion. Tamoxifen and endometrial cancer. Number 169, February 1996. Committee on Gynecologic Practice. American College of Obstetricians and Gynecologists. *Int J Gynaecol Obstet* 1996;53:197–199.

echogenic tissue with small cystic spaces; heterogeneous tissue with small cystic spaces; and solid heterogeneous tissue and polyps. When 5 mm is used as the upper limit of normal endometrial thickness, the sensitivity of transvaginal sonography for the detection of endometrial abnormalities is 91% to 100%. An endometrial thickness of greater than 10 mm is almost always associated with some type of endometrial abnormality, such as hyperplasia or polyps. Figures 14–3A and 14–3B show an endometrial polyp as seen on vaginal sonography and hysteroscopy, respectively.

Some investigators have utilized transvaginal pulse Doppler color flow imaging and have concluded that it does not contribute to the assessment of asymptomatic postmenopausal breast cancer patients treated with tamoxifen. Another technique often utilized is sonohysterography. This involves filling the endometrial cavity with saline under sonographic visualization, thus distending the cavity and allowing more effective analysis. Sonohysterography is particularly useful for delineating polyps and space-occupying lesions, such as submucosal myomas, and for identifying a thickened endometrium (Figure 14–4).

At M. D. Anderson, patients scheduled to begin tamoxifen therapy are frequently referred to the Gynecologic Oncology Center for transvaginal sonography before starting tamoxifen therapy. The likelihood of detecting endometrial pathology in the asymptomatic patient is very small, usually between 0.6% and 4%, and most abnormal findings do not require specific treatment. If a patient has no symptoms and sonography shows an endometrial thickness greater than 10 mm, an endometrial biopsy is generally performed, although outcome data from our center are currently being examined. If sonography shows a thickened endometrium (5–10 mm) and the patient is asymptomatic, repeat transvaginal sonography should be performed within 12 months. Any patient who has vaginal bleeding or a bloody vaginal discharge while taking tamoxifen should undergo immediate endometrial biopsy regardless of the thickness of the endometrial lining on sonography.

UTERINE OR OVARIAN ENLARGEMENT

Enlargement of the uterus or ovaries is a frequent reason for referral of breast cancer patients to the Gynecologic Oncology Center. In many cases, the enlargement is detected on an abdominal-pelvic computed tomography scan obtained for staging or follow-up purposes.

Uterine Enlargement

The most common cause of uterine enlargement is leiomyoma, which is found in approximately 20% to 25% of women of reproductive age and is detected in about 50% of postmenopausal women. Leiomyomata are usu-

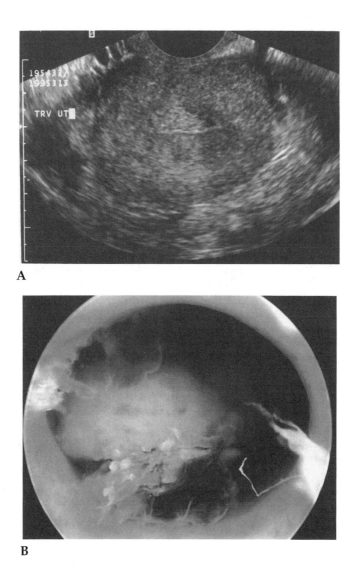

Figure 14–3. Endometrial polyp as seen on vaginal sonography (A) and hysteroscopy (B).

ally asymptomatic. Unless the disease is symptomatic or the size of the uterus has increased rapidly, the patient with leiomyoma should simply be reassured and should not be subjected to surgical intervention. A sudden increase in the size of the uterus or pain associated with leiomyoma should raise concern about the possibility of leiomyosarcoma. However, such tumors are rare, occurring in less than 0.2% of all patients with leiomyoma. If leiomyoma causes enlargement of the uterus or excessive

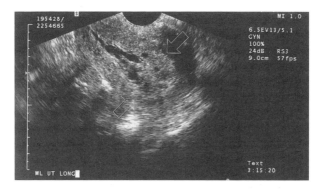

Figure 14–4. Thickened endometrium as seen on sonohysterography.

bleeding, a total hysterectomy may be required for therapeutic and diagnostic purposes.

Ovarian Enlargement

The most common cause of ovarian enlargement is an ovarian cyst. Ovarian cysts can be classified as either nonneoplastic or neoplastic. Nonneoplastic ovarian cysts include physiologic cysts, such as corpus luteum and endometriotic cysts. The most common types of neoplastic ovarian cyst are cystic teratoma (dermoid cyst), which is usually found in younger patients, and serous or mucinous cystadenoma, which occurs in patients of all ages.

In women of reproductive age, the ovaries may enlarge slightly in parallel with physiologic effects of pituitary-ovarian stimulation. Physiologic cysts are simple cysts (usually unilocular on sonography). Physiologic cysts may regress by the next cycle but sometimes persist for 2 or more cycles. When enlargement is greater than 5 cm or if there is any palpable enlargement after the menopause, the possibility of a neoplastic event should be considered.

The initial evaluation should include a thorough history that specifically addresses menstrual history, sexual history, and associated symptoms. This is followed by a comprehensive physical examination, with the pelvic examination being the primary focus. The goal is to assess the evidence of a pelvic mass and the consistency (solid or cystic), mobility (mobile or fixed), and size of any such mass. Dysmenorrhea, dyspareunia, or pain that radiates to the upper thigh, with or without a prior history of endometriosis, may suggest a diagnosis of endometriosis. Pain associated with an enlarged ovary is usually related to a benign process except in the case of a rapidly growing or necrotic neoplasm of the ovary, such as a sarcoma or granulosa cell tumor.

Vaginal sonography can provide useful information about the size and complexity of an ovarian mass (Figure 14–5). Multiloculation, excrescences, and increased Doppler flow (low impedance) should increase the suspicion of a neoplasm. Even in the case of ovarian cysts less than 5 cm in diameter, sonography may be helpful in determining whether the cyst is simple, unilocular, or multilocular.

An elevated serum CA-125 value may also be helpful in suggesting underlying pathology, although the CA-125 value is normal in up to 50% of early-stage ovarian cancers. Moreover, even though CA-125 is used as a marker for ovarian cancer, levels of this marker may also be significantly elevated in patients who have a diagnosis of uterine fibroids, adenomyosis, or endometriosis; in patients with cirrhosis of the liver; and in 5% to 7% of normal women.

Ovarian cysts less than 5 cm in diameter that do not appear to be multiloculated on sonography can be managed conservatively. Conservative management should include serial clinical examinations and vaginal sonography, generally repeated after approximately 8 weeks.

Ovarian cysts larger than 5 cm in diameter and ovarian cysts that increase in size usually require surgical exploration, primarily to rule out a neoplastic cause. In patients who have had breast reconstruction with a transverse rectus abdominis myocutaneous flap, appropriate surgical intervention may be carried out using a laparoscopic approach or midline abdominal laparotomy approach. It should be emphasized that these are general guidelines and do not replace clinical judgment in individual patients.

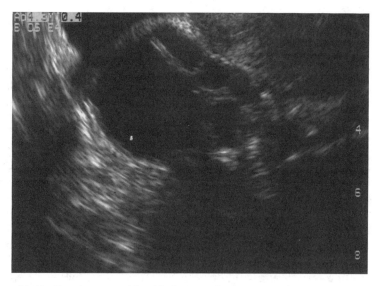

Figure 14–5. Ovarian mass identified on vaginal sonography.

It is important to recognize that the ovaries and other genital-tract organs can be the site of metastases from breast cancer. If one or both ovaries are replaced by solid masses, especially when radiologic findings indicate metastases in the abdomen or elsewhere, percutaneous needle biopsy of the ovaries under computed tomographic guidance provides rapid and useful information without the need for surgical intervention. If ovarian metastases from breast cancer cause symptoms (pain, bladder pressure, or constipation) or contribute to obstruction of the small or large bowel, abdominal surgery may be necessary to correct the problem. If the patient is asymptomatic and ovarian metastases from breast cancer are confirmed, tumor-reductive surgery is not generally favored over additional systemic therapy unless it can be demonstrated with high certainty that the cancer is localized to pelvic organs and that hysterectomy or oophorectomy alone will remove most or all of the metastatic disease.

Prophylactic Oophorectomy

Over the past few years, knowledge of genetic susceptibility to ovarian and breast cancer has increased substantially. Testing for mutations in the *BRCA1* and *BRCA2* genes is becoming increasingly available to women in whom the chance of a familial predisposition is believed to be elevated. At the same time, more patients are turning to gynecologists, gynecologic oncologists, and other health care providers for estimates of their own and their daughters' risks of developing ovarian cancer and for information about options for surveillance and prevention. In discussions of these issues, patients must be provided with information on a well-researched pedigree of the family, factors associated with oral contraceptives and hormone replacement therapy, risks of surgery, and the possibility that peritoneal carcinoma may develop subsequent to prophylactic oophorectomy. These issues are discussed in more detail in chapter 3.

Indications

Some authors suggest that prophylactic bilateral oophorectomy in patients undergoing hysterectomy or coincidental pelvic surgery may reduce the incidence of ovarian cancer by approximately 2000 cases per year. This potential benefit, however, has to be balanced against the long-term risks of estrogen withdrawal, including a possible increased risk of cardiovascular disease and predisposition to osteoporosis. These potential risks are particularly important in patients with breast cancer, in whom exogenous estrogens are usually contraindicated.

Prophylactic oophorectomy is also sometimes considered in women with familial cancer risk. The lifetime risk of ovarian cancer in women who are known to have mutations in *BRCA1* or *BRCA2* is 44% to 56%.

However, the risk is unclear for women with "breast/ovarian cancer syndrome" because the term remains inadequately defined. In many studies, the number of family members affected with either breast or ovarian cancer has been assigned arbitrarily. Available information suggests that it is reasonable to offer prophylactic oophorectomy to a woman who has 2 or more first- or second-degree relatives with ovarian cancer or breast cancer provided the woman does not wish to bear children in the future.

Hereditary ovarian cancers tend to present at an earlier age, but the optimum age at which to perform prophylactic oophorectomy remains unknown. The Gilda Radner Familial Ovarian Cancer Registry recommends oophorectomy when fertility is no longer a factor or by the age of 35 years. At the M. D. Anderson Gynecologic Oncology Center, we recommend that the procedure be performed 5 to 10 years earlier than the age when cancer developed in the closest affected relative.

Patient Counseling and Treatment Selection

The surgical approach to oophorectomy must be discussed carefully with the patient. Laparoscopic oophorectomy is the preferred treatment method in the absence of contraindications such as multiple prior abdominal surgeries, morbid obesity, history of severe endometriosis, pelvic inflammatory disease, or tubo-ovarian abscesses. Laparoscopic oophorectomy has several advantages: the procedure can be performed on an outpatient basis; there is minimal blood loss and decreased need for postoperative analgesia; and the patient can return more quickly to normal daily activities. Given the possibility of encountering undiagnosed early-stage ovarian cancer during laparoscopic surgery, the patient should be informed that the procedure might require conversion to a laparotomy in the event that a diagnosis of ovarian cancer is made.

The disadvantages and benefits associated with performing a hysterectomy at the time of the oophorectomy also need to be addressed. The disadvantages include an increase in overall morbidity due to increased duration of the surgical procedure and increased blood loss. The cost of the procedure is also higher when hysterectomy is performed at the same time as oophorectomy. *BRCA1* mutations may be associated with increased risk of fallopian tube carcinoma, and complete excision of the fallopian tube requires hysterectomy. Moreover, women in high-risk families may have an overall lifetime risk of greater than 10% of developing uterine cancer, which is considerably higher than the 2% risk documented in the general population. Patients should also be informed that peritoneal carcinoma develops in 1.8% to 10.7% of patients after oophorectomy.

Many patients choose not to undergo surgical excision of the ovaries and choose close observation instead. With these patients, it is important to discuss the preventive measures available to decrease the chances of developing ovarian cancer. However, it is not known whether any of these

---

KEY PRACTICE POINTS

- Women undergoing standard or high-dose chemotherapy are at increased risk for vulvar and vaginal infections.

- Any vaginal bleeding in a patient with breast cancer should be fully evaluated to rule out endometrial carcinoma.

- Patients receiving tamoxifen or other hormonal agents should be monitored for the development of endometrial carcinoma.

- Urinary incontinence and prolapse occur most commonly in women of advanced age or following previous birth trauma. Urinary incontinence may also be an early symptom of an undiagnosed pelvic mass.

- Vaginal sonography and hysteroscopy are very useful diagnostic tools in patients who have vaginal bleeding or other pelvic symptoms.

- Prophylactic oophorectomy may be warranted in certain patients who are genetically predisposed to the development of ovarian cancer.

---

suggestions will provide the same benefit to carriers of the *BRCA1* mutation as they will for the general population.

Oral contraceptives have been shown to reduce the risk of ovarian cancer development by 50%, with the protective effect persisting for 10 to 15 years after the oral contraceptive has been stopped. Unfortunately, there is also evidence that use of oral contraceptives may increase the risks of breast cancer. At this time, oral contraceptives cannot be recommended for patients who have been diagnosed with breast cancer.

Surveillance and screening for ovarian cancer need to be addressed, particularly for known carriers of *BRCA1* mutations. The best available tools for early detection of ovarian cancer are physical examination combined with determination of the serum CA-125 level and transvaginal sonography; however, these methods remain only marginally effective as screening approaches. Both CA-125 and transvaginal sonography have a very high false-positive rate, particularly in premenopausal women. Even among patients with known first- or second-degree relatives with a history of ovarian cancer, Bourne et al (1993) found that 10 surgical explorations were required to identify 1 patient with ovarian cancer. An even higher number of unnecessary procedures would have to be performed in patients whose only risk factor was a personal history of breast cancer. While we await tests with higher sensitivity and specificity, patients at risk are offered annual physical examination, a rectovaginal examination combined with serum CA-125 determination, and transvaginal sonography. More attention is being focussed on the psychological impact of increased susceptibility for ovarian cancer. Recent studies have highlighted the importance of providing personalized feedback and counseling interventions tailored to the individual's psychological profile.

Suggested Readings

ACOG committee opinion. Tamoxifen and endometrial cancer. Number 169, February 1996. Committee on Gynecologic Practice. American College of Obstetricians and Gynecologists. *Int J Gynaecol Obstet* 1996;53:197–199.

Boike G, Averette H, Hoskins W, et al. National survey of ovarian carcinoma. IV. Women with prior hysterectomy: a failure of prevention? *Gynecol Oncol* 1993;A22:112.

Bourne TH, Campbell S, Reynolds KM, et al. Screening for early familial ovarian cancer with transvaginal ultrasonography and colour blood flow imaging. *BMJ* 1993;306:1025–1029.

Cancer and Steroid Hormone Study of the Centers for Disease Control and the National Institute of Child Health and Human Development. The reduction in risk of ovarian cancer associated with oral-contraceptive use. *N Engl J Med* 1987;316:650–655.

Cohen I, Beyth Y, Tepper R. The role of ultrasound in the detection of endometrial pathologies in asymptomatic postmenopausal breast cancer patients with tamoxifen treatment. *Obstet Gynecol Surv* 1998;53:429–438.

Cohen I, Rosen DJ, Tepper R, et al. Ultrasonographic evaluation of the endometrium and correlation with endometrial sampling in postmenopausal patients treated with tamoxifen. *J Ultrasound Med* 1993;12:275–280.

Exacoustos C, Zupi E, Cangi B, Chiaretti M, Arduini D, Romanini C. Endometrial evaluation in postmenopausal breast cancer patients receiving tamoxifen: an ultrasound, color flow Doppler, hysteroscopic and histological study. *Ultrasound Obstet Gynecol* 1995;6:435–442.

Fisher B, Costantino JP, Wickerham L, et al. Tamoxifen for prevention of breast cancer: report of the National Surgical Adjuvant Breast and Bowel Project P-1 Study. *J Natl Cancer Inst* 1998;90:1371–1388.

Ford D, Easton DF, Bishop DT, Narod SA, Goldgar DE. Risk of cancer in BRCA1-mutation carriers. Breast Cancer Linkage Consortium. *Lancet* 1994;343:692–695.

Goldstein SR, Scheele WH, Rajagopalan SK, Wilkie JL, Walsh BW, Parsons AK. A 12-month comparative study of raloxifene, estrogen, and placebo on the postmenopausal endometrium. *Obstet Gynecol* 2000;95:95–103.

Ismail SM. Gynecological effects of tamoxifen. *J Clin Pathol* 1999;52:83–88.

Jaiyesimi IA, Buzdar AU, Decker DA, Hortobagyi GN. Use of tamoxifen for breast cancer: twenty-eight years later. *J Clin Oncol* 1995;13:513–529.

Jishi MF, Itnyre JH, Oakley-Girvan IA, Piver MS, Whittemore AS. Risks of cancer among members of families in the Gilda Radner Familial Ovarian Cancer Registry. *Cancer* 1995;76:1416–1421.

Miller SM, Fang CY, Manne SL, Engstrom PF, Daly MB. Decision making about prophylactic oophorectomy among at-risk women: psychological influences and implications. *Gynecol Oncol* 1999;75:406–412.

Pepper JM, Oyesanya OA, Dewart PJ, Howell A, Seif MW. Indices of differential endometrial:myometrial growth may be used to improve the reliability of detecting endometrial neoplasia in women on tamoxifen. *Ultrasound Obstet Gynecol* 1996;8:408–411.

Piver MS, Jishi MF, Tsukada Y, Nava G. Primary peritoneal carcinoma after prophylactic oophorectomy in women with a family history of ovarian cancer: a report of the Gilda Radner Familial Ovarian Cancer Registry. *Cancer* 1993;71: 2751–2755.

Simard J, Tonin P, Durocher F, et al. Common origins of BRCA1 mutations in Canadian breast and ovarian cancer families. *Nat Genet* 1994;8:392–398.

Struewing JP, Watson P, Easton DF, Ponder BA, Lynch HT, Tucker MA. Prophylactic oophorectomy in inherited breast/ovarian cancer families. *J Natl Cancer Inst Monogr* 1995;17:33–35.

Tepper R, Cohen I, Altaras M, et al. Doppler flow evaluation of pathologic endometrial conditions in postmenopausal breast cancer patients treated with tamoxifen. *J Ultrasound Med* 1994;13:635–640.

Tobacman JK, Greene MH, Tucker MA, Costa J, Kase R, Fraumeni JF Jr. Intra-abdominal carcinomatosis after prophylactic oophorectomy in ovarian-cancer-prone families. *Lancet* 1982;2:795–797.

Zweemer RP, van Diest PJ, Verheijen RH, et al. Molecular evidence linking primary cancer of the fallopian tube to BRCA1 germline mutations. *Gynecol Oncol* 2000;76:45–50.

15 SPECIAL CLINICAL SITUATIONS IN PATIENTS WITH BREAST CANCER

Karin M. Gwyn and Richard L. Theriault

CHAPTER OVERVIEW

A number of special clinical situations can arise during the management of a patient with breast cancer, including pregnancy, leptomeningeal carcinomatosis, epidural spinal cord compression, hypercalcemia, and second primary malignancy. For women diagnosed with breast cancer during pregnancy, modified radical mastectomy with axillary lymph node dissection is the preferred surgical option. At M. D. Anderson Cancer Center, pregnant women with breast cancer have been safely treated during the second and third trimesters of pregnancy with combination chemotherapy consisting of 5-fluorouracil, doxorubicin, and cyclophosphamide. Leptomeningeal carcinomatosis, a life-threatening complication of breast cancer even when treated, is diagnosed by analysis of the cerebrospinal fluid and gadolinium-enhanced magnetic resonance imaging. Treatment involves intrathecal chemotherapy via an Ommaya reservoir with agents such as methotrexate or newer agents such as sustained-release cytarabine plus radiation therapy for focal areas of bulky disease. Epidural spinal cord compression is usually diagnosed with magnetic resonance imaging, and treatment includes the use of corticosteroids and surgery with or without radiation therapy or radiation therapy alone. The primary agents used in the treatment of hypercalcemia are the bisphosphonates, particularly pamidronate disodium. Patients with breast cancer are already at risk for a second breast cancer, and those who are exposed to chemotherapy, hormonal therapy, radiation therapy, or a combination of these are at increased risk for second primary malignancies, including lung cancer, myelodysplastic syndrome, acute myeloid leukemia, and endometrial cancer. Regular follow-ups with thorough histories and physical examinations as well as yearly mammograms and chest radiographs for those women exposed to radiation therapy are important for the detection of second malignancies in patients with breast cancer.

INTRODUCTION

While caring for the patient with breast cancer, the clinician may encounter some unusual and relatively infrequent clinical situations, such as breast cancer diagnosed during pregnancy, leptomeningeal carcinomatosis, epidural spinal cord compression (ESCC), hypercalcemia, and second malignancies occurring in the background of a primary breast cancer. Some of these clinical situations can be managed with relative ease; others require extensive clinical acumen and experience to provide patients with the most appropriate care. However, because of their relative rarity, there may not be any guidelines supported by appropriately powered randomized clinical trials to help the clinician in the decision process. This chapter reviews these special clinical situations and offers suggestions for diagnosing, treating, and monitoring patients.

BREAST CANCER DURING PREGNANCY

Pregnancy-associated breast cancer is defined as breast cancer that is diagnosed during pregnancy or within the year after delivery. Breast cancer is the most common cancer associated with pregnancy, and its prevalence increases with increasing maternal age. As more women delay childbearing, there may be an increase in the incidence of pregnancy-associated breast cancer. Approximately 2% of women with breast cancer are pregnant at the time of diagnosis. In two studies conducted at M. D. Anderson Cancer Center and Memorial Sloan-Kettering Cancer Center, the prevalence of pregnancy-associated breast cancer in patients with breast cancer who were under the age of 30 was found to be 25.6% and 9.7%, respectively.

Diagnosis

The most common clinical manifestation of breast cancer during pregnancy is a mass in the breast or a thickening of the breast. The physiologic changes that occur in the breast during pregnancy and subsequent lactation (i.e., increased size and density) are thought to delay the recognition of symptoms by both the patient and the physician and therefore delay the cancer diagnosis. Delays of 6 months or more in diagnosis are common. As a result, women with pregnancy-associated breast cancer are more likely to have larger tumors and involved axillary lymph nodes at diagnosis.

Mammography has been thought to be of little value in the diagnosis of breast cancer during pregnancy because of the increased water content and loss of contrasting fat in the breasts of pregnant women. A small series by Max and Klamer (1983) reported normal mammograms in 6 of 8 pregnant women with a palpable mass that was later diagnosed as carcinoma of the breast. However, Liberman et al (1994) reported that 78% of mammograms in pregnant women with breast cancer were abnormal, with findings such as masses, calcifications, and diffuse increases in parenchymal density. In 6 of 6 patients in this series, sonography demonstrated focal abnormalities. At M. D. Anderson, pregnant women with a breast mass undergo a clinical breast examination in conjunction with sonography, mammography with abdominal shielding, or both. If there is appropriate abdominal shielding, mammography can be performed with little risk of exposing the fetus to radiation.

To further evaluate a suspicious breast mass in a patient who is pregnant, fine-needle aspiration biopsy may be performed. This technique is useful and accurate in assessing the cytologic features of breast masses. Fine-needle aspiration and core needle biopsy of the breast are associated with low rates of false-positive and false-negative diagnoses. If necessary, a surgical breast biopsy can be performed without significant risk to a pregnant patient even in the first trimester. The general approach used at M. D. Anderson to establish a diagnosis of breast cancer in a pregnant patient is outlined in Figure 15–1.

Staging

A framework for assessing the presence and extent of local, regional, and disseminated disease in the pregnant patient with a diagnosis of breast cancer is the tumor-node-metastasis staging system. This staging system can be used to assess prognosis as well as to plan treatment. A thorough physical examination of the breast and regional lymph node–bearing areas with careful documentation of any abnormalities found is important. Clinically suspicious regional nodal disease may warrant a more detailed evaluation for metastases. Diagnostic mammography with abdominal shielding, sonography of the breast and regional nodal basins, or both may direct a clinician to those areas that warrant fine-needle aspiration for cytologic confirmation of disease.

At M. D. Anderson, routine assessment for pregnant women includes 2-view chest radiography with abdominal shielding, a complete blood cell count, and renal and liver function tests. Alkaline phosphatase is frequently elevated during pregnancy and thus would be of limited usefulness in diagnosing breast cancer. If there are concerns that a patient has symptoms of metastatic disease or is at high risk for metastatic disease based on initial staging, additional tests may be performed. In general, computed tomography (CT) scanning should not be performed because of the risk of fetal radiation exposure. Magnetic resonance imaging (MRI) may be used to document marrow and visceral-organ involvement, particularly of the liver, which can become quite fatty during pregnancy and thus more difficult to assess by sonography. Studies have shown that bone scans in early-stage breast cancer have a low true-positive yield of bone metastases. However, in patients with symptoms of bone pain, a bone scan may be of use because a 25% true-positive yield has been reported in clinical stage III disease. Bone scans should be deferred if possible until the later stages of pregnancy or until after delivery because of the risk of exposing the fetus to radiation. Magnetic resonance imaging of thoracic and lumbar spine may be a useful screening test for occult bone metastases.

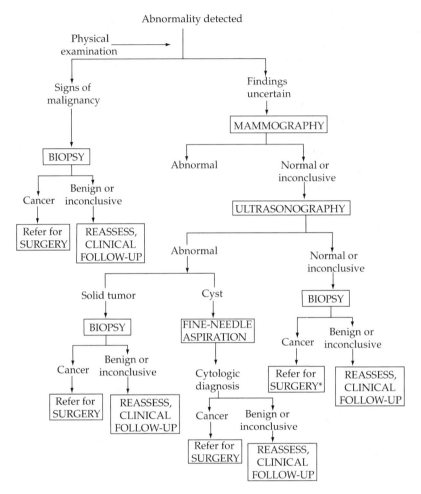

Figure 15–1. General approach to diagnosis of breast cancer in pregnant patients at M. D. Anderson. * Depending on stage and trimester, neoadjuvant chemotherapy may be appropriate.

Only a small number of studies have assessed and compared the pathologic features of primary breast tumors in pregnant and nonpregnant patients. One study by Tobon and Horowitz (1993) reported infiltrating ductal carcinoma in 13 of 14 patients, negative estrogen receptor (ER) status in 7 patients, and positive progesterone receptor (PR) status in 5 patients. In a separate study of 14 patients, 3 were both ER and PR positive, 6 were ER and PR negative, 1 was ER positive and PR negative, and 4 were ER negative and PR positive (Jackisch et al, 1995). In a study of 15 pregnant women with breast cancer, one third of the tumors were ER positive, and approximately half were PR positive (Elledge et al, 1993). It is important to measure ER and PR status immunohistochemically and not by the ligand-binding assay (LBA). During pregnancy, there are 2 mechanisms by which the LBA can produce false-negative results. First, the increase in estrogen and progesterone levels can downregulate ER levels to the point at which they are no longer detectable by the LBA. Second, LBA depends on the availability of the unbound receptor, and in a pregnant woman, it is possible that all binding sites could be occupied because of the increase in estrogen levels. HER-2/*neu* status should also be determined, although there are few studies of this biomarker in pregnant women. Elledge et al (1993) found 7 of 12 tumors to be positive for HER-2/*neu* in a series of women with breast cancer diagnosed during pregnancy. Only 16% of age-matched, nonpregnant patients had HER-2/*neu*–positive tumors.

Monitoring the Pregnancy

The pregnant woman with breast cancer should be continually and carefully monitored during her pregnancy. A medical team highly skilled in the management of maternal and fetal health should assess and monitor the health of both mother and fetus in conjunction with the oncologist. Gestational age and the expected date of delivery should be determined by sonography. As the pregnancy progresses, fetal maturity should be monitored by sonography; in some cases amniocentesis may be necessary to determine pulmonary maturity, particularly if induction of labor is being considered.

Treatment

The treatment goal for the pregnant woman with breast cancer is the same as that for a nonpregnant breast cancer patient: to control local and systemic disease. Although the treatment strategies for pregnant and nonpregnant women with breast cancer are similar, in the pregnant patient, the impact of treatment on the fetus and the outcome of the pregnancy must be considered.

Surgery

Mastectomy with axillary lymph node dissection can be performed with minimal risk to the developing fetus or the continuation of the pregnancy and is the usual surgical treatment for pregnant women with breast cancer. Although breast-conserving surgery (lumpectomy or quadrantectomy) with axillary lymph node dissection is technically feasible in the pregnant patient with breast cancer, the radiation therapy required to complete local therapy for the breast is contraindicated during pregnancy because of the risks associated with exposure of the fetus to radiation. The developing fetus may be exposed to radiation doses in excess of 15 cGy if breast irradiation is performed in the first trimester and even higher doses if the radiation is given later in the pregnancy. Although there are situations in which radiation therapy could be delayed until after delivery, if surgery is indicated, modified radical mastectomy is the treatment of choice for breast cancer diagnosed in the first or second trimesters. In a recent report from M. D. Anderson on the results of a standardized protocol for the management of pregnancy-associated breast cancer, the majority of patients (18 of 22) had a modified radical mastectomy, with only 2 patients having segmental resection with postpartum radiation therapy (Berry et al, 1999).

Systemic Therapy

The indications for systemic therapy in the pregnant patient with breast cancer are similar to those for the nonpregnant breast cancer patient. All patients with tumors 1.0 cm or larger as well as women with node-positive disease should be offered systemic therapy. Little is known about the pharmacokinetics of individual cytotoxic agents in the pregnant patient. Physiologic changes during pregnancy, including alterations of renal and hepatic function, increases in plasma volume, and the appearance of a "third space" of the amniotic sac, may influence the pharmacology of antineoplastic drugs.

Most of the information about cytotoxic chemotherapy for pregnancy-associated breast cancer has been derived from case studies and case-control studies that are primarily retrospective in nature. Researchers at M. D. Anderson recently published a standardized protocol for the treatment of breast cancer during pregnancy (Berry et al, 1999). Women with breast cancer diagnosed during pregnancy were treated with chemotherapy consisting of 500 mg/m^2 5-fluorouracil intravenously on days 1 and 4, 50 mg/m^2 doxorubicin by continuous infusion over 72 hours, and 500 mg/m^2 cyclophosphamide intravenously on day 1 (FAC) during the second and third trimesters of pregnancy. At M. D. Anderson, we have found that administration of doxorubicin over 72 hours is associated with less cardiac toxicity (Hortobagyi et al, 1989). A median of 4 cycles of chemotherapy were administered during pregnancy. The mean gestational age at delivery was 37.6 weeks, and no neonatal complications or subsequent developmental delays were reported. Berry and colleagues concluded that a multimodality approach to breast cancer treatment for the pregnant patient is feasible. Although the cytotoxic agents used in this protocol are rated pregnancy risk factor D (Code of Federal Regulations, 1997), the researchers concluded that chemotherapy can be administered for the treatment of breast cancer during the second and third trimesters with minimal complications. There are no published studies in which taxanes or tamoxifen have been used in the treatment of pregnant women with breast cancer. Most reports do not recommend the use of methotrexate in the management of breast cancer during pregnancy because methotrexate is an abortifactant and causes severe fetal malformations when given during the first trimester (Doll et al, 1989).

Because many cytotoxic drugs, especially the alkylating agents, are known to be or thought to be excreted in breast milk, women in the M. D. Anderson studies were not permitted to breast-feed their newborns. In addition, a number of the antiemetics are rated as pregnancy risk factor C, and breast-feeding is not recommended when patients are taking these medications. The newer antiemetics, such as ondansetron and granisetron, are rated as pregnancy risk factor B, and these agents have been used to manage nausea in pregnant women with breast cancer who are undergoing chemotherapy.

Impact of Pregnancy on Recurrence and Survival

When pregnant and nonpregnant women with breast cancer who are the same age and have the same stage of disease are compared, pregnancy does not appear to be associated with a higher risk of breast cancer recurrence or death from breast cancer. A number of studies have concluded that women who have had chemotherapy for the treatment of breast cancer do not appear to have adverse fetal outcomes if they become pregnant after the treatment (Gallenberg and Loprinzi, 1989; Theriault, 2000). In these women, pregnancy did not appear to affect breast cancer recurrence risk or patient survival. Others are more cautious in their interpretation of the available data and conclude that the effect of posttreatment pregnancy on breast cancer prognosis is unclear (Petrek, 1996).

LEPTOMENINGEAL CARCINOMATOSIS

Leptomeningeal carcinomatosis or carcinomatous meningitis is the result of malignant solid tumor cells seeding the leptomeninges. Approximately 5% of all patients with breast cancer will have this complication, but most will have widely disseminated cancer at the time leptomeningeal carcinomatosis is diagnosed. Increasingly successful breast cancer treatment regimens enable patients to live long enough for leptomeningeal carcinomatosis to become clinically apparent. This diagnosis is serious, and without treatment, the median survival duration is 4 to 6 weeks. Death in untreated patients is secondary to progressive neurological dysfunction, and the majority of treated patients will succumb to systemic disease. At M. D. Anderson, the diagnostic and treatment procedures used in the management of patients with breast cancer who have leptomeningeal carcinomatosis are very similar to the guidelines recommended by the National Comprehensive Cancer Network (Grossman and Spence, 1999).

Clinical Presentation

Patients with leptomeningeal carcinomatosis typically present with a combination of signs and symptoms that suggest dysfunction at multiple levels of the neuraxis (i.e., cranial nerve, cerebral, and spinal). The most frequent findings are multiple cranial nerve deficits resulting in diplopia, dysphagia, dysarthria, and hearing loss. Other focal neurological deficits may include radiculopathies, stroke-like syndromes, and seizures. Patients may also present with symptoms of increased intracranial pressure, such as headache, nausea and vomiting, or symptoms of encephalopathy. Only 15% of patients with leptomeningeal carcinomatosis exhibit nuchal rigidity and mechanical difficulties. The differential diagnosis of a breast cancer patient with cranial nerve findings, particularly involvement of cranial nerve VI, includes base-of-skull syndrome. This condition is best diagnosed by thin-cut CT of the skull base and is often treated with radiation therapy.

Diagnosis

A combination of radiologic studies and cerebrospinal fluid examination is used to diagnose leptomeningeal carcinomatosis.

Radiologic Studies

To determine whether parenchymal brain metastases are present and to estimate the risk of herniation following lumbar puncture, contrast-enhanced CT or gadolinium-enhanced MRI scans of the brain should be performed. To identify leptomeningeal enhancement, gadolinium-enhanced MRI is a more sensitive approach and is the preferred test at M. D. Anderson. Scans should also be made of all regions of the neuraxis where the patient is symptomatic. Of note is that lumbar puncture alone can produce leptomeningeal contrast enhancement, which could make the interpretation of MRI more difficult if MRI is performed after diagnostic lumbar puncture (DeAngelis, 1998; Grossman and Krabak, 1999).

Abnormal findings on imaging studies are seen in approximately 50% of patients with leptomeningeal carcinomatosis. The most common imaging findings are enhancement of the basilar cisterns, cortical convexities or cauda equina, and hydrocephalus without an identifiable mass lesion. However, most of the imaging abnormalities provide information that is only consistent with or suggestive of leptomeningeal disease; thus, a diagnosis of leptomeningeal carcinomatosis requires the demonstration of malignant cells in the cerebrospinal fluid (CSF).

Cerebrospinal Fluid Examination

After studies to determine the risk of herniation in a patient with neurological signs and symptoms of leptomeningeal carcinomatosis, a lumbar puncture should be performed for diagnosis. Positive findings on cytologic examination of the CSF are found in 50% of individuals with leptomeningeal carcinomatosis on the first lumbar puncture, and 85% of those who undergo 3 high-volume (6 cc) lumbar punctures will have a positive finding (Grossman and Krabak, 1999). Patients with focal involvement of the leptomeninges are less likely to have positive findings on cytologic examination of the CSF than are patients with extensive meningeal involvement (38% vs 66%) (Glass et al, 1979).

Poor sensitivity and specificity have limited the use of biochemical markers in the analysis of the CSF in patients with leptomeningeal carcinomatosis. Beta-glucuronidase and lactic acid dehydrogenase isoenzymes can be elevated abnormally in the presence of leptomeningeal carcinomatosis, but these are nonspecific markers that can also be elevated in a number of other neurological diseases. Although the use of biomarkers such as carcinoembryonic antigen may be more reliable, the serum level of a particular biomarker can influence the level in the CSF, particularly if the blood-brain barrier has been disrupted (DeAngelis, 1998). At M. D. Anderson, tumor biomarkers are not routinely analyzed in the CSF of patients with breast cancer who have leptomeningeal carcinomatosis. Rather, the CSF is examined for the level of protein because the protein level is often elevated in leptomeningeal carcinomatosis. A low CSF glucose level can reflect a high disease burden in the leptomeninges and is thought to be a poor prognostic factor (Yap et al, 1978).

Treatment

The treatment goal for patients with leptomeningeal carcinomatosis is to prevent permanent neurological disabilities. Extant neurological deficits rarely improve. In deciding how aggressively the disease should be treated in the patient with breast cancer, several factors must be considered, including the patient's performance status, the extent of systemic disease, the extent and types of prior therapy, the presence of fixed neurological deficits, the natural history of the underlying malignancy, and the presence of any abnormalities in CSF flow. The goals of the therapeutic plan, the associated risks, and the potential complications must be carefully considered and explained in detail to the patient.

Radiation Therapy

At M. D. Anderson, most patients with breast cancer in whom leptomeningeal carcinomatosis develops receive radiation therapy to all areas of the neuraxis that appear on radiographs to have bulky disease. Focal radiation therapy is given to relieve pain and stabilize symptoms but is unlikely to produce significant neurological recovery. Nonbulky leptomeningeal disease is treated with intrathecal chemotherapy (see the section Intrathecal Chemotherapy below).

Although women with breast cancer who have leptomeningeal carcinomatosis are likely to have tumor disseminated throughout the subarachnoid compartment, irradiation of the whole neuraxis is not routinely done. Radiation therapy is often very morbid, associated with significant myelosuppression, and not curative, and it does not prevent further neurological deficits from developing.

Intrathecal Chemotherapy

Intrathecal chemotherapy is most reliably administered through an implanted subcutaneous reservoir and ventricular catheter (an Ommaya reservoir). There are several advantages to this approach: the device is well suited to outpatient care, the administration of chemotherapy is virtually painless, drug distribution may be more uniform following intraventricular administration, and the drugs are more likely to reach the CSF. Only 85% to 90% of chemotherapy is thought to be delivered to the subarachnoid space using lumbar administration. Because CSF taken from an Ommaya reservoir is less likely to demonstrate positive cytology compared with CSF sampled at the same time from the lumbar region, periodic lumbar punctures are required to monitor the efficacy of therapy in patients with an Ommaya reservoir.

Abnormalities of CSF flow are common in patients with leptomeningeal carcinomatosis. These abnormalities may influence the distribution of intrathecal chemotherapy and its subsequent efficacy and toxic effects. A CSF flow study using indium In 111 diethylenetriamine pentaacetic acid (111Indium-DTPA) is recommended before the initiation of Ommaya reservoir–administered intrathecal chemotherapy. Should abnormalities in flow be detected, radiation therapy to all areas in question is recommended.

Traditionally, only 3 chemotherapeutic agents have been used routinely in the intrathecal treatment of leptomeningeal carcinomatosis: methotrexate, cytarabine, and thiotepa. Methotrexate has been used as the first-line agent. This agent can be administered intrathecally twice a week for a total of 8 treatments or until the CSF is clear of disease cells. If the CSF clears, patients can be treated once a week and then monthly as maintenance therapy. This regimen can produce myelosuppression in patients with limited bone marrow reserve, renal insufficiency, or "third-spacing" (effusions or ascites). Folinic acid can be administered systemically to prevent possible myelosuppression or mucositis because folinic acid does not enter the CSF. At M. D. Anderson, we do not use folinic acid prophylactically for patients undergoing intrathecal methotrexate therapy. New drugs such as sustained-release cytarabine (DepoCyt) are being added to the small list of chemotherapeutic agents suitable for the treatment of leptomeningeal carcinomatosis. This formulation of cytarabine maintains cytotoxic concentrations in the CSF for more than 14 days after a single 50-mg intrathecal injection. In a recent randomized controlled trial comparing sustained-release cytarabine with methotrexate in the treatment of leptomeningeal carcinomatosis in patients with solid tumors, the 2 drugs were found to have similar response rates. Although patients treated with sustained-release cytarabine had a significantly increased time to neurological progression compared with those treated with methotrexate, there was no significant difference in survival between the 2 groups (Glantz et al, 1999).

At M. D. Anderson, our neuro-oncology colleagues are evaluating other new agents for their efficacy in the treatment of leptomeningeal carcinomatosis. Mafosfamide is currently being evaluated in a phase I trial. Mafosfamide is a chemically stable thioethane sulfonic acid salt of cyclophosphamide that spontaneously degrades to 4-hydroxycyclophosphamide, the active metabolite of cyclophosphamide. A phase I study of intrathecal topotecan, a topoisomerase I inhibitor, in the treatment of leptomeningeal carcinomatosis is also under way, and a phase II study of this drug will open soon.

Systemic Chemotherapy

The use of systemic chemotherapy in the treatment of solid-tumor leptomeningeal carcinomatosis has been limited because most patients have chemotherapy-resistant metastatic disease by the time the complication develops. We do not routinely use systemic therapy in the treatment of leptomeningeal carcinomatosis at M. D. Anderson; however, systemic chemotherapy is used concomitantly with intrathecal chemotherapy when appropriate.

Surgery

Surgery is rarely used in the treatment of leptomeningeal carcinomatosis other than for the placement of Ommaya reservoirs. In rare instances, patients with leptomeningeal carcinomatosis may benefit from the placement of a ventriculo-peritoneal shunt if there are symptoms of increased intracranial pressure that do not respond to other therapies. However, placement of such a shunt is for palliative purposes, and it interferes with subsequent administration of intrathecal chemotherapy.

Treatment-Related Toxic Effects

The placement of an Ommaya reservoir can cause perioperative complications, migration of the catheter tip from the ventricle into adjacent brain tissue, and infections. Radiation therapy may contribute to myelosuppression and to the neurotoxicity resulting from intrathecal chemotherapy. Intrathecally administered methotrexate has a number of possible toxic effects, including acute arachnoiditis with associated nausea, vomiting, and changes in mental status and the aforementioned mucositis and myelopsuppression. Seizures have been reported with high levels of methotrexate in the CSF. Common adverse events associated with the use of sustained-release cytarabine are headache and arachnoiditis. The most significant toxic effect seen in the treatment of leptomeningeal carcinomatosis is necrotizing leukoencephalopathy, which is most common in patients who receive intrathecal chemotherapy after cranial irradiation. Patients develop progressive dementia and other neurological complications, which lead to progressive, irreversible disability and ultimately death.

Prognosis

Of all solid tumors, breast cancer responds best to treatment for leptomeningeal carcinomatosis, with many patients experiencing an improvement in symptoms and some experiencing a remission with regard to this complication. The median survival duration for breast cancer patients from time of diagnosis of leptomeningeal carcinomatosis is 6 months, with 11% to 25% of patients alive 1 year after diagnosis (DeAngelis, 1998).

EPIDURAL SPINAL CORD COMPRESSION

Epidural spinal cord compression is an oncologic emergency requiring prompt diagnosis and treatment. The incidence of ESCC in patients with breast cancer is approximately 4%, and the overall incidence of ESCC in patients with cancer is 5%. Of all cases of ESCC diagnosed, 7% to 32% occur in patients with breast cancer (Freilich and Foley, 1996). Most of the patients with breast cancer who develop ESCC have known bony metastases at the time of onset of neurological symptoms. In their study of 70 patients with breast cancer, Hill et al (1993) reported that the median time from breast cancer diagnosis to the onset of ESCC was 42 months (range, 0–336 months). The median time from a diagnosis of bony metastasis to the development of ESCC in this series was 11 months (range, 0–90 months).

Epidural metastases arise most commonly from the vertebral column, although approximately 10% to 15% arise from metastases to the paravertebral space. Rarely do epidural metastases arise from direct hematogenous spread to the epidural space or to the parenchyma of the spinal cord. Breast cancer patients with metastases to their spine typically have multilevel involvement. Epidural spinal cord compression in breast cancer patients usually occurs in the thoracic spine, the narrowest part of the spinal canal.

Clinical Presentation

The most common complaint of patients with ESCC is pain. Most patients with ESCC will have pain for more than 1 week before a diagnosis is made, with the mean duration of pain being 6 weeks. Pain can precede other symptoms by a median of 7 weeks. Increasing back pain is an ominous sign of the possibility of ESCC in a woman with breast cancer. There are 3 types of pain associated with ESCC: local, radicular, and referred. Almost all patients have local pain that presents as a constant ache. Radicular pain, usually described as a shooting pain, is less common with thoracic lesions and is more common with cervical or lumbosacral disease. In the case of cervical and lumbosacral epidural metastases, radicular pain is usually unilateral, whereas in the case of thoracic disease, it is usually bilateral. Thoracic epidural metastases may produce pain in the lateral or anterior chest wall more commonly than pain in the back itself. Referred pain occurs distant to the lesion in question, and this type of pain does not radiate. Patients with epidural metastases typically complain of increased pain when they are in the supine position and during Valsalva maneuvers such as coughing, sneezing, and straining with bowel movements. Certain stretching maneuvers (e.g., neck flexion in the case of cervical or upper thoracic lesions and straight leg raising with thoracic or lumbosacral lesions) may also increase the pain from ESCC.

Another characteristic clinical finding in patients with ESCC is myelopathy. Patients may complain of limb weakness, numbness, and paresthesia as well as sphincter disturbance, which may manifest as urinary retention, urinary urgency, urge incontinence, and constipation. In one report, at the time of diagnosis of ESCC, 76% of patients complained of weakness, 87% were weak on examination, 57% had autonomic dysfunction, 51% had sensory symptoms, and 78% had sensory deficits on examination (Gilbert et al, 1978). Some studies have reported that fewer than 50% of patients with ESCC are ambulatory at diagnosis, and up to 25% are paraplegic at diagnosis. On examination, patients with a myelopathy may have paraparesis or quadriparesis, increased muscle tone, clonus, hyperreflexia, extensor plantar responses, a distended bladder, and a sensory level. Although the sensory, motor, and reflex levels may indicate the level of disease, the sensory level may be several segments below the actual ESCC, and there may be multiple sites of epidural disease (Freilich and Foley, 1996).

In the case of ESCC at the conus medullaris or the cauda equina, pain is still a prominent feature, but the neurological signs and symptoms are quite different. Lesions at the conus medullaris usually produce early and marked sphincter disturbance as well as perineal sensory loss. Cauda equina lesions produce patchy lower-motor-neuron signs, including hyporeflexia or areflexia, myotomal leg weakness, and dermatomal sensory loss. The loss of sphincter tone is usually a late event in cauda equina lesions and is typically less marked than what is seen with lesions of the conus medullaris.

Diagnosis

A thorough history and physical examination should be performed to elicit signs and symptoms suggestive of spinal cord compression. Patients whose signs and symptoms are suggestive of ESCC require emergency evaluation.

Radiologic evaluation is used to confirm the presence of ESCC and determine its extent. In 72% of patients with ESCC, bony abnormalities can be detected on plain radiographs. In cancer patients with back pain, plain radiographs can be used to detect the presence and location of epidural metastases in 83% of cases. However, if there is significant suspicion of ESCC based on clinical findings, negative findings on plain radiographs should not preclude further investigation. At M. D. Anderson, MRI with gadolinium is the imaging method of choice for the detection of epidural metastases. Magnetic resonance imaging is noninvasive, is more sensitive and more specific than bone scintigraphy for the detection of spinal metastases, and is as accurate as myelography or CT in detecting spinal cord compression. In addition, MRI may be superior to myelography and CT in the identification of epidural metastases between myelographic blocks and in the detection of additional sites of bony metastases. It is also useful for identifying paravertebral tumors. Computed tomography or myelography is used when MRI is not diagnostic, when MRI is unavailable, when patients are unable to remain still during the MRI, or when the patient is claustrophobic or has severe scoliosis. Computed tomography is superior to MRI in the evaluation of vertebral stability and cortical bone destruction and thus is performed before surgical intervention.

Treatment

The treatment of ESCC at M. D. Anderson is a multidisciplinary effort that involves the neurology, neurosurgery, and radiation oncology services. In consultations between these services, clinicians determine the best treatment plan for the patient. Treatment should be given promptly to preserve or recover neurological function or prevent further deterioration in neurological function. In patients with cancer and ESCC, the amount of neurological dysfunction is the strongest determinant of treatment outcome. For example, approximately 20% to 60% of cancer patients who are paraparetic secondary to ESCC recover ambulation, whereas 80% of patients who have little to no difficulty with ambulation retain the ability to walk. Fewer than 10% of patients with cancer who have paraplegia at presentation improve with treatment (Freilich and Foley, 1996). Improvement or preservation of neurological function is one of the primary goals of treatment in patients with ESCC. Other goals include the palliation of pain, prevention of local recurrence, and preservation of spinal stability.

Systemic Therapy

Dexamethasone should be administered when a diagnosis of ESCC has been made as well as in cases in which there is a high clinical suspicion of ESCC but definitive radiographic investigation is pending. The optimal dose and schedule of dexamethasone have not been determined, and there is some controversy with regard to the benefit of low-dose versus high-dose steroids. Patients may obtain greater pain relief with higher-dose steroids. Most clinicians administer a loading dose of at least 10 mg of dexamethasone with subsequent doses of 4 to 24 mg every 6 hours. Depending on the individual treatment plan and response, dexamethasone should eventually be given orally, and the dose should be tapered after definitive treatment is completed.

After initial treatment of ESCC with steroids, radiation therapy, or surgery (with or without radiation therapy), consideration should be given to systemic therapy for the patient's breast cancer. Systemic therapy consisting of chemotherapy with or without hormonal therapy may also be used as initial treatment for patients in whom radiation therapy or surgery is not an option. For individuals who develop ESCC as a result of breast cancer metastasis to bone, the use of pamidronate disodium (Aredia) should be considered.

Surgery

There are no published prospective randomized studies that compare surgery alone with radiation therapy alone in the treatment of ESCC. There are certain situations in which surgery is the preferred treatment modality for ESCC. Spinal instability, redevelopment of epidural compression at a previously irradiated site, rapid progression of neurological dysfunction during radiation therapy, and cord compression secondary to retropulsion of bony fragments are examples of situations in which surgery should be the first option.

Anterior decompression of the spinal cord with mechanical stabilization is the treatment of choice for epidural metastases arising from the vertebral body. Laminectomy is reserved for the removal of posterior tumors. Walsh et al (1997) reported the results of 61 patients at M. D. Anderson (the majority of whom had metastatic cancer) in whom thoracic spine tumors were removed by anterior resections to alleviate critical spinal cord compromise. Most of the patients had improvement in pain control (90%) and recovery of ambulatory function (75%). After surgery, patients may be assessed to determine whether radiation therapy is needed. Patients who have residual tumor after surgery may derive significant benefit from postoperative radiation therapy (Loblaw and Laperriere, 1998).

Radiation Therapy

Radiation therapy is the treatment of choice for ESCC in patients who have not previously been irradiated in the area in question, do not have spinal instability, and do not have compression from retropulsed bone. Radiation therapy has been found to decrease pain in 70% of patients with cancer and ESCC. Motor function is improved in 45% to 60% of patients, and in 11% to 16% of patients, paraplegia is reversed. Neurological function before treatment is the most important measure of neurological recovery.

The radiation fields should be centered on the site of epidural compression. Radiation portals usually extend 2 vertebral bodies above and 2 below the site of compression because it has been demonstrated that recurrent epidural disease will usually occur within 2 vertebral bodies of the initial site of spinal cord compression. The treatment port should also include any adjacent sites of bone involvement as well as any paravertebral masses.

HYPERCALCEMIA

Hypercalcemia is the most common metabolic cancer-associated emergency. Hypercalcemia of malignancy is estimated to occur in 10% to 20% of cancer patients, with lung and breast being the 2 tumor sites most commonly associated with this complication. The main cause of hypercalcemia of malignancy is the increased amount of calcium released from the bone. The tumor secretes humoral and paracrine factors that markedly stimulate osteoclast activity and proliferation and often inhibit osteoblast activity. The result is an uncoupling between bone resorption and bone formation. The parathyroid hormone-related protein is integral to the development of hypercalcemia from a number of tumor types (Grill et al, 1991).

Patients with hypercalcemia of malignancy can have profound intravascular volume depletion secondary to the polyuria from hypercalciuria. Saline infusion is the most effective means of restoring intravascular volume. The volume required to establish a brisk diuresis can be as much as 4 to 6 liters, which should be administered as quickly as possible (for example, starting at 250 cc/h). However, the manner in which rehydration is conducted is influenced by the patient's symptoms, the patient's known or presumed cardiac function, and the degree of hypercalcemia. Although some trials have reported the use of loop diuretics to increase calciuresis, the use of such diuretics should be limited to the relief of volume overload resulting from vigorous rehydration.

The bisphosphonates have become front-line agents in the treatment of hypercalcemia of malignancy. These agents bind avidly to hydroxyapatite crystals and inhibit bone resorption. The use of bisphosphonates in individuals whose corrected serum calcium level is 12 mg/dL (3.0 mmol/L) or greater is accepted as standard treatment. Patients who are symptomatic and whose corrected serum calcium level is less than 12 mg/dL should also be treated with bisphosphonates. Although there is some controversy in the literature regarding the treatment of asymptomatic patients whose corrected serum calcium level is less than 12 mg/dL, at M. D. Anderson, such patients are usually treated with bisphosphonates. Because many of our patients with known bony metastases are on monthly infusions of pamidronate disodium, severe, life-threatening hypercalcemia is an uncommon occurrence among patients with breast cancer at our institution.

The bisphosphonate most commonly used in the treatment of hypercalcemia at M. D. Anderson is pamidronate disodium at a dose of 90 mg administered intravenously over 2 hours (Hortobagyi et al, 1996; Theriault et al, 1999). In randomized clinical trials, pamidronate disodium has been shown to be more effective than etidronate disodium in the treatment of hypercalcemia of malignancy. Clodronate disodium, an oral bisphosphonate, is not approved for use in the United States for the treatment of hypercalcemia. Studies of newer and more potent bisphosphonates, such as zoledronate, are under way.

Calcitonin binds directly to osteoclast receptors and inhibits osteoclastic bone degradation. This agent acts rapidly to lower serum calcium, but the duration of the hypocalcemic effect is short, with tachyphylaxis developing within 72 hours. Calcitonin has been shown to be effective in 60% to 80% of patients treated. Since the development of the bisphosphonates, the use of calcitonin is primarily limited to the first 48 hours of the treatment of severe, life-threatening hypercalcemia.

In cases of hormone-sensitive breast cancer, corticosteroids have been reported to be of value in restoring normal calcium levels. At M. D. Anderson, corticosteroids are used in patients with hormone-sensitive breast cancer for the treatment of severe and life-threatening hypercalcemia.

The use of other agents, such as gallium nitrate and plicamycin, has been supplanted by the use of bisphosphonates in the treatment of hypercalcemia of malignancy.

SECOND MALIGNANCIES

Women who have a history of breast cancer are at increased risk for other malignancies, either as a result of treatment for their breast cancer or because of genetic susceptibility. As part of their routine follow-up, a thorough medical history and physical examination are conducted for all women with a history of breast cancer. Any signs or symptoms noted should be considered suggestive of a second malignancy and should be appropriately investigated.

Treatment-Related Second Malignancies

Treatment-related second malignancies in women with a history of breast cancer include lung cancer, leukemia, endometrial cancer, and contralateral breast cancer.

Lung Cancer

A number of studies have examined the risk for lung cancer among women with breast cancer who are treated with local radiation therapy.

Women who are exposed to radiation are at highest risk for lung cancer if it has been at least 10 years past their initial diagnosis of breast cancer, and the risk is greater among smokers. Not surprising, lung cancer develops most often in the ipsilateral lung, where radiation exposure is the greatest. At M. D. Anderson, all patients with breast cancer are encouraged to stop smoking. Patients can be referred to smoking cessation programs offered at our institution. For women treated with radiation therapy, a yearly chest radiograph is performed. Any signs or symptoms that cause concern, such as shortness of breath and cough, are investigated.

Leukemia

There is an increased risk for treatment-induced myelodysplastic syndrome (MDS) and acute myeloid leukemia (AML) in patients with breast cancer who are treated with adjuvant chemotherapy. Diamandidou et al (1996) reported the incidence of treatment-related leukemia in patients with breast cancer who were treated with FAC chemotherapy. The 10-year estimated incidence of leukemia was 1.5% (95% confidence interval [CI], 0.75%–2.9%) for all patients treated. The chemotherapy-only group had a 10-year estimated incidence of leukemia of 0.5% (95% CI, 0.1%–2.4%), and in the radiation-therapy-plus-chemotherapy group, the rate was 2.5% (95% CI, 1.0%–5.1%). The difference in the estimated 10-year incidence of leukemia between these 2 groups was statistically significant. Other studies have also noted that the combination of chemotherapy and radiation therapy has a multiplicative effect on the overall risk for leukemia in patients with breast cancer. DeCillis et al (1997) reported the incidence of MDS or AML in the National Surgical Adjuvant Breast and Bowel Project (NSABP) trial B-25, a trial designed to assess the effectiveness of higher doses of cyclophosphamide in combination with standard-dose doxorubicin. The cumulative 4-year incidence of MDS or AML in the NSABP B-25 study was 0.87%. This incidence was higher than the rate seen in other NSABP trials that used the more standard dose of cyclophosphamide (600 mg/m^2). The combination regimen of cyclophosphamide, epirubicin, and 5-fluorouracil (CEF) was compared with the combination of cyclophosphamide, methotrexate, and 5-fluorouracil (CMF) in patients with node-positive breast cancer. The epirubicin-containing regimen was associated with a significantly greater risk of leukemia (1.42% of patients in the CEF group vs no patients in the CMF group, with a median latency period of 66 months) (Levine et al, 1998).

There is some controversy as to whether high-dose chemotherapy with stem cell support is associated with an increased risk for MDS or AML. A number of investigators have suggested that it is the chemotherapy given for the primary malignancy rather than that given for the transplant that increases the risk for MDS or AML.

Physicians caring for patients with a history of breast cancer who have been exposed to alkylating agents such as cyclophosphamide or topoisomerase II inhibitors (e.g., doxorubicin or epirubicin) should be aware of the increased risk for MDS and AML in these patients, particularly those also treated with radiation therapy. Signs and symptoms suggestive of MDS or AML should be thoroughly investigated.

Endometrial Cancer

The use of tamoxifen is associated with an increased risk for endometrial cancer, and this risk increases with prolonged duration of use. Fisher et al (1994) reported that the use of tamoxifen as adjuvant therapy for breast cancer in the NSABP B-14 trial was associated with a relative risk of 2.2 for development of endometrial cancer. Although most of the endometrial cancers that occurred were of good to moderate histologic grade and were stage I, 4 patients died from uterine cancer. Despite the fact that a number of other studies have also reported increased risk for uterine cancer among women exposed to tamoxifen, the benefits of tamoxifen for the adjuvant treatment of primary breast cancer are thought to outweigh the risk.

A recent study concluded that routine transvaginal sonograpy in asymptomatic women being treated with tamoxifen was not worthwhile because of a high rate of false-positive diagnoses and a low frequency of significant findings (Love et al, 1999). At M. D. Anderson, we do not perform routine transvaginal sonography in patients undergoing tamoxifen therapy. All women with an intact uterus have a yearly pelvic examination as well as a Papanicolaou smear. A history of vaginal spotting would indicate the need for prompt and thorough evaluation, including transvaginal sonography and a gynecologic consultation.

Contralateral Breast Cancer

A number of population-based studies have concluded that breast cancer survivors have a 2- to 5-fold increased risk for contralateral breast cancer compared with women with no history of breast cancer. Women with a breast cancer history have an average annual risk of approximately 0.5% to 0.7% of developing a second breast cancer. Known breast cancer risk factors such as family history and nulliparity are associated with a further increased risk of a contralateral breast cancer.

There is some controversy in the literature as to whether exposure to radiation therapy for local treatment of breast cancer increases the risk of contralateral breast cancer. The literature has been difficult to evaluate because a number of the population-based studies were unable to control for factors known to influence the risk of breast cancer, and there may have been inaccuracies in the data. In a retrospective study of patients with stage II and III breast cancer at M. D. Anderson who received postoperative radiation therapy, it was concluded that the patients treated with radiation therapy were at increased risk for a second primary breast cancer compared with patients who did not receive radiation therapy.

KEY PRACTICE POINTS

- Modified radical mastectomy with axillary lymph node dissection is the surgical treatment of choice in pregnant women with breast cancer.
- The experience at M. D. Anderson indicates that FAC chemotherapy can be safely administered during the second and third trimesters of pregnancy.
- Leptomeningeal carcinomatosis is diagnosed using a combination of clinical presentation, cytologic examination of the CSF, and MRI. The primary treatment is intrathecal methotrexate administered via an Ommaya reservoir, although sustained-release cytarabine appears promising.
- Epidural spinal cord compression is usually diagnosed by MRI and is treated with corticosteroids, radiation therapy, or surgery with or without radiation therapy.
- Hypercalcemia is best treated with bisphosphonates, particularly pamidronate disodium.
- Women with breast cancer who are treated with radiation therapy, chemotherapy, hormonal therapy, or a combination of these are at increased risk for second malignancies, particularly lung cancer (especially in smokers who are exposed to radiation therapy), MDS and AML, endometrial cancer, and contralateral breast cancer.

All women with a history of breast cancer followed at M. D. Anderson have a thorough clinical breast examination at every follow-up appointment. They also have yearly diagnostic mammography of the contralateral breast and the remaining breast if breast-conserving surgery was performed. Any clinically or radiographically suspicious masses are further investigated.

Second Malignancies Caused by Genetic Susceptibility

For information about second malignancies resulting from hereditary breast or ovarian cancer syndromes, please see chapter 3.

Suggested Readings

Berry DL, Theriault RL, Holmes FA, et al. Management of breast cancer during pregnancy using a standardized protocol. *J Clin Oncol* 1999;17:855–861.

Body JJ, Bartl R, Burckhardt P, et al. Current use of bisphosphonates in oncology. International Bone and Cancer Study Group. *J Clin Oncol* 1998;16:3890–3899.

Buzdar A, Hortobagyi GN, Kau S, Singletary E. Increased risk of second primary breast cancer (SPBC) after radiotherapy for treatment of breast cancer. *Proceedings of the American Association for Cancer Research* 1993;34:227. Abstract 1358.

Code of Federal Regulations: Title 21, Volume 4, Parts 200–299, revised April 1, 1997.

Collins JC, Liao S, Wile AG. Surgical management of breast masses in pregnant women. *J Reprod Med* 1995;40:785–788.

DeAngelis LM. Current diagnosis and treatment of leptomeningeal metastasis. *J Neurooncol* 1998;38:245–252.

DeCillis A, Anderson S, Bryant J, Wickerham DL, Fisher B. Acute myeloid leukemia (AML) and myelodysplastic syndrome (MDS) on NSABP B-25: an update. *Proceedings of the American Society of Clinical Oncology* 1997;130A. Abstract 459.

Diamandidou E, Buzdar AU, Smith TL, Frye D, Witjaksono M, Hortobagyi GN. Treatment-related leukemia in breast cancer patients treated with fluorouracil-doxorubicin-cyclophosphamide combination adjuvant chemotherapy: The University of Texas M. D. Anderson Cancer Center experience. *J Clin Oncol* 1996;14:2722–2730.

DiFronzo LA, O'Connell TX. Breast cancer in pregnancy and lactation. *Surg Clin North Am* 1996;76:267–278.

Doll DC, Ringenberg QS, Yarbro JW. Antineoplastic agents and pregnancy. *Semin Oncol* 1989;16:337–346.

Elledge RM, Ciocca DR, Langone G, McGuire WL. Estrogen receptor, progesterone receptor, and HER-2/neu protein in breast cancers from pregnant patients. *Cancer* 1993;71:2499–2506.

Fisher B, Costantino JP, Redmond CK, Fisher ER, Wickerham DL, Cronin WM. Endometrial cancer in tamoxifen-treated breast cancer patients: findings from the National Surgical Adjuvant Breast and Bowel Project (NSABP) B-14. *J Natl Cancer Inst* 1994;86:527–537.

Flickinger FW, Sanal SM. Bone marrow MRI: techniques and accuracy for detecting breast cancer metastases. *Magn Reson Imaging* 1994;12:829–835.

Freilich RJ, Foley KM. Epidural metastasis. In: Harris JR, Lippman ME, Morrow M, Hellman S, eds. *Diseases of the Breast*. Philadelphia: Lippincott-Raven; 1996:779–789.

Fuller BG, Heiss J, Oldfield EH. Spinal cord compression. In: DeVita VT Jr, Hellman S, Rosenberg SA, eds. *Cancer: Principles and Practice of Oncology*. Vol. 2. 5th ed. Philadelphia: Lippincott-Raven; 1997:2476–2486.

Gallenberg MM, Loprinzi CL. Breast cancer and pregnancy. *Semin Oncol* 1989; 16:369–376.

Gilbert RW, Kim JH, Posner JB. Epidural spinal cord compression from metastatic tumor: diagnosis and treatment. *Ann Neurol* 1978;3:40–51.

Glantz MJ, Jaeckle KA, Chamberlain MC, et al. A randomized controlled trial comparing intrathecal sustained-release cytarabine (DepoCyt) to intrathecal methotrexate in patients with neoplastic meningitis from solid tumors. *Clin Cancer Res* 1999;5:3394–3402.

Glass JP, Melamed M, Chernik NL, Posner JB. Malignant cells in cerebrospinal fluid (CSF): the meaning of positive CSF cytology. *Neurology* 1979;29:1369–1375.

Grill V, Ho P, Body JJ, et al. Parathyroid hormone-related protein: elevated levels in both humoral hypercalcemia of malignancy and hypercalcemia complicating metastatic breast cancer. *J Clin Endocrinol Metab* 1991;73:1309–1315.

Grossman SA, Krabak MJ. Leptomeningeal carcinomatosis. *Cancer Treat Rev* 1999;25:103–119.

Grossman SA, Spence A. NCCN clinical practice guidelines for carcinomatous/lymphomatous meningitis. *Oncology* 1999;13:144–152,

Hill ME, Richards MA, Gregory WM, Smith P, Rubens RD. Spinal cord compression in breast cancer: a review of 70 cases. *Br J Cancer* 1993;68:969–973.

Hortobagyi GN, Frye D, Buzdar AU, et al. Decreased cardiac toxicity of doxorubicin administered by continuous intravenous infusion in combination chemotherapy for metastatic breast carcinoma. *Cancer* 1989;63:37–45.

Hortobagyi GN, Theriault RL, Porter L, et al. Efficacy of pamidronate in reducing skeletal complications in patients with breast cancer and lytic bone metastases. Protocol 19 Aredia Breast Cancer Study Group. *N Eng J Med* 1996;335:1785–1791.

Jackisch C, Schwenkhagen A, Louwen F, Brandt B, Holzgreve W, Schneider HPG. Breast cancer in pregnancy. *Proceedings of the American Society of Clinical Oncology* 1995;14:132A. Abstract 228.

Levine MN, Bramwell VH, Pritchard KI, et al. Randomized trial of intensive cyclophosphamide, epirubicin, and fluorouracil chemotherapy compared with cyclophosphamide, methotrexate, and fluorouracil in premenopausal women with node-positive breast cancer. National Cancer Institute of Canada Clinical Trials Group. *J Clin Oncol* 1998;16:2651–2658.

Liberman L, Giess CS, Dershaw DD, Deutch BM, Petrek JA. Imaging of pregnancy-associated breast cancer. *Radiology* 1994;191:245–248.

Loblaw DA, Laperriere NJ. Emergency treatment of malignant extradural spinal cord compression: an evidence-based guideline. *J Clin Oncol* 1998;16:1613–1624.

Love CD, Muir BB, Scrimgeour JB, Leonard RC, Dillon P, Dixon JM. Investigation of endometrial abnormalities in asymptomatic women treated with tamoxifen and an evaluation of the role of endometrial screening. *J Clin Oncol* 1999;17:2050–2054.

Max MH, Klamer TW. Pregnancy and breast cancer. *South Med J* 1983;76:1088–1090.

Neugut AI, Weinberg MD, Ahsan H, Rescigno J. Carcinogenic effects of radiotherapy for breast cancer. *Oncology (Huntingt)* 1999;13:1245–1256.

Petrek JA. Breast cancer and pregnancy. In: Harris JR, Lippman ME, Morrow M, Hellman S, eds. *Diseases of the Breast.* Philadelphia: Lippincott-Raven; 1996:883–892.

Sanal SM, Flickinger FW, Caudell MJ, et al. Detection of bone marrow involvement in breast cancer with magnetic resonance imaging. J Clin Oncol 1994; 12:1415–1421.

Sobecks RM, Le Beau MM, Anastasi J, Williams SF. Myelodysplasia and acute leukemia following high-dose chemotherapy and autologous bone marrow or peripheral blood stem cell transplantation. *Bone Marrow Transplant* 1999;23:1161–1165.

Theriault RL. Breast cancer during pregnancy. In: Singletary ES, Robb GL, eds. *Advanced Therapy of Breast Disease.* Hamilton: B. C. Decker; 2000:167–173.

Theriault RL. Hypercalcemia of malignancy: pathophysiology and implications for treatment. *Oncology (Huntingt)* 1993;7:47–50.

Theriault RL, Lipton A, Hortobagyi GN, et al. Pamidronate reduces skeletal morbidity in women with advanced breast cancer and lytic bone lesions: a randomized, placebo-controlled trial. Protocol 18 Aredia Breast Cancer Study Group. *J Clin Oncol* 1999;17:846–854.

Tobon H, Horowitz, LF. Breast cancer during pregnancy. *Breast Disease* 1993;6:127–134.

Walsh GL, Gokaslan ZL, McCutcheon IE, et al. Anterior approaches to the thoracic spine in patients with cancer: indications and results. *Ann Thorac Surg* 1997;64:1611–1618.

Yap HY, Yap BS, Tashima CK, DiStefano A, Blumenschein GR. Meningeal carcinomatosis in breast cancer. *Cancer* 1978;42:283–286.

16 REHABILITATION OF PATIENTS WITH BREAST CANCER

Anne N. Truong

CHAPTER OVERVIEW

Growing concern exists regarding the impact of breast cancer and its treatment on patients' quality of life. Sequelae of modified radical mastectomy or segmental mastectomy with axillary lymph node dissection may include pain, shoulder dysfunction, and lymphedema. A rehabilitation team consisting of a physiatrist, a physical therapist, and an occupational therapist can comprehensively and appropriately assess physical disabilities and prescribe an individual treatment plan. Early mobilization of the affected arm with supervision by the therapist can accelerate return of range of motion, decrease pain, and reduce emotional trauma without increasing the risk of postsurgical complications. Restoration of function of the patient's extremity produces a sense of recovery and control in the patient's life. Lymphedema can be managed with complex decongestive therapy performed by a physical therapist under the physiatrist's supervision. The rehabilitation team can assist the patient in correcting self-care and mobility deficits and transitioning from an inpatient to an outpatient setting. The physical and emotional recovery course is proportional to the extent of the surgery. Early intervention by the rehabilitation team can minimize long-term disability, thereby improving quality of life.

INTRODUCTION

Advances in early cancer detection and improved multimodality treatments are increasing the number of breast cancer survivors. Issues of quality of life are becoming ever more relevant and critical in the spectrum of cancer treatment. Survivors often face physical and psychosocial impairments that adversely affect their quality of life. Recognition of potential complications from breast cancer treatment can minimize these traumatic insults to the patient.

Prevention and restoration of function should be addressed as early in the treatment course as possible. In general practice, a multidisciplinary team approach is utilized only after complications develop. At M. D. Anderson Cancer Center, however, the multidisciplinary rehabilitation team assesses the patient soon after surgery and suggests early preventive measures designed to help the patient reach maximal functional recovery. Members of the rehabilitation team include a physiatrist (physician specializing in physical medicine and rehabilitation), a physical therapist, and an occupational therapist.

At M. D. Anderson, we have the unique opportunity to work with physicians from multiple specialties, such as surgical oncology, radiation oncology, and medical oncology, who provide preventive and comprehensive measures to ensure that breast cancer patients reach their maximal potential. This chapter describes the rehabilitation approach used at M. D. Anderson to minimize morbidity associated with breast cancer treatment and accelerate patients' recovery to the best possible quality of life. Most of the chapter focuses on rehabilitation after modified radical mastectomy or segmental mastectomy with axillary lymph node dissection (ALND). The last part of the chapter discusses rehabilitation issues in patients with metastatic disease and psychosocial and vocational rehabilitation after breast cancer treatment.

Integration of Rehabilitation and Breast Cancer Treatment

Cancer rehabilitation is a subspecialty of physical medicine and rehabilitation concerned with many broad areas of human function, including physical, psychological, social, and vocational activities. The goal of cancer rehabilitation is to help each patient achieve maximum function in all these areas within the limitations imposed by the disease or its treatment. Patients can benefit from a physical medicine and rehabilitation referral when they are not functioning at their maximal level, regardless of the extent of their disease. A physician can begin this process by evaluating the several components of function (physical, psychological, and vocational) in each cancer patient before treatment and referring patients to a physiatrist when there are deficits in any of these functional components. The physiatrist will evaluate the patient and determine an appropriate setting for rehabilitation (hospital, subacute hospital, home care, or ambulatory care) and an individualized therapeutic program.

Until recently, the typical role of physiatrists in the treatment of breast cancer patients was to consult on patients with shoulder dysfunction years after the surgery. With this delayed approach, therapeutic measures designed to improve the scarred tissue and the arthrosclerotic joint often brought about little improvement. In recent years, recognizing that musculoskeletal and soft-tissue reparative responses to surgery are amenable to manual therapy before the tissue becomes scar tissue, physiatrists have begun to see patients soon after surgery. As a result, patients now regain shoulder function more rapidly, have less pain, and are better able to resume activities of daily living.

Potential Physical Sequelae of Modified Radical Mastectomy or Segmental Mastectomy with Axillary Lymph Node Dissection

After surgical treatment of breast cancer, physical impairments of varying degrees can develop that affect survivors' quality of life. The risk of physical impairment and the degree of impairment are similar in patients who undergo modified radical mastectomy and patients who undergo segmental mastectomy with ALND. Unfortunately, the physical problems that may ensue after surgery are frequently not fully discussed with the patient before surgery.

Modified radical mastectomy and segmental mastectomy with ALND can lead to disabling shoulder dysfunction, swelling, lymphedema, and pain. Such sequelae lead to limitations in activities of daily living and reduction in the overall level of physical activity. Common findings after modified radical mastectomy or segmental mastectomy with ALND include disorganized fibrous tissue deposits (described as "cordlike" bands) in the axillary area that restrict range of motion of the shoulder in all planes (Figures 16–1 and 16–2); myofascial or soft tissue contractures; and adhesions to nearby structures (Figure 16–2).

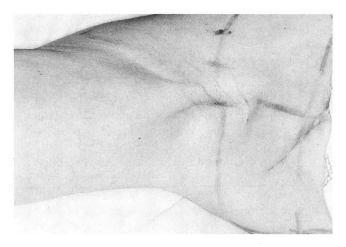

Figure 16–1. Cording in the axilla in a patient who received radiation therapy.

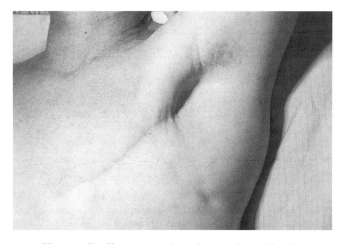

Figure 16–2. Chest wall adhesions and cording in the axilla after mastectomy.

Ganz and colleagues (1987) studied the immediate (1 month) physical and constitutional problems that occur after modified radical mastectomy. Their main findings are summarized in Table 16–1. After surgery, patients have mechanical limitation in shoulder movement and have pain in the axilla with shoulder movement. Shoulder immobility, weakness, and pain are common sequelae of mastectomy. Because neurogenic pain can be exacerbated by myofascial inflexibility due to immobility, pain is a common complaint long after modified radical mastectomy. In a 1994 survey of breast cancer survivors 16 months to 32 years after surgery, the reported incidence of physical impairments was as follows: arm numbness, 81%; arm and forearm pain, 65%; limitations in activities of daily living, 52%; arm weakness, 36%; and arm swelling, 34% (Polinsky, 1994).

ASSESSMENT OF THE PATIENT AFTER SURGERY

In assessment of the patient after breast cancer surgery, the extremity, the upper trunk, and the rest of the body are considered together as a closed kinetic chain. Impairment in 1 structure leads to an imbalance in the rest of the structures, and this imbalance leads to compensation and, consequently, overuse and decompensation. The goal of rehabilitation is to recognize this biomechanical imbalance and reset the involved structures to the previous or a new equilibrium.

At M. D. Anderson, patients are referred to physical medicine and rehabilitation soon after breast cancer surgery. The physical medicine and rehabilitation team can screen for premorbid problems of the upper trunk, which may affect the postsurgical recovery of the extremity. Examples of such premorbid conditions include cervical neck disorders, radiculopathy, arthritis, bursitis, rotator cuff derangements, and adhesive capsulitis.

Immediately after modified radical mastectomy or segmental mastectomy with ALND, functional problems that may be seen include postural

Table 16–1. Physical Problems Experienced by Patients 1 Month After Modified Radical Mastectomy

Tightness of chest wall	85%
Fatigue	80%
Limited upper extremity mobility	68%
Arm weakness	65%
Lymphedema	40%
Arm numbness	30%

Source: Ganz PA, Schag CC, Polinsky ML, Heinrich RL, Flack VF. Rehabilitation needs and breast cancer: the first month after primary therapy. *Breast Cancer Res Treat* 1987;10:243–253.

abnormality, range-of-motion deficits in the glenohumeral joint, and elbow problems due to cording (Figure 16–3). Limited chest wall movement, pectoralis muscle spasm, abnormal scapular movement, and a winged scapula due to long thoracic or thoracodorsal nerve neurapraxia might also be seen shortly after surgery.

Patients who have undergone immediate breast reconstruction are at risk for additional problems. Patients who have undergone reconstruction with a transverse rectus abdominis myocutaneous (TRAM) flap may be at risk for back pain or sacroiliac joint dysfunction because of the harvesting of muscle and subcutaneous tissue from the abdominal wall. This biomechanical imbalance of a weakened abdominal wall can increase the risk of other problems after breast cancer surgery. Patients who have undergone reconstruction with a latissimus dorsi pedicled flap can have significantly altered glenohumeral and scapular rhythm, leading to severe shoulder mobilization problems. For these patients, longer duration of treatment with an experienced therapist is crucial to recovery.

Timing of Physical Therapy

An important issue in rehabilitation of the breast cancer patient is how soon after surgery to initiate physical therapy. Recommendations in the literature regarding the timing of therapeutic interventions after modified radical mastectomy or segmental mastectomy with ALND are quite varied. Some authors advocate shoulder immobilization in the immediate postoperative period, others advocate early mobilization of the shoulder,

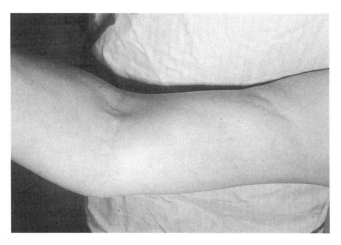

Figure 16–3. Cording in the right arm and forearm.

and still others report that the timing of shoulder mobilization has no effect on outcome.

Past studies advocated shoulder immobilization in the early postoperative period to prevent postoperative complications. However, these studies that advocate shoulder immobilization have several deficiencies. These studies did not evaluate total drain output prior to removal of drains and did not measure range of motion before and after breast cancer surgery. Furthermore, in these studies, mobilization of the shoulder was not performed by or supervised by therapists.

Jansen and colleagues (1990) compared the effect of immediate and delayed (postoperative day 8) shoulder exercises on rehabilitation after ALND and found that the 2 approaches produced similar outcomes. They measured range of motion of the shoulder before and immediately after surgery and found that range of motion decreased by half after surgery. Range of motion improved with both early and delayed mobilization; however, at 6 months after surgery, range of motion was still slightly reduced (by 20 degrees) in both groups as compared with presurgery measurements. The investigators postulated that shoulder and arm motion pump lymphatic fluid into the axillary fossa and dead space. This motion may also create a shearing force that might damage flaps used for breast reconstruction.

The effect of early or delayed physical therapy on seroma formation is another important question. Seromas are accumulations of lymphatic fluid that form under the skin flaps after drains are removed. Seromas interfere with wound healing, often require prolonged treatment, and can delay further adjuvant therapy. They are also associated with lymphedema. The reported incidence of seromas after modified radical mastectomy or segmental mastectomy with ALND ranges widely, from 15% to 40%. Tadych and Donegan (1987) found that immobilization of the arm did not alter the frequency of seromas. Two parameters that did correlate directly with the frequency of seromas were drainage during the last 24 hours prior to removal of suction drains and total drain output. Seromas were minimized if drains were removed when output was less than 30 cc within 24 hours. Drain output was greater in the early-mobilization group than in the delayed-mobilization group. Analysis of seroma fluid revealed that it was indeed lymph output. The risks of seromas and other postoperative complications in relationship to early mobilization of the upper extremity after surgery need to be further explored.

Recent randomized controlled studies suggest that immediate postoperative exercises do not complicate recovery after breast cancer surgery (Wingate et al, 1989; Na et al, 1999). These recent studies suggest that early physical therapy (therapy beginning on postoperative day 1) facilitates postoperative shoulder mobility. Addressing flexibility of fibrotic tissues is easier before joint contractures develop, which usually occurs within 1 week (Trudel and Uhthoff, 2000). In contrast, these studies suggest that delaying postoperative exercises until drains have been removed, which can take weeks and possibly even as long as a month, is associated with poor range of motion as well as prolonged pain and suffering. In these recent studies, the time to recovery of presurgery range of motion and functional activity was longer in the delayed-therapy group than in the early-therapy group.

No information is available in the literature about the effects of early physical therapy on rehabilitation after modified radical mastectomy and immediate TRAM flap reconstruction. At M. D. Anderson, physical therapy in patients who have undergone TRAM flap reconstruction is initiated as soon as drains are removed. Patients are evaluated by a physiatrist, who determines what level of physical therapy is most appropriate for the patient. The intensity of the therapy program depends on the patient's pain, swelling, myofascial inflexibility, and premorbid conditions. The patient undergoes treatment and receives education about arm and skin care practices designed to prevent further swelling. The physical therapy lasts for an average of 12 sessions given 3 times a week. No increase in post-surgical complications has been observed with this type of supervised physical therapy.

M. D. ANDERSON APPROACH TO REHABILITATION OF THE POSTMASTECTOMY EXTREMITY

At M. D. Anderson, we are proactive in our approach to rehabilitation of the postmastectomy extremity. We recognize common problems and treat these problems before they become complications.

Reach for Recovery Exercises and Physical Therapy

At M. D. Anderson, patients scheduled to undergo breast cancer surgery are visited by a Reach for Recovery volunteer prior to surgery. Reach for Recovery is a volunteer organization composed of women who have undergone breast cancer surgery. They talk to the patient about what to expect during the recovery period and share their own experiences. They also show each woman a set of exercises that can be done to improve range of motion in the affected shoulder. After surgery, while drains are still in place, patients continue with the Reach for Recovery exercises with the following restrictions: flexion and abduction of the shoulder are limited to between 45° and 90°, and internal and external rotations are limited to what the patient can tolerate.

Occasionally, a physically active, motivated, pain-free woman without other premorbid shoulder problems can regain function of the shoulder with Reach for Recovery exercises alone. However, these exercises may not be effective for cording in the axilla and the arm, and they may not be sufficient to fully restore scapular rhythm. Any postoperative pain, muscle guarding, or fear of harming the wound can prevent the patient from fully performing the suggested Reach for Recovery exercises. Hence, range of motion of the shoulder may not be fully restored with these exercises. Full range of motion requires the upper extremity to be in flexion (elevated) such that the extended elbow is parallel to the ipsilateral ear.

Drains are removed approximately 7 to 10 days after surgery or when output is less than 30 cc per day for 2 days. At this time, the restrictions on range of motion of the shoulder are lifted, and the patient is seen by a physiatrist. At institutions where such evaluation is not routine, patients should be evaluated by a physiatrist if they lack full range of motion or continue to have pain or swelling 1 month after drain removal. Soft tissue and muscle become more inflexible after this period. Patients who undergo segmental mastectomy with ALND may not need supervised therapy because this surgery is typically associated with less severe soft tissue and myofascial contractures.

The physiatrist performs a thorough history and a physical examination before generating the specific therapeutic prescription. The physical examination includes a neurological examination, circumferential measurements of both arms and forearms, and range-of-motion measurements performed using a goniometer. Patients who present with any of the following symptoms are referred to physical therapy: swelling greater than 2 cm on the ipsilateral arm, range of motion less than 90^0 in shoulder abduction and flexion, cording and pectoral tightness, or shoulder pain with or without movement.

The basic goals of physical therapy are to increase flexibility of the myofascial and soft tissues of the shoulder, the chest wall scar, and scapula thoracic rhythm prior to shoulder mobilization. Overhead pulleys used in the home setting further facilitate increase in range of motion. Pain control measures, including warm and cold packs and transcutaneous electrical nerve stimulation, are added to reduce muscle splinting. Postural education is given to decrease strain on axial structures. Deep breathing and relaxation methods can be added. If the patient underwent reconstruction with a TRAM flap, gentle abdominal activity is necessary to bring the pelvis forward, thereby decreasing lower back strain. Postural education is added to prevent further strain on the upper back and neck. If the patient underwent reconstruction with a latissimus dorsi flap, a cautious shoulder exercise regimen is recommended to avoid disruption of the flap. Patients who underwent reconstruction with a latissimus dorsi flap may take longer to regain full range of motion than patients who underwent reconstruction with a TRAM flap.

Prior to discharge from the hospital, patients who did not undergo reconstruction are given a temporary prosthesis (a cotton fluff). Assuming minimal swelling and a well-healed incision, patients are usually ready to be fitted for a permanent prosthesis 3 to 6 weeks after surgery.

Each of the above-mentioned physical therapy interventions can be accomplished on an outpatient basis. The intensity and duration of therapy depend on the patient's symptoms and clinical presentation, as well as the oncology treatment course. A median of 12 physical therapy sessions is prescribed when patients begin therapy after their drains are discontinued. Most patients experience a complete recovery with this type of therapeutic program.

These interventions can benefit not only patients who are in the early postoperative period but also patients who are several years out from their surgical treatment. Some improvement in soft tissue mobility and hence shoulder range of motion can be expected. Pain can be improved with increased soft tissue flexibility and adjunctive modalities such as moist heat and cold and transcutaneous electrical nerve stimulation.

Home Exercise Program and Instructions for Arm and Skin Care

Once physical therapy is complete, patients are given a recommended home exercise program to be performed at least 3 to 5 times a week. In addition, patients are given written instructions regarding arm care and skin care after a mastectomy (Table 16–2). The goal of the recommended precautions is to prevent lymphedema. These precautions are recommended indefinitely. Education and the recommended precautions are key to the continued effectiveness of the therapy regimen and avoidance of lymphedema.

Treatment of Neural and Musculoskeletal Complications

When a patient has preexisting musculoskeletal abnormalities, such as arthritis or rotator cuff tears or impingement, the postoperative recovery will be complicated. These abnormalities impede physical therapy interventions unless the underlying comorbid condition is correctly diagnosed. M. D. Anderson's practice of routinely referring patients for a consultation with a physiatrist is a proactive step designed to ensure that at-risk patients have as complete a recovery as possible. A treatment plan cannot be prescribed unless the physician has a thorough knowledge of the patient's shoulder biomechanics.

In patients with neural and musculoskeletal complications, the physical therapy plan involves resolving the soft tissue and muscle tightness to increase range of motion and then cautious shoulder and scapula stabilization exercises. The goal is often to relieve pain that occurs with shoulder movement rather than to obtain full range of motion of the shoulder.

Table 16–2. Guidelines for Prevention of Lymphedema after Modified Radical Mastectomy or Segmental Mastectomy and Axillary Lymph Node Dissection

- Avoid needle puncture and sphygmomanometry on affected extremity.
- Keep the skin moist and clean to prevent skin from cracking, drying, and tearing.
- Wear long sleeves and gloves when outdoors to reduce the risk of cuts, scrapes, insect bites, and sunburn.
- Do not wear shirts with tight elasticized cuffs, tight-fitting jewelry, or a tight-fitting bra.
- Use an electric razor when shaving the affected extremity.
- Use protective hand and finger covering when washing dishes, cooking, or sewing.
- Refrain from carrying heavy loads (> 10 pounds) and excessive repetitive use of the arm.
- Inspect skin and arm daily for swelling, pain, or color changes.
- Drink adequate water daily (6 glasses a day).
- Avoid rapid weight gain.
- If a handbag must be carried, carry a lightweight handbag (minimize contents) and carry it on the unaffected arm.
- Avoid dangling the affected arm when walking; swing the arms with elbows bent.
- Elevate the affected arm above heart level during prolonged sitting. Flex and extend the elbow, and perform circular arm motions.
- Limit the weight used for arm-strengthening exercises to 3 to 5 pounds, and discontinue any painful exercises.
- Do not cut nails too closely to the nail bed.
- Avoid saunas, solariums, and cold temperatures.
- An elastic compression sleeve is recommended during travel by airplane.

The earlier the treatment for shoulder dysfunction after mastectomy, the better the response to treatment.

Peripheral Nerve Damage

Neurapraxia of the long thoracic nerve will cause weakness of the serratus anterior muscle and, as a consequence, winging of the medial border of the scapula (Figure 16–4). The therapeutic approach is to strengthen residual serratus anterior muscle and other muscles that stabilize the scapula (rhomboid, levator scapula, and trapezius muscles), thus reducing further muscle atrophy and progression of shoulder girdle imbalance. Electrical stimulation is used to maintain muscle bulk. The weakness usually improves in 3 months in the case of neurapraxia. Electromyography is often needed to differentiate neurapraxia from neurotmesis (partial or complete severance of a nerve). The chances for neurological recovery are less in the case of neurotmesis.

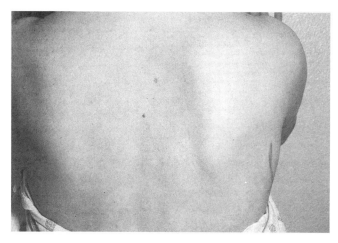

Figure 16–4. Scapular winging due to weakness of the serratus anterior muscle.

Radiation Plexopathy

Factors that predispose to the development of adhesive capsulitis (frozen shoulder) are immobility, older age (40–60 years), female gender, diabetes, thyroid disease, history of humeral trauma, and prior irradiation of the region. Adhesive capsulitis is characterized by shoulder pain and deficits in all ranges of shoulder motion.

Radiation fibrosis may injure the brachial plexus. Clinically, differentiation of recurrent tumor and radiation plexopathy can be challenging. A comparison of the 2 entities is presented in Table 16–3. Radiation plexopathy classically presents as aching pain around the shoulder region, radiating from the scapula to the forearm. Paresthesias can also occur from the arm to the hand, resulting in weakness of the hand muscles. Various studies indicate that patients with recurrent tumors are more likely to experience significant pain. Tumor plexopathy usually affects the lower trunk (cervical roots c_8, T_1) of the plexus, whereas radiation plexopathy usually affects the upper trunk (cervical roots c_5, c_6). Radiation-induced fibrosis can occur as long as 5 years after therapy. Magnetic resonance imaging and computed tomography scans may be beneficial in distinguishing radiation plexopathy from recurrent tumor; however, these scans must be interpreted carefully, and the findings on clinical examination must be taken into account. Electromyography is helpful for distinguishing between radiation plexopathy and recurrent tumor plexopathy. Surgical exploration of patients with radiation plexopathy reveals fibrosis affecting the neural tissue, with secondary constriction of the vasa nervorum and other vascular tissue in the region and subsequent ischemic damage to the axons.

Table 16–3. Comparison between Radiation Plexopathy and Recurrent
             Tumor Plexopathy

Characteristic	Radiation Plexopathy	Tumor Plexopathy
Pain	Frequently absent	Frequently present
Onset	Insidious	Fairly rapid progression
Location	Upper trunk of the brachial plexus	Lower trunk of the brachial plexus
Location of weakness	Mainly in the shoulder	Mainly in the hand
Paresthesia	Present in the hand	Present in the neck and shoulder
Findings on electromyography	Diagnostic for "myokymia"	Not distinguishable from other processes

Brachial plexopathy can be managed with therapeutic strengthening, electrical stimulation, and appropriate orthotic prescription. The goal is to maximize function within the constraints of the neuronal damage.

Peripheral Neuropathy

Postoperative chemotherapy and endocrine therapy may cause peripheral neuropathy. Distal extremities are affected first. The first nerves affected are small sensory afferent nerve endings conveying pain and temperature; later, nerves affecting touch, proprioception, and vibration are affected. Dysesthesias may occur in the extremities and can be quite disabling with respect to activities requiring fine hand movements. If such dysesthesias are not managed successfully, patients could be unable to resume any work that requires fine hand dexterity.

In patients with peripheral neuropathy, amitriptyline or gabapentin might be helpful for symptom management. If the neuropathy interferes with activities of daily living, an occupational therapist can suggest compensation strategies and adaptive equipment. The work environment can be ergonomically modified to compensate for weakness in the extremities. A physical therapist can address gait disturbances resulting from lack of proprioception in the lower extremities.

Pain

Disruption of the intercostobrachial nerve during surgery can cause neuralgia, known as "postmastectomy pain syndrome." The mastectomy scar can cause adhesions of the chest wall, irritating the nerves as well as surrounding muscles and soft tissue. Approximately 43% of patients who undergo mastectomy experience postmastectomy pain long after the mastectomy (Smith et al, 1999). Young age, tall stature, and increased body weight are associated risk factors.

Phantom breast pain affects approximately 10% of patients who undergo mastectomy. Phantom breast pain is an uncomfortable sensation of the missing breast in patients who have not undergone reconstruction. Phantom breast pain is common in women who had pain prior to mastectomy. Symptoms usually improve as shoulder range of motion and scar flexibility increase. Trials of transcutaneous electrical nerve stimulation, medications, or both may be helpful during the initial treatment phase. Use of oral pain medications during therapy can increase patients' tolerance for range-of-motion exercises.

TREATMENT OF LYMPHEDEMA

Lymphedema results from functional overload of the lymphatic system—i.e., the situation in which lymph volume exceeds transport capabilities. When lymph flow stops ("lymphostasis"), fluid and proteins collect in the interstitium, promoting chronic inflammation and subsequent proliferation of connective tissue, which can result in the development of fibrosclerosis. Fibrosclerosis increases the risk of infection. Lymphedema can begin insidiously at any interval after ALND. Risk factors for lymphedema are receipt of ALND, receipt of radiation therapy, higher body weight, older age, and complex surgery. The pathophysiology of lymphedema is not fully understood. An intimate relationship exists between the lymphatic system, the vascular system, and the surrounding soft tissues. This complex relationship plays a significant role in the development of lymphedema and ultimately the response to treatment.

Various methods for measuring the edematous arm have been described in the literature, and there is currently no consensus about what degree of enlargement constitutes lymphedema. Therefore, the incidence of lymphedema varies in the medical literature. A review by Petrek and Heelan (1998) suggested an incidence of 15% to 20%. The appearance of arm swelling can be more distressing for the patient than the mastectomy and perhaps the cancer itself. Approximately 80% of cases of lymphedema manifest within 2 years after primary surgery and radiation therapy.

The 4 types of lymphedema are early, acute, erysipeloid, and delayed. The early type occurs immediately after the operation and is characterized by pitting edema within the extremity. This is resolved with elevation and hand exercises within 1 week. The acute type is characterized by painful edema, which usually occurs 2 to 6 weeks after surgery. The preferred treatment is elevation and anti-inflammatory medication within 2 weeks of onset. The erysipeloid type is characterized by a chronically edematous arm, evidenced by an erythematous, painful course. Treatment consists of elevation and antibiotic medications. A compression pump is contraindicated in the case of erysipeloid lymphedema as use of a pump might lead to proximal spread. Patients with all types of lymphedema will have normal findings on neurological examination.

Delayed lymphedema is the most common presentation of lymphedema. This type presents with insidious, painless, nonerythematous swelling with sustained pitting. Lymphedema starts at the base of the extremity. Swelling usually begins in the trunk, spreading to the dorsal aspect of the arm and forearm. Patients experience tension and heaviness, followed by pain and reduced arm mobility. Protein-rich interstitial edema increases the activity of macrophages, fibroblasts, and lymphocytes. Fibrosis and sclerosis develop, leading to local flow disturbances that affect the ligaments and tendons of the shoulder. Sequelae of chronic lymphostasis are recurrent infections, arthropathy, arterial and venous insufficiency, elephantiasis, and skin pigmentation. Lymphangiosarcoma (Stewart-Treves syndrome) can also develop as a result of chronic lymphedema.

Pfaff (1988) identified several diseases that commonly coexist with lymphedema (Table 16–4). The differential diagnosis of lymphedema includes venous stasis swelling, venous thrombosis, reflex sympathetic dystrophy (complex regional pain syndrome), chronic inflammatory arthritis, and recurrent tumor.

Diagnosis

The diagnosis of lymphedema is made by history and physical examination. Lymphoscintigraphy is recommended if autogenous transplantation of lymph vessels is planned. Blood tests are not needed to diagnose lymphedema, and lymphographic examinations are usually not required. Phlebography should be performed only if the results will affect therapeutic management. Computed tomography and magnetic resonance imaging are usually not helpful in the evaluation of lymphedema except in the case of a search for recurrent tumor.

Complex Decongestive Therapy

Even though complex decongestive therapy (CDT) for lymphedema has been described since the late 19th century, it is only within the past 25 years that this treatment has become widely accepted. Complex deconges-

Table 16–4. Diseases that Commonly Coexist with Lymphedema

Disease	Incidence in Patients with Lymphedema (%)
Radiation fibrosis	48
Erysipelas	35
Shoulder range-of-motion deficit	30
Paresis	22
Venous flow disturbances	22
Ulcer	5

Source: Pfaff A. Unilateral secondary postmastectomy arm lymphedema. Study of inpatient physical therapy [in German]. Z Lymphol 1988;12:19–23.

tive therapy is well tolerated and has almost no side effects. Many studies have proven the effectiveness of this treatment.

The therapeutic goal of CDT is to achieve faster lymph transport in the edematous area and thus reduce the accumulation of proteins in the interstitium. Complex decongestive therapy combines several treatments that synergistically promote reduction of lymphostasis. These treatments include manual lymph drainage, compression bandaging to avoid new fluid accumulation in the treated area, hygienic measures, and decongestive exercises for the bandaged extremity. The texture of the swelling of the affected arm and the volume correlate with the response to treatment. The response to CDT is greater in patients with edema volume of less than 500 cc than in those with greater edema volume.

Manual lymph drainage consists of massage with slow, rotating, mild tissue compression (Figure 16–5). The massage is begun at the central portion of the arm and proceeds to the peripheral extremity. Manual lymph drainage results in a "sucking effect" on the lymphatic, which increases the transport capacity of the lymphatic system. Increased lymph drainage promotes the protein-degrading activity of macrophages and therefore reduces the volume of lymph. These processes facilitate fragmentation of subcutaneous collagen fibers. The arm must be bandaged with low-stretch bandages after manual lymph drainage (Figure 16–6). This technique maintains pressure on the arm and thus resists the accumulation of more fluid. Once lymphedema reduction is stabilized, a compression garment with compression pressures of 30 mm to 60 mm Hg is necessary for maintenance (Figure 16–7).

Compression bandages and garments increase tissue pressure, which reduces abnormal ultrafiltration and improves reabsorption. The pressure

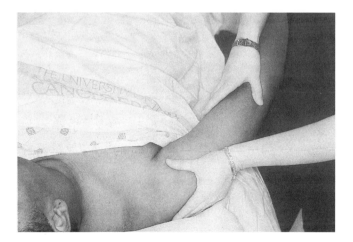

Figure 16–5. Therapist performing manual lymph drainage.

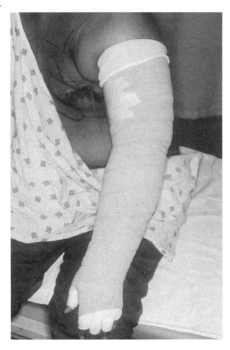

Figure 16–6. Compression bandaging of the extremity after manual lymph drainage.

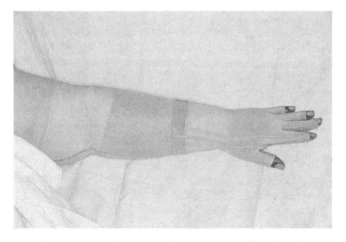

Figure 16–7. Compression sleeve and glove worn on the extremity.

causes the joint and muscle to pump more effectively, which increases lymph motoricity and reduces fibrosis and sclerosis.

Maintenance and prevention are essential to successful treatment of lymphedema. The patient should be instructed to perform manual lymph drainage 3 times a week, to elevate the extremity daily, to apply or have someone else apply compression bandaging, and to perform arm and skin care assessments. Incomplete treatment, compliance problems, occult infection, tumor recurrence, or an incorrect diagnosis can result in failure of CDT.

Complex decongestive therapy is usually performed on an outpatient basis. Each stage of CDT must be meticulously completed for success, and only specially trained therapists should perform CDT. Complex decongestive therapy is contraindicated in patients with thrombosis, cardiac failure, active local infection, or regional metastasis.

Use of Pneumatic Compression Pump

Controversy exists in the literature regarding the usefulness of compression pumps in the treatment of lymphedema. Compression pumps promote temporary movement of fluid from the distal to the proximal end of the extremity. Stasis of proximal edema may lead to the development of fibrosis, creating a "bottleneck" appearance of the extremity. Increased lymphatic transport capacity requires the proximal trunk to be free of edema to facilitate clearance. Only manual lymph drainage can produce this outcome. The compression pump is not suitable as an exclusive decongestive therapy for chronic lymphedema, and it cannot replace manual lymph drainage. The compression pump cannot be used without risk in any situation and should only be used by experienced lymphedema therapists.

Medications

Currently, lymphedema cannot be treated effectively with medications. Administering diuretics would cause water extraction, resulting in a higher protein concentration in the tissues and the promotion of fibrosclerotic processes. Benzopyrones might seem promising because they stimulate macrophage activity and increase lymph transport. However, currently available data indicate no therapeutic effects of benzopyrones on chronic lymphedema, and benzopyrones have not been approved for treatment of lymphedema in the United States.

Surgical Management

Surgical treatment of lymphedema is considered only if a trial of conservative treatment fails and the patient has a correct diagnosis. Lymphatic-to-lymphatic or lymphatic-to-venous anastomosis can be performed with the goal of improving drainage. Another method is eradication of excess subcutaneous tissue to reduce the swelling. However, available data do not show promising results with these procedures.

Inpatient Rehabilitation

Breast cancer patients undergoing rehabilitation can be divided into 2 groups: those with local disease and disability and those with systemic disease and disability. For patients with localized breast cancer, rehabilitation can usually be accomplished on an outpatient basis. However, in patients with metastatic breast cancer, rehabilitation may need to take place in an inpatient setting.

Metastatic disease involving the central nervous system, bone, liver, or lungs is often accompanied by significant pain, mobility problems, self-care deficits, and fatigue. The medical consequences of this metastatic involvement can include fractures, neurological compromise from spinal cord compression or neuropathy, and metabolic complications. Rehabilitation professionals can manage nonsurgical fractures with gait aids, orthotics, protective ambulating devices, and weight-bearing compensation techniques. Functional sequelae of neurological complications can include weakness or paraparesis with bladder or bowel involvement. The patient's uncertainty regarding the disease can result in anxiety, depression, and sleep disturbances.

Inpatient rehabilitation is a multidisciplinary approach, led by a physiatrist who coordinates medical and therapeutic treatment for the patient. Other members of the rehabilitation team include a physical therapist, occupational therapist, speech and language pathologist, social worker, case manager, dietician, rehabilitation nurse, and chaplain. The major goals of rehabilitation in patients with metastatic breast cancer are to achieve optimal pain relief and comfort; to enable self care and resumption of mobility as much as possible; to increase endurance and strength; to provide education for patients and their families to prepare them to continue care in the home; to ensure a safe discharge to home; and to provide support while being realistically hopeful.

Various studies have shown that inpatient rehabilitation is effective for cancer patients. Cancer patients make gains in function comparable with those of noncancer patients. Chemotherapy, radiation therapy, and specific tumor types have not been shown to adversely affect the outcome of rehabilitation. Poor long-term prognosis should not preclude inpatient rehabilitation if functional gains—even short-term gains—are likely to be made.

Psychological and Vocational Issues

From the time of diagnosis to the time of modified radical mastectomy or segmental mastectomy with ALND, a patient with breast cancer and her family experience a wide range of feelings. Throughout this period, the

---

KEY PRACTICE POINTS

- A multidisciplinary approach to the care of the breast cancer patient is crucial for recovery following a mastectomy or segmental mastectomy with ALND.

- Shoulder dysfunction due to modified radical mastectomy or segmental mastectomy with ALND can be treated or minimized with early supervised physical therapy.

- Relevant comorbid conditions should be identified prior to therapy.

- Brachial plexopathy and neurapraxia and muscle atrophy may be present after a mastectomy.

- Lymphedema can be managed with CDT.

- The rehabilitation team can comprehensively address and treat the physical disabilities that result from metastatic disease.

- Recognizing, minimizing, and preventing physical and psychological insults can dramatically improve the quality of life of breast cancer survivors.

---

patient undergoes physical and emotional trauma and recuperation. She experiences varying degrees of depression, mourning, anger, and fear—all of which require time to be resolved.

Although coping styles differ among individuals, several common psychological issues arise after modified radical mastectomy or segmental mastectomy and ALND. The patient may have a worsened self-image because of the loss of her breast and her sense of loss of a body part that is sexually significant. The patient may also have a demeaned self-worth as a woman, whereby she sees herself as unattractive; she may withdraw from mates. The patient may believe that shoulder dysfunction and lymphedema are unavoidable consequences of breast cancer surgery; thus she may believe that she should be able to endure these side effects without help. The patient may feel embarrassed at having had a mastectomy. As a means of moving toward a healthy denial of her breast cancer experience, she may try to keep others from knowing about her surgery. Other common themes are fear and anxiety at possible recurrence of disease, further surgery, and possibly death and concerns regarding the family and burdening them with the stress associated with the cancer.

From the moment of the mastectomy, the patient's vocation is disrupted. Side effects of chemotherapy and radiation therapy hinder resumption of work. These sequelae may prevent the woman from returning to her previous occupation. In one study, only 74% of patients returned to full-time work within 3 months of their mastectomies (Winick and Robbins, 1977). This affects not only the woman's psychological well-being but also her financial stability. These stressors and the cancer itself may result in maladaptive or dysfunctional behavior.

Rehabilitation interventions not only facilitate physical recovery but also direct the patient towards psychological recovery strategies. A multidisciplinary approach combining comprehensive rehabilitation with psychiatric and psychological support has been shown to improve outcomes in the management of breast cancer. Therapies address difficulties with activities of daily living, sleep, work, and driving. Relaxation techniques are helpful and can give the patient a sense of mastery and control. The identification and treatment of these dysfunctions will maximize the patient's performance, thereby reducing anxiety and symptoms of depression.

The interventions of the rehabilitation team improve or restore function and preserve independence to assure quality of life for cancer survivors. We must look at the whole patient and not divorce emotional care from physical care. Problems such as a frozen shoulder or a partially functioning arm should be the exception rather than common postsurgical sequelae. Physicians have the moral responsibility to prescribe preventive as well as curative treatment.

SUGGESTED READINGS

Atkins H, Hayward JL, Klugman DJ, Wayte AB. Treatment of early breast cancer: a report after ten years of a clinical trial. *BMJ* 1972;2:423–429.

Brennan MJ, DePompolo RW, Garden FH. Focused review: postmastectomy lymphedema. *Arch Phys Med Rehabil* 1996;77(suppl 3):S74–S80.

Dorval M, Maunsell E, Deschenes L, Brisson J, Masse B. Long-term quality of life after breast cancer: comparison of 8-year survivors with population controls. *J Clin Oncol* 1998;16:487–494.

Flew TJ. Wound drainage following radical mastectomy: the effect of restriction of shoulder movement. *Br J Surg* 1979;66:302–305.

Ganz PA, Coscarelli A, Fred C, Kahn B, Polinsky ML, Petersen L. Breast cancer survivors: psychosocial concerns and quality of life. *Breast Cancer Res Treat* 1996;38:183–199.

Ganz PA, Rowland JH, Desmond K, Meyerowitz BE, Wyatt GE. Life after breast cancer: understanding women's health-related quality of life and sexual functioning. *J Clin Oncol* 1998;16:501–514.

Ganz PA, Schag CC, Polinsky ML, Heinrich RL, Flack VF. Rehabilitation needs and breast cancer: the first month after primary therapy. *Breast Cancer Res Treat* 1987;10:243–253.

Gutman H, Kersz T, Barzilai T, Haddad M, Reiss R. Achievements of physical therapy in patients after modified radical mastectomy compared with quadrantectomy, axillary dissection, and radiation for carcinoma of the breast. *Arch Surg* 1990;125:389–391.

Jansen RF, van Geel AN, de Groot HG, Rottier AB, Olthuis GA, van Putten WL. Immediate versus delayed shoulder exercises after axillary lymph node dissection. *Am J Surg* 1990;160:481–484.

Knight CD Jr, Griffen FD, Knight CD Sr. Prevention of seromas in mastectomy wounds. The effect of shoulder immobilization. *Arch Surg* 1995;130:99–101.

Lotze MT, Duncan MA, Gerber LH, Woltering EA, Rosenberg SA. Early versus delayed shoulder motion following axillary dissection: a randomized prospective study. *Ann Surg Oncol* 1981;193:288–295.

Marciniak CM, Sliwa JA, Spill G, Heinemann AW, Semik PE. Functional outcome following rehabilitation of the cancer patient. *Arch Phys Med Rehabil* 1996;77: 54–57.

Na YM, Lee JS, Park JS, Kang SW, Lee HD, Koo JY. Early rehabilitation program in postmastectomy patients: a prospective clinical trial. *Yonsei Med J* 1999;40:1–8.

Petrek JA, Heelan MC. Incidence of breast carcinoma-related lymphedema. *Cancer* 1998;83(suppl 12 American):2776–2781.

Pfaff A. Unilateral secondary postmastectomy arm lymphedema. Study of inpatient physical therapy [in German]. *Z Lymphol* 1988;12:19–23.

Polinsky ML. Functional status of long-term breast cancer survivors: demonstrating chronicity. *Health Soc Work* 1994;19:165–173.

Pollard R, Callum KG, Altman DG, Bates T. Shoulder movement following mastectomy. *Clin Oncol* 1976;2:343–349.

Price J, Purtell JR. Prevention and treatment of lymphedema after breast cancer. *Am J Nurs* 1997;97(9):34–37.

Schultz I, Barholm M, Grondal S. Delayed shoulder exercises in reducing seroma frequency after modified radical mastectomy: a prospective randomized study *Ann Surg Oncol* 1997;4:293–297.

Smith WC, Bourne D, Squair J, Phillips D, Alastair Chambers W. A retrospective cohort study of post mastectomy pain syndrome. *Pain* 1999;83:91–95.

Swedborg I, Wallgren A. The effect of pre- and postmastectomy radiotherapy on the degree of edema, shoulder-joint mobility, and gripping force. *Cancer* 1981;47:877–881.

Tadych K, Donegan WL. Postmastectomy seromas and wound drainage. *Surg Gynecol Obstet* 1987;165:483–487.

Trudel G, Uhthoff HK. Contractures secondary to immobility: is the restriction articular or muscular? An experimental longitudinal study in the rat knee. *Arch Phys Med Rehabil* 2000;81:6–13.

Truong A, Singletary SE, Bruera E. Early rehabilitation improves extremity function and decreases postoperative complications in cancer patients undergoing modified radical mastectomy: a preliminary report. *Proceedings of the American Society of Clinical Oncology* 2000;19:614. Abstract 2416.

van der Horst CM, Kenter JA, de Jong MT, Keeman JN. Shoulder function following early mobilization of the shoulder after mastectomy and axillary dissection. *Neth J Surg* 1985;37:105–108.

Wingate L, Croghan I, Natarajan N, Michalek AM, Jordan C. Rehabilitation of the mastectomy patient: a randomized, blind, prospective study. *Arch Phys Med Rehabil* 1989;70:21–24.

Winick L, Robbins GF. Physical and psychologic readjustment after mastectomy: an evaluation of Memorial Hospital's PMRG program. *Cancer* 1977;39:478–486.

Winick L, Robbins GF. The Post-Mastectomy Rehabilitation Group program. Structure, procedure, and population demography. *Am J Surg* 1976;132:599–602.

17 MENOPAUSAL HEALTH AFTER BREAST CANCER

Rena Vassilopoulou-Sellin

CHAPTER OVERVIEW

The gradual decline in estrogen production that follows menopause often contributes to significant climacteric symptoms, accelerated bone loss, and cardiovascular morbidity. Estrogen replacement can prevent or reverse many postmenopausal morbidities and has been widely used for several decades. The concern that researchers in early studies may have been hasty in their conclusions about the safety of estrogen replacement has prompted the reassessment of old data and further analyses of large groups of women. These new analyses take into consideration age, estrogen formulation, and duration of estrogen administration as risk factors for breast cancer. An emerging consensus is that very prolonged estrogen use may contribute to breast cancer risk. The suggestion that women who have previously undergone treatment for breast cancer should not receive exogenous estrogen has constituted one area of general agreement for many years. Accordingly, alternative strategies have been developed to address postmenopausal health needs for breast cancer survivors. However, this proscription has been challenged in recent years because both the population characteristics and health needs of women with a prior diagnosis of breast cancer have been changing. Recent information about the outcome of women who elect to take estrogen after breast cancer as well as those who develop breast cancer while taking estrogen is contributing to the emerging opinion that decisions regarding estrogen may be individualized in some cases.

INTRODUCTION

As a group, women with a history of breast cancer are exposed to estrogen deficiency more often and for longer periods of time than women who have not had breast cancer. One reason for the increased likelihood of estrogen deficiency in this patient population is that chemotherapy, which is increasingly advocated as treatment for localized breast cancer, generally precipitates premature ovarian failure and thus early menopause. Hormone replacement therapy (HRT) is effective as a treatment for estrogen deficiency; however, HRT is contraindicated in women with breast cancer or a history of this disease because breast cancer is considered a hormone-responsive disease. In fact, women who are receiving HRT following the onset of menopause are almost always taken off the treatment if they later develop breast cancer. For breast cancer patients, then, it may be necessary to delineate nonhormonal alternatives for managing the health problems caused by estrogen deficiency.

CONSEQUENCES OF ESTROGEN DEFICIENCY

Ovarian estrogen production gradually declines after about age 50 years. During the decades that follow, estrogen deficiency causes complex metabolic changes that characterize the menopausal years (Greendale and Judd, 1993; Utian and Schiff, 1994; Speroff et al, 1994). Hot flashes and vasomotor instability are the most frequent and most distressing health problems resulting from estrogen deficiency, and they are the conditions that typically motivate women to seek treatment. Genitourinary atrophy may also occur. This condition often leads to dyspareunia and may predispose the patient to bladder infections. Another consequence of estrogen deficiency is accelerated bone loss, which leads to clinically significant osteoporosis in many women. Osteoporosis is the most common metabolic bone disease in postmenopausal women, and it is responsible for more than 1 million hip fractures per year. The most serious health problem associated with estrogen deficiency is the progressive increase in the risk of cardiovascular disease, which is the leading cause of death among older women.

Effect of Hormone Replacement Therapy on Sequelae of Estrogen Deficiency

The efficacy of HRT in preventing or ameliorating the many sequelae of estrogen deficiency and in reducing mortality caused by estrogen deficiency has been well established (Grady et al, 1992; Grodstein et al, 1997). Many population-based retrospective analyses have shown that HRT reduces cardiovascular mortality overall in postmenopausal women, partly because HRT improves the lipid profile but mostly because estrogen has direct beneficial effects on the heart and vasculature. Recently published data, however, have dampened earlier enthusiasm for the efficacy of HRT by suggesting that its apparent protective effect may not apply to women who have established heart disease. The wisdom of caution is reinforced by an early, interim analysis of data from the Women's Health Initiative, a large ongoing prospective trial. The investigators, however, have indicated that any changes in clinical practice (based on the findings of earlier, retrospective analyses) would be premature at this time.

The most common reason that postmenopausal women pursue HRT is for relief or prevention of climactic symptoms. Vasomotor and genitourinary symptoms are readily corrected with HRT, and HRT can reduce or prevent the development of osteoporosis and its related morbidity and mortality. In contrast, apprehension that HRT may increase the risk of developing breast cancer is the most frequent reason for avoiding estrogen.

Breast Cancer Survivors' Attitudes about Hormone Replacement Therapy

In any discussion with a breast cancer survivor who is considering HRT, the health professional must carefully examine the woman's views and opinions regarding HRT, because the woman needs to be a thoughtful partner in all health care decisions.

In recent years, opinion pieces, editorials, scientific studies, and philosophical analyses of menopause and its "management" have been prominent in both the medical and lay literature. Women also receive advice about HRT from their health care providers, their relatives, and their friends. Opinions about HRT shift in response to new studies, personal experiences, and anecdotes. Well-intended yet contradictory information underscores the uncertainty about this treatment. Breast cancer survivors are often reluctant to receive HRT despite considerable climacteric discomfort they may be experiencing due to menopause. Likewise, the long-standing position of regulatory agencies and those in medical practice that HRT is contraindicated in breast cancer survivors makes clinicians hesitant to recommend the treatment for these patients. However, a number of women conclude that the potential benefits of HRT override the potential risks, and they make a personal decision to begin taking estrogen (Vassilopoulou-Sellin and Zolinski, 1992; Couzi et al, 1995).

NONESTROGEN INTERVENTIONS FOR MANAGEMENT OF MENOPAUSE

For women who cannot use HRT or who choose not to, alternative approaches are available to correct or palliate some of the sequelae of estrogen deficiency (Table 17–1).

Table 17–1. Nonestrogen Alternatives for Treatment of Symptoms of Estrogen Deficiency in Postmenopausal Women with a History of Breast Cancer

Symptom	Intervention
Cardiovascular disease	Smoking cessation
	Weight regulation
	Physical fitness
	Control of comorbid conditions (e.g., hypertension and diabetes)
	Lipid-lowering agents
	Selective estrogen receptor modulators
Osteoporosis	Exercise (weight bearing)
	Calcium and vitamin D supplements
	Bisphosphonates
	Calcitonin
	Sodium fluoride
	Selective estrogen receptor modulators
Climacteric vasomotor instability	Bellergal-S
	Clonidine
	Venlafaxine
	Progesterone
Genitourinary symptoms	Nonhormonal lubricants
	Low-dose topical estrogen

Cardiovascular Disease

The fact that cardiovascular disease is the most serious health threat for aging women has been amply emphasized in recent years. Constitutional factors that increase the risk for cardiovascular disease include a family history of coronary disease at a young age, hypertension, a history of claudication or stroke, diabetes mellitus, and hyperlipidemia. Lifestyle factors such as smoking, obesity, and physical inactivity are also important. Clearly, smoking cessation, weight regulation, and physical fitness are important nonhormonal strategies for preserving cardiovascular health and for maintaining a sensible, healthy lifestyle in general. Likewise, meticulous control of hypertension and diabetes is critically important for avoiding vascular complications in affected patients, regardless of age or sex. A variety of medications and therapeutic algorithms for treatment of cardiovascular disease are outlined in standard medical textbooks.

Osteoporosis

Progressive bone loss occurs naturally with advancing age, and in women, the rate of bone loss is accelerated after menopause. Nevertheless, clinically significant osteoporosis with disabling vertebral or hip fractures is far from inevitable. Whereas estrogen deficiency remains an important correlate with osteoporosis, the effect of hereditary and racial factors on loss of bone mass are increasingly apparent. Having a thin frame, living a sedentary lifestyle, being of the white race, and being a smoker are all important risk factors for osteoporosis. Nonhormonal treatments for established osteoporosis include exercise, calcium and vitamin D supplementation, bisphosphonates, calcitonin, and sodium fluoride (Hodgson and Johnston, 1996).

In the past few years, the bisphosphonates have emerged as an effective and well-tolerated group of compounds that support and even enhance bone mineral density. Available data indicate that the benefits of bisphosphonates persist during several years of continuous therapy. The potential impact of bisphosphonates on the long-term morbidity and mortality related to skeletal fractures is still under investigation but appears promising on the basis of results of initial studies of several years of continued use. Alendronate sodium has been approved by the Food and Drug Administration for use in the prevention and treatment of osteoporosis. The most significant side effect of this drug is esophageal irritation, which can be minimized when the patient follows the insert instructions carefully. Other bisphosphonates are currently available for treatment of hypercalcemia and Paget's disease of the bones and may be useful for treating osteoporosis in patients who cannot tolerate alendronate sodium. Additional bisphosphonates are also under development.

Calcitonin has also been approved for treatment of osteoporosis. It prevents bone loss and has important analgesic properties; however, there is no good evidence that it reduces the incidence of hip fracture. Calcitonin administered for many years as an injection frequently causes nausea and flushing. These side effects can be especially disturbing for women with a history of cancer and prior exposure to chemotherapy. The recently formulated calcitonin nasal spray appears to produce fewer symptoms than the injections.

Sodium fluoride has been used as a treatment for osteoporosis because it appears to accelerate bone formation. Several studies have demonstrated that administration of sodium fluoride increases bone mineral density. However, controversy continues as to whether sodium fluoride may paradoxically increase the risk of fractures. Most recently, low-dose and slow-release sodium fluoride in combination with calcium has been shown to reduce the risk of vertebral fractures. If this finding is confirmed, this relatively safe drug may provide another promising therapeutic alternative for women with osteoporosis.

Preventing calcium and vitamin D deficiency is an important measure in maintaining skeletal integrity. Calcium supplementation significantly slows bone loss in healthy postmenopausal women, and it is generally included in menopause-treatment regimens. Whether pharmacologic administration of vitamin D can significantly reduce the risk of vertebral or hip fracture remains controversial; however, 2 recent studies have shown that low-dose vitamin D and calcitriol were associated with decreased rates of hip and vertebral fractures, respectively.

The benefit of exercise in the prevention of osteoporosis is a presumption that has been difficult to document. Whereas immobilization and weightlessness result in significant bone loss, neither endurance nor weight-bearing-exercise programs can easily be shown to prevent or reverse menopause-induced osteopenia. Perhaps the single most important measure that can reduce the cost and suffering associated with osteoporosis is the prevention of accidental falls, which are the most frequent and immediate causes of hip fractures.

Climacteric Vasomotor Instability

Hot flashes are the most prominent peri- and postmenopausal condition experienced by women. Hot flashes affect more than 70% of women and may persist for several years, although the condition usually abates spontaneously after 2 years. Hot flashes are characterized by a sensation of heat, sweating, flushing, and anxiety. The cause of hot flashes remains unclear, but they are considered to be a result of dysfunctional thermoregulation, which may be mediated by changes of central catecholamine secretion. This presumed etiology has guided the design of nonhormonal therapies, most of which have been discovered by serendipity.

Bellergal-S, a combination of phenobarbital, ergotamine tartrate, and belladonna, has been moderately effective in treating hot flashes for many years. However, blurred vision, dry mouth, and gastrointestinal problems are frequent side effects that lead many women to abandon this drug.

Clonidine, a centrally active α-agonist, is also used to treat hot flashes (Goldberg et al, 1994). Initially developed as an antihypertensive medication, clonidine has been shown in several studies to alleviate both the frequency and severity of hot flashes associated with estrogen deficiency or tamoxifen administration. Drowsiness and dry mouth are frequent side effects but are usually not severe enough to interrupt therapy. Orthostatic symptoms, however, may become limiting and should be monitored closely, especially at the beginning of treatment. Other centrally acting and antidopaminergic agents (e.g., venlafaxine or veralipride) have also been used with moderate success.

Progestational agents are often considered in the management of hot flashes (Loprinzi et al, 1994). However, since progesterone is an ovarian hormone with significant potential to cause the proliferation of breast tissue, these agents should not be used until carefully designed studies have determined their safety. Estriol, a relatively weak estrogen, has been used to relieve hot flashes and to improve genitourinary symptoms. It is popular among clinicians, especially in Europe, and is frequently recommended for women in menopause. Estriol is often discussed as an attractive alternative to HRT for women with a history of breast cancer. However, appropriate and sufficient data regarding the safety of estriol in this population are not available at this time, and estriol should be considered another estrogenic preparation. Similarly, the safety of dehydroepiandrosterone sulfate, an adrenal steroid frequently discussed as an alternate to estrogen, is not defined for this group of women.

Other Climacteric Symptoms

Genitourinary atrophy, bladder dysfunction resulting in stress incontinence and infections, dyspareunia, and decreased libido frequently develop at the time of menopause. These symptoms may become increasingly troublesome with time and are attributed to estrogen deficiency. Nonhormonal lubricants are often used to improve dyspareunia but do not relieve bladder problems. Vaginal estrogen in the form of an ointment or a slow-release-delivery ring can be very helpful when used judiciously and at doses low enough to prevent significant systemic absorption but high enough to correct genitourinary symptoms. It is generally possible to monitor systemic levels of estrogen and gonadotropin and to adjust the dose of topical estrogen with good results. Other hormone preparations that may be used to relieve genitourinay atrophy can be obtained without prescription; however, as with topical estrogen, concerns regarding systemic absorption apply, and caution should be exercised regardless of whether these compounds require medical prescription.

Emotional symptoms such as irritability, nervousness, depression, insomnia, and inability to concentrate are also described by many menopausal women; however, the causal association between these symptoms and estrogen deficiency is still being debated. A number of herbal remedies, such as St. John's wort, are advocated by the health food industry and are widely used although information about their efficacy remains anecdotal.

Dietary Supplements

Nonprescription dietary supplements are popular remedies for climacteric symptoms. For example, estrogenic compounds are widely distributed in natural foodstuffs and herbal remedies used to treat menopausal symptoms. In fact, the symptomatic benefit derived from supplements such as Chinese herbs and soy products may well be related to their estrogenic properties. Phytoestrogens have been used for centuries by many cultures to relieve climacteric symptoms and are the subject of discussions and investigations regarding their potentially protective effect against the development of several cancers, including breast cancer. Phytoestrogens clearly interact with estrogen receptors, both in vitro and in vivo, but their safety in patients with breast cancer remains unestablished. Among other dietary supplements, vitamin E was recently examined in a randomized trial and soy protein was examined in a recent placebo-controlled study. Both were found ineffective in controlling climacteric symptoms.

Selective Estrogen Receptor Modulators

A number of compounds have been developed that act as estrogens on some tissues but have an antiestrogenic effect on other tissues. These compounds are known as selective estrogen receptor modulators (SERMs). Tamoxifen, the oldest SERM, is a very effective antineoplastic agent that is used widely and for prolonged periods of time in postmenopausal women with breast cancer. Early concerns that this antiestrogen might have deleterious effects on the cardiovascular and skeletal systems have fortunately proved unwarranted. Tamoxifen administration is associated with a fall of total cholesterol and low-density lipoprotein cholesterol levels. The effects of tamoxifen on high-density lipoprotein cholesterol levels are less consistent. The beneficial effects of tamoxifen persist for at least 2 years of continuous use and may be accompanied by improvements of clinical cardiovascular morbidity. The possibility of benefit is supported by recent reports that among patients randomly assigned to receive either tamoxifen or no treatment, fewer tamoxifen-treated patients were admitted to the hospital for cardiac disease or suffered a fatal heart attack (Love et al, 1991; Rutqvist and Mattsson, 1993).

Equally promising is evidence that tamoxifen may exert a weak estrogenic effect on the skeleton and thus prevent postmenopausal bone loss (Fornander et al, 1990). However, long-term reduction in the rate of vertebral and hip fractures has yet to be clearly demonstrated. On the other hand, tamoxifen may exacerbate climacteric vasomotor symptoms and depression and may cause additional side effects, especially endometrial proliferation. At this time, tamoxifen is used most effectively as adjuvant therapy for breast cancer or for breast cancer chemoprevention rather than as an intervention for management of menopause.

More recently, raloxifene has been approved for use in preventing osteoporosis (Delmas et al, 1997). Like tamoxifen, raloxifene decreases total cholesterol and low-density lipoprotein cholesterol levels. Unlike tamoxifen, however, raloxifene does not appear to induce endometrial hyperplasia. It is not clear whether raloxifene will be shown to protect against cardiovascular disease. A large randomized, prospective trial (the Study of Tamoxifen and Raloxifene) has been initiated to examine whether raloxifene is useful in breast cancer prevention and how it compares with tamoxifen in terms of efficacy and side effects. At this time, however, the safety of raloxifene in women with prior breast cancer is unknown, and it is recommended that caution be practiced in the use of this drug. Additional SERMs, including tibolone and droloxifene, are under investigation or are available for use outside the United States for management of menopausal symptoms.

USE OF HORMONE REPLACEMENT THERAPY AFTER BREAST CANCER DIAGNOSIS AND TREATMENT

Hormone replacement therapy is generally avoided in women with a history of breast cancer, although considerable skepticism about this practice is reflected in many recent editorials and commentaries. Many investigators have discussed the importance of developing appropriate guidelines for use of HRT in women with a history of breast cancer and have emphasized the need for clinical trials specifically designed to evaluate the use of HRT in this population. In the absence of data from randomized, prospective trials, information on the safety of HRT in women with a history of breast cancer can be obtained from recently presented or published retrospective or prospective single-arm and pilot studies, which are outlined in Table 17–2. In general, these studies included women with localized disease with different combinations of hormone receptor status and lymph node status. It is difficult to reach meaningful conclusions about the safety of HRT from such limited reports. Still, the rates of recurrence reported in these studies are fairly low and similar to what might be generally expected among HRT nonusers. From such reports, one can reasonably infer that HRT does not have a pronounced adverse effect on cancer recurrence in select former patients rendered disease-free after treatment for localized disease. Nevertheless, in routine clinical practice, it is not appropriate to deviate from the widely held, established standards of care unless appropriate safety data become available.

Table 17–2. Hormone Replacement Therapy after Breast Cancer: Published and Presented Studies

Study	Number of Patients	Median Duration of HRT, Months (range)	Follow-up, Months (range)	Number of Breast Cancer Cases
Powles et al (1993)	35	15 (1–238)	43 (NA)	2
Eden et al (1995)	90	18 (4–144)	84 (4–360)	7
DiSaia et al (1996)	77	27 (1–233)	59 (10–425)	7
Vassilopoulou-Sellin et al (1997)	43	31 (24–142)	144 (46–342)	1
Peters and Jones (1996)	67	37 (2–192)	94 (1–454)	0
Decker et al (1996)	61	26 (3–198)	NA	6
Gorins et al (1997)	28	33 (NA)	NA	1
Bluming et al (1997)	146	28 (1–52)	NA	4
Marsden and Sacks (1997)	50	6 (NA)	<6 (NA)	0
Guidozzi (1999)	24	48 (42–61)	68 (32–134)	0

HRT, hormone replacement therapy; NA, not available.

We recently had the opportunity to prospectively analyze the oncologic outcome of 319 women who were potential participants in our ongoing randomized, prospective trial of HRT in breast cancer survivors. A minimum 2 years of follow-up was required for eligibility. Women with estrogen receptor–positive breast cancer were not eligible for the trial (Vassilopoulou-Sellin et al, 1999). Thirty-nine women were receiving HRT, and the remaining 280 were controls; the prognostically significant patient and disease characteristics of the 2 groups were similar. Among the HRT recipients, a new, contralateral tumor developed in 1 patient. Among the controls, a new or recurrent breast cancer developed in 14 patients, and other cancers developed in 6 patients. Therefore, HRT did not appear to increase the incidence of breast cancer events in this subset of patients with localized disease. In a different report from another institution, a nonsignificant trend of increased risk of breast cancer recurrence was reported in women with a history of ductal carcinoma in situ who were receiving HRT, but information regarding clinical outcome was not noted in that study.

Prospective randomized trials of HRT in breast cancer survivors are now beginning or are under way (HABITS trial: L. Holmberg, personal communication, December 1998; ECOG trial: M. Cobleigh, personal communication, July 1997: Tibolone trial: I. S. Fentiman, personal communication, September 1997; The University of Texas M. D. Anderson Cancer Center trial), but results will not be mature for some time. Until such time, HRT should be considered only in very special, individual cases or within the context of clinical trials.

In the absence of definitive safety data, we continue to counsel our patients that a history of breast cancer remains a contraindication for HRT. We do, however, analyze the menopausal health of the individual patient, and we occasionally conclude with the patient that estrogen replacement is the preferred choice. Rather than attempt to construct arbitrary criteria for such a decision, we weigh the anticipated benefits against the potential risks and consider the inherent uncertainties. We do, however, discourage patients with recent, hormone-responsive disease from taking HRT.

Course of Women Who Develop Breast Cancer while Receiving Hormone Replacement Therapy

If estrogen stimulates the growth of malignant breast cells, one might be concerned that subclinical disease might be fueled by HRT and that such disease might grow rapidly, resulting in a worse clinical outcome than if HRT were not used. We have no information on the outcome of recurrent disease in women who have already had breast cancer and then begin to take estrogen. In the general population, however, this concern has been the focus of several recent studies, all of which have provided reassuring evidence that the prognosis of women who develop initial breast cancer while receiving HRT is similar to if not better than that of women not receiving HRT when they develop breast cancer.

Hormone replacement therapy appears to beneficially affect the biological characteristics of breast tumors (Dupont et al, 1989; Squitieri et al, 1994; Harding et al, 1996; Bonnier et al, 1998; Gapstur et al, 1999). Breast tumors diagnosed in women receiving HRT behave less aggressively than other breast tumors (Bergkvist et al, 1989; Magnusson et al, 1996; Holli et al, 1998), and the overall mortality rate of the disease in women receiving HRT at diagnosis has been reported to be either unchanged (Hunt et al, 1990; Strickland et al, 1992; Yuen et al, 1993; Fowble et al, 1999) or improved (Willis et al, 1996; Sellers et al, 1997; Jernstrom et al, 1999; Schairer et al, 1999). It is possible that the improved outcome of HRT recipients is due to a combination of a health-conscious lifestyle, including conscientious screenings, plus the favorable effect of HRT on the biology of the disease.

CONCLUSIONS

Many menopausal women, including breast cancer survivors, experience mild and self-limiting climacteric symptoms but, by virtue of their individual health profiles, are not at risk for heart or bone disease. For these women, no medical interventions are needed. Other individuals have an increased risk of heart disease or osteoporosis but not both, and for some women, the climacteric symptoms are overwhelming and overshadow all other considerations. The therapeutic and palliative approaches in these varying scenarios must be individualized for each patient.

For many years, it has generally been agreed that women who have been treated for breast cancer should avoid exogenous estrogen, and this belief, which is based on theoretical considerations and experimental data, has been the basis for standard practice. This proscription has been challenged recently because both the population characteristics and the health needs of women with a prior diagnosis of breast cancer have been changing. The emerging skepticism about our current practice in this group of patients is reflected in many recent editorials and commentaries; however, carefully designed clinical trials are still needed. A consensus statement regarding treatment of estrogen deficiency symptoms in women surviving breast cancer was released recently after a conference of scientists and survivors (Hormone Foundation et al, 1998). Their recommendation discourages the use of HRT and encourages appropriate studies to explore alternatives.

At M. D. Anderson Cancer Center, we feel that appropriate nonhormonal measures should be carefully and vigorously explored as a first approach to relieving menopausal symptoms in breast cancer survivors.

KEY PRACTICE POINTS

- Estrogen deficiency is often accompanied by climacteric symptoms, bone loss, and cardiovascular morbidity, which can be prevented or reversed by estrogen replacement.

- A history of breast cancer is considered a contraindication for use of estrogen as treatment for menopausal symptoms; accordingly, alternative strategies have been developed to meet the postmenopausal health needs of breast cancer survivors.

- Emerging information from recent studies indicates that women who take estrogen after breast cancer may not experience more recurrences and that women who develop breast cancer while taking estrogen may have a better clinical outcome.

However, if climacteric symptoms or skeletal and cardiovascular morbidity coexist and compromise the patient's health or quality or life, estrogen use may be considered in the context of clinical trials and after thoughtful discussions with the patient.

SUGGESTED READINGS

Bergkvist L, Adami HO, Persson I, Bergstrom R, Krusemo UB. Prognosis after breast cancer diagnosis in women exposed to estrogen and estrogen-progestogen replacement therapy. *Am J Epidemiol* 1989;130:221–228.

Bluming AZ, Waisman JR, Dosik GM, et al. Hormone replacement therapy (HRT) in women with previously treated primary breast cancer. Update II. *Proceedings of the American Society of Clinical Oncology* 1997;16:131A.

Bonnier P, Bessenay F, Sasco AJ, et al. Impact of menopausal hormone-replacement therapy on clinical and laboratory characteristics of breast cancer. *Int J Cancer* 1998;79:278–282.

Couzi RJ, Helzlsouer KJ, Fetting JH. Prevalence of menopausal symptoms among women with a history of breast cancer and attitudes toward estrogen replacement therapy. *J Clin Oncol* 1995;13:2737–2744.

Decker D, Cox T, Burdakin I, et al. Hormone replacement therapy (HRT) in breast cancer survivors. *Proceedings of the American Society of Clinical Oncology* 1996;15:136A.

Delmas PD, Bjarnason NH, Mitlak BH, et al. Effects of raloxifene on bone mineral density, serum cholesterol concentrations, and uterine endometrium in postmenopausal women. *N Engl J Med* 1997;337:1641–1647.

DiSaia PJ, Grosen EA, Kurosaki T, Gildea M, Cowan B, Anton-Culver H. Hormone replacement therapy in breast cancer survivors: a cohort study. *Am J Obstet Gynecol* 1996;174:1494–1498.

Dupont WD, Page DL, Rogers LW, Parl FF. Influence of exogenous estrogens, proliferative breast disease, and other variables on breast cancer risk. *Cancer* 1989;63:948–957.

Eden JA, Bush T, Nand S. A case-control study of combined continuos estrogen-progestin replacement therapy among women with a personal history of breast cancer. *Menopause* 1995;2:67–72.

Fornander T, Rutqvist LE, Sjoberg HE, Blomqvist L, Maltsson A, Glas U. Long-term adjuvant tamoxifen in early breast cancer: effect on bone mineral density in postmenopausal women. *J Clin Oncol* 1990;8:1019–1024.

Fowble B, Hanlon A, Freedman G, et al. Postmenopausal hormone replacement therapy: effect on diagnosis and outcome in early-stage invasive breast cancer treated with conservative surgery and radiation. *J Clin Oncol* 1999;17:1680–1688.

Gapstur SM, Morrow M, Sellers TA. Hormone replacement therapy and risk of breast cancer with a favorable histology: results of the Iowa Women's Health Study. *JAMA* 1999;281:2091–2097.

Goldberg RM, Loprinzi CL, O'Fallon JR, et al. Transdermal clonidine for amelio-rating tamoxifen-induced hot flushes. *J Clin Oncol* 1994;12:155–158.

Gorins A, Cremieu A, Espie M, et al. Hormone replacement therapy (HRT) in women with previously treated primary breast cancer. Update III. *Proceedings of the American Society of Clinical Oncology* 1997;5:131A.

Grady D, Rubin SM, Petitti DB, et al. Hormone therapy to prevent disease and prolong life in postmenopausal women. *Ann Intern Med* 1992;117:1016–1037.

Greendale GA, Judd HL. The menopause: health implications and clinical man-agement. *J Am Geriatr Soc* 1993;41:426–436.

Grodstein F, Stampfer MJ, Colditz GA, et al. Postmenopausal hormone therapy and mortality. *New Engl J Med* 1997;336:1769–1775.

Guidozzi F. Estrogen replacement therapy in breast cancer survivors. *Int J Gynaecol Obstet* 1999;64:59–63.

Harding C, Knox WF, Faragher EB, Baildam A, Bundred NJ. Hormone replacement therapy and tumour grade in breast cancer: prospective study in screening unit. *BMJ* 1996;312:1646–1647.

Hodgson SF, Johnston CC. AACE Clinical Practice Guidelines for the Prevention and Treatment of Postmenopausal Osteoporosis. *Endocrine Practice* 1996;2:155–170.

Holli K, Isola J, Cuzick J. Low biologic aggressiveness in breast cancer in women using hormone replacement therapy. *J Clin Oncol* 1998;16:3115–3120.

Hormone Foundation, Canadian Breast Cancer Research Initiative, National Cancer Institute of Canada, Endocrine Society, and the University of Virginia Cancer Center and Women's Place. Treatment of estrogen deficiency symp-toms in women surviving breast cancer. *J Clin Endocrinol Metab* 1998;83:1993–2000.

Hunt K, Vessey M, McPherson K. Mortality in a cohort of long-term users of hormone replacement therapy: an updated analysis. *Br J Obstet Gynaecol* 1990;97:1080–1086.

Jernstrom H, Frenander J, Ferno M, Olsson H. Hormone replacement therapy before breast cancer diagnosis significantly reduces the overall death rate compared with never-use among 984 breast cancer patients. *Br J Cancer* 1999;80:1453–1458.

Loprinzi CL, Michalak JC, Quella SK, et al. Megestrol acetate for the prevention of hot flashes. *N Engl J Med* 1994;331:347–352.

Love RR, Wiebe DA, Newcomb PA, et al. Effects of tamoxifen on cardiovascular risk factors in postmenopausal women. *Ann Intern Med* 1991;115:860–864.

Magnusson C, Holmberg L, Norden T, Lindgren A, Persson I. Prognosis charac-
teristics in breast cancers after hormone replacement therapy. *Breast Cancer Res Treat* 1996;38:325–334.

Marsden J, Sacks NPM. Hormone replacement therapy and breast cancer. *Endocrine-Related Cancer* 1997;4:269–279.

Peters GN, Jones SE. Estrogen replacement therapy in breast cancer patients. A time for change? *Proceedings of the American Society of Clinical Oncology* 1996;15:121A.

Powles TJ, Hickish T, Casey S, O'Brien M. Hormone replacement after breast cancer. *Lancet* 1993;342:60–61.

Rutqvist LE, Mattsson A. The Stockholm Breast Cancer Study Group. Cardiac and thromboembolic morbidity among postmenopausal women with early-stage breast cancer in a randomized trial of adjuvant tamoxifen. *J Natl Cancer Inst* 1993;85:1398–1406.

Schairer C, Gail M, Byrne C, et al. Estrogen replacement therapy and breast cancer survival in a large screening study. *J Natl Cancer Inst* 1999;91:264–270.

Sellers TA, Mink PJ, Cerhan JR, et al. The role of hormone replacement therapy in the risk for breast cancer and total mortality in women with a family history of breast cancer. *Ann Intern Med* 1997;127:973–980.

Speroff L, Glass RH, Kase NG. Menopause and postmenopausal hormone therapy. In: *Clinical Gynecologic Endocrinology and Infertility.* 5th Ed. Baltimore: Williams and Wilkins; 1994:583–650.

Squitieri R, Tartter PI, Ahmed S, Brower ST, Theise ND. Carcinoma of the breast in postmenopausal hormone user and nonuser control groups. *J Am Coll Surg* 1994;178:167–170.

Strickland DM, Gambrell RD Jr, Butzin CA, Strickland K. The relationship between breast cancer survival and prior postmenopausal estrogen use. *Obstet Gynecol* 1992;80:400–404.

Utian WH, Schiff I. NAMS-Gallup Survey on women's knowledge, information sources, and attitudes to menopause and hormone replacement therapy. *Menopause* 1994;1:39–48.

Vassilopoulou-Sellin R, Asmar L, Hortobagyi GN, et al. Estrogen replacement therapy after localized breast cancer: clinical outcome of 319 women followed prospectively. *J Clin Oncol* 1999;17:1482–1487.

Vassilopoulou-Sellin R, Theriault R, Klein MJ. Estrogen replacement therapy in women with prior diagnosis and treatment for breast cancer. *Gynecol Oncol* 1997;65:89–93.

Vassilopoulou-Sellin R, Zolinski C. Estrogen replacement therapy in women with breast cancer: a survey of patient attitudes. *Am J Med Sci* 1992;304:145–149.

Willis DB, Calle EE, Miracle-McMahill HL, Heath CW Jr. Estrogen replacement therapy and risk of fatal breast cancer in a prospective cohort of postmenopausal women in the United States. *Cancer Causes Control* 1996;7:449–457.

Yuen J, Persson I, Berkvist L, Hoover R, Schairer C, Adami HO. Hormone replacement therapy and breast cancer mortality in Swedish women: results after adjustment for 'healthy drug-user' effect. *Cancer Causes Control* 1993;4:369–374.

18 Management of Sexual Problems in Women with Breast Cancer

Jennifer G. Gotto

Chapter Overview

Breast cancer and its treatment can diminish or change sexual function, sexual feeling, and sexual self-image. Women with breast cancer may experience loss of sexual desire, decreased arousability, diminished orgasmic capacity, impaired vaginal physiology, depression, and a lessened sense of "femaleness." Untreated sexual problems negatively affect intimate relationships, self-confidence, and physical well-being. Addressing the issue of sexual function before treatment begins alerts the patient to the clinician's interest and increases the chance that the patient will bring future sexual problems to the attention of the treatment team. Depending on the nature of the problem and the disease context, interventions are available for treatment of sexual problems in women with breast cancer, including vaginal moisturizers, lubricants, medications or therapy to alleviate depression-related sexual dysfunction, and couples therapy to address sexual and more general issues. Encouraging vaginal health in at-risk patients may prevent some sexual problems.

Introduction

Sexual health may suffer during and after treatment for breast cancer. Breast cancer and breast cancer treatment can cause changes in hormone status, appearance, overall physical well-being, emotional health, and interpersonal relationships, and these changes in turn can lead to sexual problems. Some women negotiate the changes in their bodies and sex life without inordinate pain and suffering, but most women suffer quietly and may regard the sexual changes as separate from their cancer, decreasing the likelihood that their problem will ever be addressed. Therefore, it is important that clinicians address issues of sexuality with breast cancer patients.

If a patient assumes that the cancer specialist is not interested in sexual problems or that nothing can be done about such problems, she may be reluctant to bring any sexual issue to the attention of her health care provider. This is a serious issue because the person living silently with a sexual problem may suffer emotional, physical, and relationship harm. It is therefore vital that the medical staff make clear to the patient that they are interested in her quality of life and sexual functioning.

Because female sexuality is a neglected area of academic study, little is known about the pathophysiology of female sexual response, and few interventions are available for the treatment of sexual problems in women. A woman's sexual experience of desire, excitement, and orgasm is measured by subjective response. Because the female sexual response is not obvious, myth, mystery, and poor understanding plague the subject of female sexuality. This brief overview is intended to aid clinicians in assessing sexual function in breast cancer patients, to heighten awareness of sexual problems that can occur in women with breast cancer, and to offer strategies for dealing with some of these sexual problems.

Assessment of Sexual Function in Breast Cancer Patients

Physicians should inquire about the patient's sexual function before treatment starts. Early indication of interest in the patient's sexual function shows the patient that her physician considers this subject worthy of discussion and increases the likelihood that the patient will tell her physician about any sexual problems that do arise.

During the intense phase of treatment, patients are focused on surviving the cancer and surviving the treatment. Some women do engage in sexual activity during this time. Regardless of whether they are sexually active, most women still enjoy the pleasure of nonsexual closeness, such as cuddling, holding, or touching.

After treatment, patients who did not receive systemic chemotherapy generally fare better than patients who did receive chemotherapy, which often causes ovarian failure. Not all women have problems resuming a satisfying sex life after treatment. However, many do, and only a fraction of women who do suffer complain about it. Thus the prudent physician will bring up the topic of sexual function again during the patient's recovery or remission phase. Complaints may range from vaginal dryness to difficulties in all phases of sexual response: desire, excitement, and orgasm. Factors that can affect the complexity of the complaint include the type of treatment, the degree of preexisting relationship conflict between the patient and her partner, the presence of depression, the presence of preexisting sexual conflict in the patient or her partner, and the use of medications or drugs that inhibit sexual response.

The sensitive physician may inquire about the patient's stamina, changes she notices in her body, her capacity to feel supported by her spouse or significant other, and other relationship dynamics that may have changed since her treatment started. If a woman is at risk for experiencing chemical menopause, the physician may choose to reinforce the concept of vaginal health and prevention of atrophy.

Management of Sexual Problems Associated with Breast Cancer and Breast Cancer Treatment

A variety of interventions are available for treatment of sexual problems in women with breast cancer.

Problems Caused by Mastectomy

Mastectomy has no direct physical effect on female sexual response since surgery does not affect the production of estrogen or androgens. However, women and their partners must adjust to the loss of the breast. Some women enjoy the sensation of being touched on the site of the breast scar. Others prefer to wear a camisole or prosthesis during sexual activity to cover the missing breast (Schover, 1988). Persistent lymphedema or pain due to mastectomy may detract from the physical pleasure of sex. This problem can be addressed by timing sexual activity when the patient is most comfortable—for example, scheduling sexual activity around pain medication.

Loss of a breast can affect the patient's sense of attractiveness and cause emotional distress. If breast reconstruction is considered to be a medically sound option, a patient may wish to pursue reconstruction, which can help restore her confidence and sense of attractiveness but will not improve her breast's sensitivity. If reconstruction is not possible, then the patient may benefit from counseling to address her loss and its effect on her self-image. If the patient is part of a couple, couples counseling may be appropriate. The goal of this approach is to facilitate communication between the couple about grief or other feelings related to the cancer and about their sex life. Couples therapy may also address any preexisting marital or sexual conflicts, thus helping the couple return to a satisfactory sex life.

The clinician should strive to prevent the patient from developing a pattern of sexual avoidance (Kaplan, 1992). This occurs when the patient anticipates that her partner will reject her because of her altered appearance (which often is not a valid assumption) and then finds ways to avoid intimate contact. If this destructive cycle continues and a pattern of sexual avoidance gets established, future attempts to repair the sexual relationship may not be successful.

Acute Side Effects of Chemotherapy

Acute side effects of chemotherapy include fatigue, hair loss, weight gain, nausea, and vomiting. Depression may be an acute or latent problem. A woman who feels tired, bald, depressed, and fat may have trouble feeling attractive. Appropriate use of makeup, wigs, and scarves can help with some confidence problems (Schover, 1988). Depression can be successfully treated if it is recognized in a timely manner. For more information, see the section Depression later in this chapter.

Hormone Deficiency

Estrogen and testosterone are both critical for female sexual function. Estrogen is responsible for maintaining female sexual organs, for providing a sense of "femaleness," and for maintaining the health and elasticity of vaginal tissue. Estrogen is also necessary for the swelling, sexual aroma, lubrication, and lengthening of the vagina that occur during sexual excitement. Testosterone is responsible for maintaining sexual vitality and interest. In women, estrogen is produced by the ovaries, and about one quarter of androgen is produced by the ovaries. The adrenal cortex produces the majority of androgen in women.

During and after menopause, the ovaries make less estrogen and testosterone, and levels of adrenal androgen may decline significantly. The hot flashes and vaginal dryness that herald menopause are caused by declining estrogen production. Testosterone deficiency (generally defined as a total testosterone level less than 20 ng/mL) may also develop (Rako, 1999). In some women, these declines in estrogen and testosterone levels can result in impairment of sexual function. Sometimes testosterone deficiency can be inadvertently induced when a menopausal woman starts taking supplemental estrogen. The supplemental estrogen induces an increase in production of sex hormone binding globulin (SHBG), and the SHBG binds to the added estrogen as well as intrinsic testosterone, thus decreasing the free fraction of testosterone and creating a situation of artificial deficiency.

In both premenopausal and postmenopausal patients, chemotherapy can impair ovarian function. Depending on the woman's age and pretreatment ovarian function, she may either experience return of ovarian function or experience "chemical menopause." In ovarian failure or chemical menopause, a woman may experience an acute drop in estrogen and testosterone. This acute drop in hormones may be experienced physically as "more severe" menopause or sexual deficiency. The alkylating agents are especially likely to impair ovarian function.

Estrogen Deficiency

Estrogen deficiency, whether it occurs naturally as a result of menopause or is chemically induced, impairs vaginal physiology. In a woman with estrogen deficiency, the vagina may not properly lubricate or expand in preparation for sexual intercourse. In the worst-case scenario, the vagina becomes dry, tight, small, and atrophic. In this situation, sexual intercourse is painful and may even be impossible if the woman's muscles tighten around the outside of her vagina and make penetration difficult. If intercourse is too painful, the woman's libido will be affected by anticipation of the pain associated with sex.

In women without a history of breast cancer, oral estrogen replacement therapy is often begun at menopause to avoid estrogen deficiency. In women with a history of breast cancer, however, estrogen replacement therapy is generally contraindicated.

To prevent vaginal atrophy, the problem of vaginal dryness should be addressed early on. In general, it is easier to prevent vaginal atrophy than to cure it. If a woman's treatment includes chemotherapy, she should start using vaginal moisturizers at the start of chemotherapy. Vaginal moisturizers such as Replens or Silken Secrets are helpful in preventing atrophy. Estrogen creams are available that can be applied to the vagina; however, use of these creams is controversial since they may increase systemic estrogen levels. The estrogen ring may be associated with less systemic absorption.

The use of water-soluble lubricants such as KY Jelly and Astroglide allows for more comfortable intercourse. The woman should apply a liberal amount to her partner and to the inside and outside of her vagina before her partner attempts penetration. A gynecologist should evaluate any complaint of painful intercourse if the cause is considered to be more complex than simple vaginal dryness. The woman with a small, tight vagina may need to use a dilator. The woman should start with a dilator of a comfortable size and work up to a dilator that approximates the size of her partner's penis. If a woman is at risk for vaginal atrophy and has sexual intercourse infrequently (less than once a week), she may want to use a dilator regularly (4–5 times a week) to "practice" good vaginal health.

Estrogen deficiency does not directly affect desire and orgasm since these are mediated by testosterone and not estrogen. Estrogen-deficient women experience desire and can get pleasure from masturbating or being touched.

Androgen Deficiency

Androgen deficiency results in a global loss of sexual function. Women with androgen deficiency complain of loss of sexual desire and a decrease in sexual feelings and thoughts. Women also complain of diminished excitability—of being less arousable in response to erotic stimuli and less responsive to partners. The clitoris may be less sensitive to stimulation. Orgasmic capacity may be entirely gone or very diminished. Orgasms, instead of being felt throughout the entire body, may feel more localized to the vagina and less intense (Schover, 1988). More direct, more intense, and longer stimulation of the clitoris may be required for the woman to achieve an orgasm. Overall vitality and energy may be reduced. The vagina may still lubricate, but the woman feels less sexually inclined. This diminished responsiveness may be misunderstood by her partner and may lead to significant marital problems and even impotence.

In a woman with suspected androgen deficiency, medications, drugs, and psychiatric status should be reviewed since certain medications and depression cause decreased sexual desire. The patient's relationship with her sexual partner should be examined for latent conflict and preexisting sexual problems. If the oncologist suspects troubled relationship dynamics, he or she may refer the couple to a couples therapist.

Treatment of androgen deficiency in patients with breast cancer is controversial. The long-term effects of replacing testosterone in healthy women are not defined. Some oncologists are wary of any hormonal manipulation in the breast cancer patient. In the androgen-deficient woman with stable disease or no evidence of disease, the use of testosterone replacement is best decided on an individual basis by the oncologist. If androgen replacement is considered acceptable, a nonvirilizing low dose of testosterone, designed to restore a normal physiologic testosterone level, may be appropriate. This treatment may improve a patient's libido and orgasmic capability. In breast cancer patients, methyltestosterone is preferred over testosterone propionate because the methyl group slows conversion of testosterone to estrogen. However, methyltestosterone confounds the testosterone blood level assay, so in women treated with this hormone, monitoring of physiologic blood levels of testosterone is not possible (Rako, 1999). Methyltestosterone is available in topical and oral forms. Methyltestosterone cream (0.25–1 mg per day) is applied to the vulva 2 days per week and to the skin of the wrist or thigh the other 5 days per week (Rako, 1999). This decreases the risk of clitoral hypertrophy. Oral methyltestosterone may be used in doses ranging from 0.25 to 0.8 mg per day.

Tamoxifen-Associated Symptoms

Tamoxifen is an antiestrogen that has fewer side effects than cytotoxic chemotherapy. It exerts both antiestrogenic and weak estrogenic effects. Little is known about the sexual side effects of tamoxifen. Depression and cognitive problems can occur in women taking tamoxifen. Not all women taking this drug experience vaginal dryness or a decline in libido or arousal. Dose reduction may alleviate any sexual side effects that do occur.

Depression

Mood disorders are common during and after treatment for breast cancer. Recognition and early treatment of depression improves the patient's overall well-being, improves her ability to tolerate and endure treatment, and enhances medical compliance. Depression is associated with a loss of sexual desire and therefore must be considered as a possible cause in cases of sexual dysfunction. In attempting to treat depression, the clinician should take care not to create a new sexual problem. Serotonergic reuptake inhibitors (such as fluoxetine [Prozac], sertraline [Zoloft], and paroxetine [Paxil]), tricyclic antidepressants, and some atypical antidepressants are associated with impaired desire, excitement, and orgasm. Antidepressants associated with less sexual impairment include nefazodone (Serzone), bupropion (Wellbutrin), mirtazapine (Remeron), and the stimulants methylphenidate (Ritalin) and dextroamphetamine (Dexedrine) (Table 18–1).

Relationship Malfunction

Breast cancer may create a situation of chronic anxiety in the patient's home. Breast cancer may also result in role reversal, in which the patient's partner assumes many caretaking and household chores previously handled by the patient. This temporary role reversal and stress can have a negative impact on a couple's communication and feeling for each other, especially if there are preexisting unaddressed relationship conflicts. The changes required for the patient's household to continue to function may cause resentment in the partner or patient, and unrecognized or unspoken anger between a couple often impairs sexual relations. Alternatively, the patient's partner may be frightened by the possibility of losing her and may be afraid to touch her. The importance of including the patient's partner in the assessment and treatment of sexual dysfunction cannot be overemphasized. This is especially true if the cause of sexual disinterest is determined to be more psychogenic than organic or if communication

Table 18–1. Potential Pharmacologic Interventions for Sexual Dysfunction

Medication	Dose	Activity	General Use	Potential Use in Treating Sexual Dysfunction
Replens	Daily	Nonestrogen vaginal moisturizer; glycerin and mineral oil	Vaginal moisturizer	Alleviate vaginal dryness
Astroglide	As needed	Nonpetroleum lubricant	Lubricant	Ease sexual intercourse
Estrogen ring	2 mg (vaginal)	Absorbed by vaginal mucosa	Treatment of postmenopausal vaginal atrophy	Treatment of vaginal atrophy
Sildenafil citrate	50–100 mg	Phosphodiesterase 5 inhibitor	Treatment of erectile dysfunction	Increase clitoral blood flow; improve arousability?
Creams (in development)	37.5–100 mg	Vasodilator	Improve genital blood flow	Improve lubrication; improve arousability?
Bupropion	37.5–100 mg	Increases central dopamine activity	Antidepressant; smoking cessation (Zyban)	Reverse serotonin reuptake inhibitor–related inhibition of erection/orgasm; improve desire
Buspirone	5–30 mg	Mixed serotonergic activity	Anxiolytin (non-benzodiazepine)	Reverse serotonin reuptake inhibitor–related sexual dysfunction
Nefazodone	100–300 mg	Serotonin agonist/antagonist	Antidepressant	Antidepressant with lower incidence/risk of sexual side effects
Methylphenidate	5–90 mg	Increases central norepinephrine and dopamine	Treatment of neurobehavioral slowing, attention deficit hyperactivity disorder, and depression due to mental conditions; augmentation of serotonin reuptake inhibitor level	Lack of sexual side effects; may improve arousal
Ginkgo biloba, ginseng,* and ma huang	Not known, varies	Not known	Increase energy; improve mental alertness	Improved energy may improve sexual arousability/desire/excitability. Watch for agitation.

*Not recommended in cancer patients.

between partners appears to be a problem. In such cases, referral to a couples or sex therapist is appropriate.

Additional Pharmacologic Treatment Options

In addition to estrogen, testosterone, vaginal moisturizers, and lubricants, which have already been discussed, a variety of other pharmacologic treatments are available that may be helpful for breast cancer patients with sexual problems.

Some of the medications used to treat impotence may be helpful in alleviating female sexual complaints. Most of these treatments are not yet established but are under study.

Sildenafil (Viagra), a phosphodiesterase type 5 inhibitor, is an oral medication used in treating impotence. Sildenafil works by inhibiting phosphodiesterase and thus prolonging the life of nitric oxide in the penile arterioles, allowing for increased genital blood flow and penile erection. In women, the expected response to sildenafil would be increased genital vasodilatation, vaginal lubrication, and swelling. There are some case reports of heightened sexual responsivity of the genitals and increased sexual arousal in women using sildenafil. This increased arousal with sildenafil is seen only in women. A cream containing sildenafil has been used experimentally in women. When applied to the vulva and clitoris, this cream may improve genital sensitivity.

Alprostadil (prostaglandin E1) is a natural vasodilator used for treatment of impotence. Alprostadil is available in 2 forms: a liquid that is injected directly into the penis and a suppository that is placed in the urethra. Alprostadil may improve vaginal lubrication when applied topically. This use of alprostadil is under investigation.

Dream Cream (Kaminetsky, 2000) is an off-label combination of 2 vasodilators: aminophylline and L-arginine. L-arginine is an amino acid available in health food stores used by some athletes to promote muscle development. Side effects include genital warmth and even heat. In evaluations of Dream Cream, women reported feeling more "full," more sexually excited, and more lubricated and reported more intense orgasms. Other combination creams containing vasodilators such as aminophylline or isosorbide dinitrate are also available and may produce effects similar to those seen with Dream Cream.

Antidepressant medications that increase dopamine levels may also be useful in promoting the sexual experience in women. Methylphenidate (5 mg) taken prior to sexual activity may enhance all phases of the sexual response cycle in women. Bupropion is an atypical antidepressant with primarily dopaminergic effects and no serotonergic effect. At higher doses (225–300 mg), bupropion may increase arousal and enhance orgasm in women. Bupropion may reverse sexual dysfunction caused by serotonin

---

KEY PRACTICE POINTS

- Before treatment begins, the clinician should inquire about the patient's current sexual function and should inform the patient about chemotherapy's potential effects on sexual function.
- Regular vaginal lubrication and moisturizing beginning at the start of chemotherapy may help prevent vaginal atrophy.
- Educating the patient and her partner about potential sexual side effects is the best prevention against incomplete recovery from breast cancer.

---

reuptake inhibitors. Other dopamine-promoting drugs that may enhance female sexual response are selegiline hydrochloride (Deprenyl), a reversible monoamine oxidase-B inhibitor used in the treatment of Parkinson's disease, and apomorphine, a dopamine agonist reported to stimulate nitric oxide and exert a local genital vasodilatation effect.

Ginseng, ephedra equisetina (ma huang), and ginkgo biloba extract are alternative therapies used by persons seeking assistance for sexual problems (Bartlik et al, 1999). These agents should all be used with extreme caution in cancer patients. Ma huang may result in sympathetic activation. The "energizing" effect of ginseng may lead to agitation, and ginseng may promote tumor growth. Ginkgo biloba is reported to improve cerebral circulation and blood flow by its inhibition of platelet-activating factor. Ginkgo biloba may improve genital blood flow by the same mechanism. However, this substance should be used with caution when bleeding or thrombocytopenia is a concern.

REFERRING PATIENTS TO A COUPLES THERAPIST OR SEX THERAPIST

If a patient's problem does not respond to education, reassurance, or simple intervention, it may be appropriate to refer her to a psychiatrist, psychologist, or sex therapist for additional treatment.

SUGGESTED READINGS

Bartlik B, Kaplan P, Kaminetsky J, Roentsch G, Goldberg J. Medication with the potential to enhance sexual responsivity in women. *Psychiatric Annals* 1999;29:46.

Chakravarti S, Collins WP, Newton JR, Oram DH, Studd JW. Endocrine changes and symptomatology after oophorectomy in premenopausal women. *Br J Obstet Gynaecol* 1977;84:769–775.

Duffy L, Greenberg D, Younger J, Ferraro M. Iatrogenic acute estrogen deficiency and psychiatric syndromes in breast cancer patients. *Psychosomatics* 1999;40:304–308.

Kaminetsky, Jed, Web site. http://www.femalesexualtherapy.com. Accessed August 17, 2000.

Kaplan H. A neglected issue: the sexual side effects of current treatment for breast cancer. *Journal of Sex and Marital Therapy* 1992;18:3–19.

Kaplan H, Owett T. The female androgen deficiency syndrome. *Journal of Sex and Marital Therapy* 1993;19:3–24.

Pesmen C. Health report: lust lotions. *Glamour*. August 1999, 60.

Rako S. Testosterone deficiency and supplementation for women: matters of sexuality and health. *Psychiatric Annals* 1999;29:23.

Sands R, Studd J. Exogenous androgens in postmenopausal women. *Am J Med* 1995;98(suppl 1A):76S–79S.

Schover L. Sexuality and cancer. American Cancer Society, 1988.

Waxenberg S, Drellich M, Sutherland A. The role of hormones in human behavior. 1. Changes in female sexuality after adrenalectomy. *J Clin Endocrinol* 1959;19:193.

INDEX